# Novel Aspects of COVID-19 after a Two-Year Pandemic

# Novel Aspects of COVID-19 after a Two-Year Pandemic

Editors

**Toshio Hattori**
**Yugo Ashino**

MDPI

Basel • Beijing • Wuhan • Barcelona • Belgrade • Novi Sad • Cluj • Manchester

*Editors*

Toshio Hattori
Research Institute of Health and Welfare
Kibi International University
Okayama
Japan

Yugo Ashino
Department of Respiratory Medicine
Sendai City Hospital
Sendai
Japan

*Editorial Office*
MDPI
St. Alban-Anlage 66
4052 Basel, Switzerland

This is a reprint of articles from the Special Issue published online in the open access journal *Reports* (ISSN 2571-841X) (available at: www.mdpi.com/journal/reports/special_issues/COVID_Aspects).

For citation purposes, cite each article independently as indicated on the article page online and as indicated below:

| |
|---|
| Lastname, A.A.; Lastname, B.B. Article Title. *Journal Name* **Year**, *Volume Number*, Page Range. |

**ISBN 978-3-7258-0498-6 (Hbk)**
**ISBN 978-3-7258-0497-9 (PDF)**
**doi.org/10.3390/books978-3-7258-0497-9**

# Contents

# Preface

Driven by the outbreak of COVID-19, this Special Issue reports on novel aspects of COVID-19, with published 14 papers on the following topics:

Development of diagnosis methods;

Therapeutic effects of new agents;

Improvements in the monitoring and managements of patients;

Characteristics of break-through infection;

Sequelae of COVID-19 infections;

Development of vaccine against COVID-19 infection;

Disasters caused by COVID-19 infection.

In this reprint, we described two types of disaster-related infectious diseases. One is a disease associated with it, and the other causes the disaster. COVID-19 is of the latter type. We also described the RNA viruses most commonly causing disaster infectious diseases. Moreover, the outcomes of persons living with HIV are discussed, and it was concluded that older age and the status of insurance are associated with more severe outcomes. We also described how Singapore was largely successful in reducing imported cases. Long-term, palliative, and hospice care strict bans on visits, particularly during end-of-life care, are associated with a strong emotional burden for patients and family members alike. Long-term care facility (LTCF), delirium, fever, and low-grade fever, alone or in clusters, should be considered in identifying and predicting the prognosis of SARS-CoV-2 infection in older patients. In the study of genitourinary (GU) malignancy, socioeconomic status has also been highlighted as part of the existing inequality.

For diagnosis, routine serum laboratory tests were examined as potentially diagnostic of COVID-19. Two PCR kits were compared, and it was clarified that each produced comparable results.

It was also proposed that SARS-CoV-2 infection upregulates GABA, protecting not only the central nervous system, but also the endothelia, pancreas, and gut microbiota.

Cases of spontaneous pneumothorax have been reported in the setting of coronavirus disease 19 (COVID-19), described as an unlikely complication, mainly occurring in critically ill patients or as a consequence of mechanical ventilation. Another case report described acute exacerbation of the disease after tocilizumab (anti-IL-6 receptor antibody) treatment. This reprint reports on the urgent medical issues brought about by the emergence of COVID-19 from clinical settings in various countries, and will be useful in responding to future COVID-19 cases that continue to increase.

**Toshio Hattori and Yugo Ashino**
*Editors*

reports

*Editorial*

# Possibility to Open Up New Areas by COVID-19 Infection

**Toshio Hattori [1,*] and Yugo Ashino [2]**

1 Research Institute of Health and Welfare, Kibi International University, Takahashi 716-8508, Japan
2 Department of Respiratory Medicine, Sendai City Hospital, Sendai 982-8502, Japan; ashino-yug@hospital.city.sendai.jp
* Correspondence: hattorit@kiui.ac.jp

The rapid increase of COVID-19 cases has brought the number of patients to 513 million. More than 6 million people have died as of 1 May 2022. Until now, epidemics of febrile infectious diseases such as dengue and malaria have occurred in the tropics. These mosquito-borne infections are also classified as disaster-related infections because people are susceptible to mosquito-borne infection when exposed to nature. Unlike these infectious diseases, COVID-19 cases predominantly spread in Western countries. A total of 15% of patients and 16% of deaths have occurred in the United States. The death toll of 6 million people worldwide indicates that COVID-19 is a disaster [1]. On the other hand, COVID-19 in developed countries has made it possible for advanced research to be conducted on acute febrile illnesses. With the latest technology, significant progress have been made in diagnosis, treatment, and prevention. In this Special Issue, we will publish the novel aspects of COVID-19 after a two-year pandemic as follows.

1. Development of diagnosis methods.
2. Therapeutic effects of new agents.
3. Improvements in monitoring and management of patients.
4. Characteristics of breakthrough infection.
5. Sequelae of COVID-19 infections.
6. Development of a vaccine against COVID-19 infection.
7. Disasters caused by COVID-19 infection.

Attempts to detect infected people by RT-PCR tests have already been attempted in dengue fever [2]. In COVID-19, automated or semi-automated kits were quickly created with promising results [3]. Since the RNA virus often causes disaster infections, it will be necessary to proceed with large-scale RT-PCR testing, not only in COVID-19, but also in other infectious diseases, to identify the risk of infection rates. In other words, the development of a diagnostic method for infectious diseases that can be performed more efficiently in disaster-stricken areas is desired. The complexity of the COVID-19 illness depends on the heterogeneities of the host's response. Patients might suddenly deteriorate into severe respiratory failure, necessitating non-invasive ventilation (NIV) or mechanical ventilation (MV). Early recognition of patients at risk of progressing to severe disease and the timely onset of targeted treatment is of the utmost importance. The production of immune mediators such as cytokines and complements is essential to fight the infection; however, these can be deleterious when produced in excess. The inhibition of virus entry and proliferation by chemical agents and antibodies may inhibit a subsequent cytokine storm. Immune therapies targeting the immune mediators of host defenses, such as corticosteroids, kinase (a Janus tyrosine kinase (JAK)) and IL-1 and IL-6 were developed. It was proposed that the early administration of a monoclonal antibody against IL-6 receptor (tocilizumab) prevented pneumonia and kidney injury caused by COVID-19 [4]. However, there is no clear indicator of which immune drugs should be given to which patients at what time. It is important to identify the patients with hyper-inflammatory syndrome who

check for updates

**Citation:** Hattori, T.; Ashino, Y. Possibility to Open Up New Areas by COVID-19 Infection. *Reports* **2022**, *5*, 16. https://doi.org/10.3390/reports5020016

Received: 13 May 2022
Accepted: 20 May 2022
Published: 22 May 2022

are suitable for anti-cytokine therapy, but it is not known which bio-makers reflect less heterogeneity of the host response.

Matricellular proteins such as galectin-9 (Gal-9) and osteopontin (OPN) are known to be markers of disaster-related febrile illnesses such as dengue, malaria, leptospirosis, and AIDS/TB [5,6]. The high AUC values of these biomarkers may indicate less heterogeneity of the host response. Furthermore, the cleaved forms of OPN and Gal-9 could be better markers in COVID-19, indicating that the proteins that aare produced by interacting with other inflammatory molecules such as proteases may show better performance as a biomarker [7]. Furthermore, thrombi occur when hypercoagulability, endothelial injury and blood stasis converge, and these conditions are frequently encountered in severe COVID-19. Subsequently, arterial and venous thromboembolisms have been frequently reported. Hyper-inflammatory syndrome may play an important role in subsequent arterial and venous thromboembolisms.

Another critical issue is the role of CT and X-ray imaging in diagnosing COVID-19—particularly those that have applied artificial intelligence to detect the disease or reach a differential diagnosis between various respiratory infections.

SARS-CoV-2 has a lower mutation rate than other RNA viruses because it encodes proofreading enzyme genes. Nevertheless, the ongoing rapid transmission between humans increases the genetic diversity of SARS-CoV-2 genomes, especially the Spike gene (or the receptor-binding domain, RBD): the latter is advantageous in virus infectivity, immune escape, and tolerance. The effects of developing vaccines or therapeutics on constantly mutating viruses need to be carefully observed. It is also interesting to clinically follow the severity of the breakthrough infection and the effect of antibody treatments.

Follow-up after treatment is also an essential issue because significant physical, psychological, and cognitive deficits following COVID-19–associated critical illness have been recognized [8]. The influence of venovenous extracorporeal membrane oxygenation (ECMO) on the outcomes of mechanically ventilated patients with COVID-19 needs to be clarified.

We are victorious in the fight against this disaster because of continuously advancing diagnostic methods, and the development of vaccines and excelletnt therapeutic agents. The technology developed for the purpose of tackling COVID-19 should also be applied to other disaster-related infectious diseases. Furthermore, it is necessary to explore the social and medical impact of this pandemic.

**Author Contributions:** Conceptualization, T.H. and Y.A.; writing T.H. All authors have read and agreed to the published version of the manuscript.

**Funding:** This work was partially supported by the Japan Society for the Promotion of Science (JSPS) Grants-in-Aid for Scientific Research (KAKENHI), Grant Number JP17H01690.

**Conflicts of Interest:** The authors declare no conflict of interest.

## References

1. Hattori, T.; Chagan-Yasutan, H.; Koga, S.; Yanagihara, Y.; Tanaka, I. Seminar Lessons: Infectious diseases associated with and causing disaster. *Report* **2022**, *5*, 7. [CrossRef]
2. Liles, V.R.; Pangilinan, L.S.; Daroy, M.L.G.; Dimamay, M.T.A.; Reyes, R.S.; Bulusan, M.K.; Dimamay, M.P.S.; Luna, P.A.S.; Mercado, A.; Bai, G.; et al. Evaluation of a rapid diagnostic test for detection of dengue infection using a single-tag hybridization chromatographic-printed array strip format. *Eur. J. Clin. Microbiol. Infect. Dis.* **2019**, *38*, 515–521. [CrossRef] [PubMed]
3. Colosimo, M.; Minchella, P.; Tallerico, R.; Talotta, I.; Peronace, C.; Gallelli, L.; Di Mizio, G.; Cione, E. Comparison of Allplex™ 2019-nCoV and TaqPath™ COVID-19 Assays. *Report* **2022**, *5*, 14. [CrossRef]
4. Ashino, Y.; Chagan-Yasutan, H.; Hatta, M.; Shirato, Y.; Kyogoku, Y.; Komuro, H.; Hattori, T. Successful Treatment of a COVID-19 Case with Pneumonia and Renal Injury Using Tocilizumab. *Reports* **2020**, *3*, 29. [CrossRef]
5. Hattori, T.; Iwasaki-Hozumi, H.; Bai, G.; Chagan-Yasutan, H.; Shete, A.; Telan, E.F.; Takahashi, A.; Ashino, Y.; Matsuba, T. Both Full-Length and Protease-Cleaved Products of Osteopontin Are Elevated in Infectious Diseases. *Biomedicines* **2021**, *9*, 1006. [CrossRef] [PubMed]
6. Iwasaki-Hozumi, H.; Chagan-Yasutan, H.; Ashino, Y.; Hattori, T. Blood Levels of Galectin-9, an Immuno-Regulating Molecule, Reflect the Severity for the Acute and Chronic Infectious Diseases. *Biomolecules* **2021**, *11*, 430. [CrossRef] [PubMed]

7. Bai, G.; Furushima, D.; Niki, T.; Matsuba, T.; Maeda, Y.; Takahashi, A.; Hattori, T.; Ashino, Y. High Levels of the Cleaved Form of Galectin-9 and Osteopontin in the Plasma Are Associated with Inflammatory Markers That Reflect the Severity of COVID-19 Pneumonia. *Int. J. Mol. Sci.* **2021**, *22*, 4978. [CrossRef] [PubMed]
8. Grigorov, V.; Grigorov, M.; Grigorov, E.; Nocheva, H. Spontaneous Post-COVID-19 Pneumothorax in a Patient with No Prior Respiratory Tract Pathology: A Case Report. *Report* **2022**, *5*, 11. [CrossRef]

reports

*Review*

# Seminar Lessons: Infectious Diseases Associated with and Causing Disaster

**Toshio Hattori [1,*], Haorile Chagan-Yasutan [2], Shin Koga [3], Yasutake Yanagihara [4] and Issei Tanaka [5,*]**

1 Research Institute of Health and Welfare, Kibi International University, Takahashi 716-8508, Japan
2 Mongolian Psychosomatic Medicine Department, International Mongolian Medicine Hospital of Inner Mongolia, Hohhot 010065, China; haorile@gjmyemail.gjmyy.cn
3 Public Interest Incorporated Foundation SBS Shizuoka Health Promotion Center, Shizuoka 422-8033, Japan; s-koga@sbs-smc.or.jp
4 Research Center for Zoonosis Control, Hokkaido University, Sapporo 001-0020, Japan; yanagihara@uv.tnc.ne.jp
5 Shizuoka Prefectural Hospital Organization, Shizuoka 420-8527, Japan
* Correspondence: hattorit@kiui.ac.jp (T.H.); issei-tanaka@i.shizuoka-pho.jp (I.T.)

**Abstract:** Disasters such as the magnitude-9 Great East Japan Earthquake occur periodically. We considered this experience while developing measures against a predicted earthquake in the Nankai Trough. This report includes a summary of 10 disastrous infectious diseases for which a countermeasures seminar was held. Thirty-five speakers from twenty-one organizations performed the lectures. Besides infectious diseases, conference topics also included disaster prevention and mitigation methods. In addition, the development of point-of-care tests, biomarkers for diagnosis, and severity assessments for infectious diseases were introduced, along with epidemics of infectious diseases affected by climate. Of the 28 pathogens that became a hot topic, 17 are viruses, and 14 out of these 17 (82%) are RNA viruses. Of the 10 seminars, the last 2 targeted only COVID-19. It was emphasized that COVID-19 is not just a disaster-related infection but a disaster itself. The first seminar on COVID-19 provided immunological and epidemiological knowledge and commentary on clinical practices. During the second COVID-19 seminar, vaccine development, virological characteristics, treatment of respiratory failure, biomarkers, and human genetic susceptibility for infectious diseases were discussed. Conducting continuous seminars is important for general infectious controls.

**Keywords:** disaster; infectious diseases; leptospirosis; tuberculosis; dengue; POCT; COVID-19



**Citation:** Hattori, T.; Chagan-Yasutan, H.; Koga, S.; Yanagihara, Y.; Tanaka, I. Seminar Lessons: Infectious Diseases Associated with and Causing Disaster. *Reports* **2022**, *5*, 7. https://doi.org/10.3390/reports5010007

Academic Editor: Ivana Kholová

Received: 8 February 2022
Accepted: 23 February 2022
Published: 28 February 2022



## 1. Introduction

In 2019, 396 natural disasters were recorded in the Emergency Events Database (EM-DAT), with 11,755 deaths, 95 million people affected, and USD 103 billion in economic losses worldwide. This burden was not shared equally since Asia suffered the highest impact, accounting for 40% of disaster events, 45% of deaths and 74% of the total affected [1]. Japan has historically suffered from large-scale natural disasters. Hojoki, one of the oldest essays in Japan, describes a great fire (A.D. 1177), a tornado followed by the relocation of the capital (A.D. 1180), a famine (A.D. 1181–2), and an earthquake (A.D. 1185). Recently, Japan endured the Great East Japan Earthquake and Tsunami (GEJET) of 11 March 2011—a magnitude-9 earthquake that attacked Sendai and neighboring cities, leaving 20,000 people missing. This area was attacked by a tsunami (Jogan) on 13 July 869, indicating that large-scale tsunamis occur within a 1000-year interval [2]. The Nankai Trough mega-earthquake (NTME) is anticipated as the next major earthquake in Japan, involving the Shizuoka prefecture. It is anticipated to cause approximately 323,000 deaths and approximately USD 1.5 trillion in direct impact, with a production and service decline amounting to approximately USD 0.4 trillion [3]. Sharing our knowledge of the disaster is one way to initiate effective measures against these disasters. For this purpose, we decided to share our knowledge with annual seminars about infectious diseases that may occur due to disasters. The participants were from the International Research Institute of Disaster Science (IRIDeS) at Tohoku University in Sendai who suffered from GEJET, and those involved in disaster countermeasures and medical treatment in the Shizuoka prefecture since 2014. It is important to enhance the resilience of national health systems for disaster risk reduction. Some approaches include integrating disaster risk management into primary, secondary, and tertiary healthcare (especially at the local level), developing health workers' understanding of disaster risks, applying and implementing disaster risk reduction approaches to healthcare, promoting and enhancing training in the field of disaster medicine, and training community health groups in disaster risk reduction through health programs in collaboration with other sectors [4]. During disasters, a lack of safe water access and inadequate sanitation facilities allow the transmission of water-borne and food-borne pathogens. Diarrheal diseases such as cholera, typhoid fever, and shigellosis cause epidemics with high mortality rates. Malaria and other vector-borne diseases in risk areas include arboviruses, such as dengue, yellow fever, Japanese encephalitis, Rift Valley fever, and tick-borne illnesses, including Crimean–Congo hemorrhagic fever and typhus. Diseases associated with overcrowding, such as measles in unvaccinated areas and tuberculosis, can occur after natural disasters. During the seminars, we discussed infectious diseases associated with disasters, such as leptospirosis [5], dengue virus infection [6], and tuberculosis [7,8]. We also discussed biomarkers for these diseases that reflect disease severity [9], and a point-of-care test (POCT) to detect pathogens, including loop-mediated thermal amplification (LAMP) in tuberculosis [10], single-tag hybridization chromatographic-printed array (STH-PAS) [11], and a nanopore technology-based sequencer called MinION [12]. We proposed that acquired immune deficiency syndrome (AIDS) co-infected with tuberculosis (TB) (AIDS/TB) constitutes a natural disaster because the deaths caused by AIDS/TB account for 47% of all deaths in South Africa [13]. Severe acute respiratory syndrome coronavirus 2 (SARS-CoV-2) [14] caused a pandemic in 2019 (COVID-19) with more than 286 million cases and 5,429,617 deaths by the end of 2021 (https://coronavirus.jhu.edu/) (accessed on 30 December 2021). The expansion of the pandemic severely damaged society. Therefore, the last two seminars were held exclusively on SARS-CoV-2 infections. In this manuscript, we introduce 10 seminars on measures against disaster-related infectious diseases and propose the role seminars play in combating infectious diseases associated with disasters.

## 2. Content of Seminars

Table 1 shows the speakers, their lecture titles, and the dates of the seminars in chronological order. The first seminar was held at Shizuoka General Hospital (SGH), followed by a second seminar hosted by the Division of Disaster-related Infectious Diseases (DRI) at IRIDeS. The third seminar was held as part of the third world conference on disaster risk reduction (DRR) in Sendai (2015) (https://www.un.org/press/en/highlights/wcdrr) (accessed on 30 December 2021). The following seminars were conducted based on the Sendai framework for disaster risk reduction [4]. The content of the seminars were classified into categories (Figure 1). Recalling the 10 seminars, 35 speakers from 21 organizations performed lectures about infectious diseases, as well as disaster prevention and mitigation methods. Five of these lectures discussed disaster risk reduction (DRR) from many aspects, including human security [2,15], the United Nations world conference [4], disaster prevention, and measures of the Shizuoka prefecture.

**Table 1.** Conference speakers and their titles in chronological order.

| No. | Date | Speaker | Affiliation | Title | Classification |
|---|---|---|---|---|---|
| 1 | 24 February 2014 | Sato T | JBCL | Examination of digestive system required for disaster infectious diseases | *E. coli* |
| | | Koga S | U. Shizuoka | Disaster infectious diseases, after earthquakes and tsunamis | DRI |
| | | Hattori T | IRIDeS | Human security program against disasters and infectious diseases | DRR |
| 2 | 19 July 2014 | Sato T | JBCL | Examination of digestive system required for disaster infectious diseases | *E. coli* |
| | | C.-Y. H | IRIDeS | Disaster-related infectious diseases in the Philippines | Tropical |
| | | Ashino Y | Tohoku U. | Actual condition of HIV infections in the Tohoku region of Japan | HIV |
| | | Egawa S | IRIDeS | Medical response in the Great East Japan Earthquake | DRHM |
| 3 | 13 March 2015 | C.-Y. H | IRIDeS | Collaborative research on disaster-related infectious diseases with Philippines | Tropical |
| | | Sumi A | SMU | Seasonal tuberculosis epidemic | MTB |
| | | Ndhlovu LC | U. Hawaii | Consideration of the HIV epidemic during disaster related events | HIV |
| | | Hakamata Y | SGH | Preparation for disaster-related infectious diseases in Shizuoka Prefecture | DRI |
| | | Suzuki Y | Hokkaido U. | Tuberculosis as a disaster-related disorders | MTB |
| 4 | 4 July 2015 | Fukuoka T | SSH | Experience of outbreak of pathogenic *Escherichia coli* O157 | *E. coli* |
| | | Kutsuna K | NCGM | Dengue fever | Tropical |
| | | Kaji M | SCHC | About infectious disease measures in Shizuoka city | DRI |
| | | Yanagihara Y | U. Shizuoka | Floods and leptospirosis in the Philippines | Tropical |
| | | Egawa S | IRIDeS | Reports of the United Nations world conference on disaster risk reduction | DRR |
| 5 | 19 November 2016 | Nakayama Y | SKH | "Chain of survival" Kumamoto earthquake, crisis of life. | DRHM |
| | | C.-Y. H | IRIDeS | Actual conditions of mosquito-borne infectious diseases and its spreading | Tropical |
| | | Sato T | JBCL | Countermeasures against norovirus infection in the event of disaster | Norovirus |
| | | Kawase M | TBA | Development of new diagnostic method STH-PAS for infectious diseases | POCT |
| | | Koga S | U. Shizuoka | Current status and countermeasures for important tick-borne infectious diseases | Tick |
| 6 | 12 December 2017 | Suzuki Y | Hokkaido U. | Tuberculosis; never-ending threat | MTB |
| | | Kawamori F | U. Shizuoka | Tick-born infectious diseases in Shizuoka prefecture | Tick |
| | | Hakamata Y | SGH | Summary of pet infectious diseases of concern at evacuation center | Pet infection |
| | | Matsui T | NIID | Risk assessment method for infectious disease at evacuation center—to facilitate 'common language' between infection control specialists and public health sectors | DRHM |
| | | Iwata K | Shizuoka U. | From disaster mitigation to disaster prevention society | DRR |

**Table 1.** *Cont.*

| No. | Date | Speaker | Affiliation | Title | Classification |
|---|---|---|---|---|---|
| 7 | 1 December 2018 | Nakagawa S | Tokai U. | How to utilize the portable DNA/RNA sequencer MiniON for disaster medical care | POCT |
| | | Mori K | SGH | Kidney disease biomarkers in disaster infectious diseases | Biomarker |
| | | Kaji M | SCHC | Measures against infectious diseases in the event of a disaster | DRI |
| | | Hattori T | KIUI | Disaster measures learned from South East Asia | Resilience |
| | | Ueda T | CMDS | Earthquake and tsunami countermeasures in Shizuoka prefecture | DRR |
| 8 | 16 November 2019 | Goka K | NIES | Fire ants, ticks, mosquitoes–biological risks caused by environmental disturbances and globalization | DRI |
| | | Kawaguchi T | KHSU | Infection prevention and control during natural disaster: lessons learned from the Kumamoto Earthquake | DRI |
| | | Tosaka N | SGH | Repones of medical institutions in infectious disease crisis management | DRHM |
| | | Ueda T | CMDS | Shizuoka prefecture disaster prevention drill | DRR |
| 9 | 20 March 2021 | Miyasaka M | Osaka U. | What did we learn from a novel coronavirus infection? | COVID-19 |
| | | Takahashi A | KIUI | Japanese immune strategy and measures against medical collapse | COVID-19 |
| | | Yano K | HMC | About new coronavirus information from CDC | COVID-19 |
| | | Iwai K | ShCH | COVID-19 from the medical side | COVID-19 |
| 10 | 27 November 2021 | Ishii K | IMS | Disruptive innovation in vaccine development research advancing COVID-19 disaster | COVID-19 |
| | | Iwatani Y | NMC | Characteristics and mutations in SARS-CoV-2 | COVID-19 |
| | | Fujimi S | OGMC | Response of the critical care center in Osaka during the COVID-19 pandemic | COVID-19 |
| | | Ashino Y | SDCH | COVID-19 treatment recommendations from Sendai city hospital | COVID-19 |
| | | Terao C | SGH | Cloned cell proliferation and infection | COVID-19 |

We must strengthen the sustainable use and management of ecosystems and implement integrated environmental and natural resource management approaches that incorporate disaster risk reduction. Through their experience and traditional knowledge, indigenous peoples provide an important contribution to the development and implementation of plans and mechanisms, including early warning and water safety [4,16]. Therefore, to increase resilience from disaster-related damage, learning to live in harmony with nature was advocated by Thai indigenous Karen peoples. The hill people can only live with intact forest. An intact forest must have seven layers, which include four aboveground layers. A tree in an intact forest must always follow this pattern: the large tree is at the center, while saplings and bushes—the living quarters of birds and insects—surround this tree. Just below the center and above the bushes and saplings are trees whose branches orchids attach to, drawing nutrients from the trees. At the lower levels are grasses and mushrooms. As for the sub-surface layers, there are roots, tubers, worms, snakes, sweet potatoes, and taros. However, if one element is missing, the system is degraded and cannot survive [17]. Living with nature appears to help recovery from disaster (Figure 2).

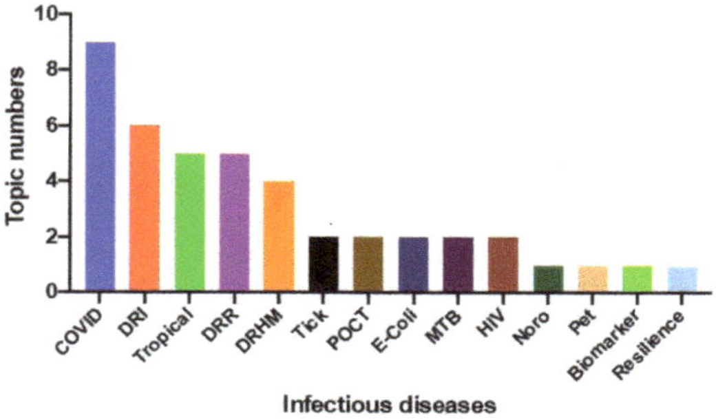


**Figure 1.** The topic classification of seminar contents. Abbreviation: COVID, COVID-19; DRI, Disaster-related infectious disease; Tropical, Tropical infectious diseases; DRR, Disaster-risk reduction; DRHM, Disaster-risk health management; Tick, Tick-borne diseases; POCT, Point of care test; *E. coli*, *Escherichia coli*; MTB, *Mycobacterium tuberculosis*; HIV, Human immunodeficiency virus; Noro, Norovirus; Pet, Pet-derived infectious diseases.

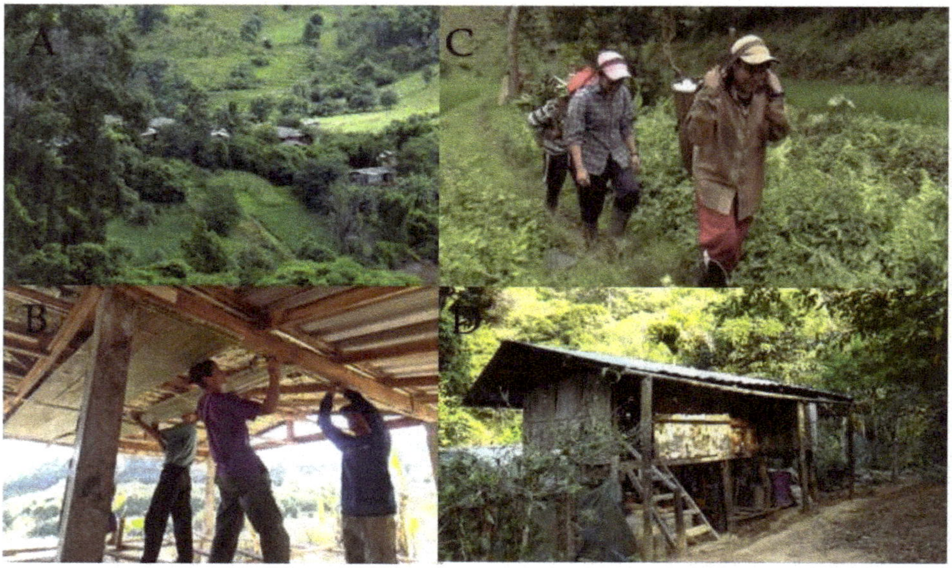


**Figure 2.** Lives of indigenous people at Ban Huai Hin Lat Nai in Chaing rai. (**A**) Houses are protected by tropical rainforest. (**B**) Houses being built by villagers. (**C**) Self-sufficiency and cultivation while protecting the forest. (**D**) Stilt food storage. (Photos are courtesy of Mr. Kunio Miyairi and Prof. Tatsuhiko Kawashima, GONGOVA, 2018).

Four lectures on disaster risk health management were also performed to understand the medical system's approach to disasters. In the Kumamoto area of Kyushu, Japan, an Mj 7.3 mainshock occurred on 16 April 2016, close to the epicenter of an Mj 6.5 foreshock that occurred about 28 h earlier [18]. How the disaster base hospitals worked against these disasters was also presented. Six lectures on disaster-related infectious diseases (DRI) shared knowledge on these diseases, including bacillary dysentery after floods [5] and norovirus outbreaks after Hurricane Katrina despite intensive public health measures [19]. Oysters in the Tohoku area carry norovirus, which causes food poisoning. Oyster contamination correlates with food poisoning and diarrhea outbreaks caused by Escherichia coli in Shizuoka [20].

Tetanus occurrence after the Aceh earthquake and tsunami in 2004 [21] and tuberculosis outbreaks after the Haiti earthquake were mentioned in another lecture [7,8]. Understanding the seasonality of tuberculosis (TB) epidemics may help identify potentially modifiable risk factors. Sumi et al. confirmed differences in the seasonality of the prevalence data for sputum smear-positive (SSP) and sputum smear-negative (SSN) pulmonary TB cases in Wuhan [22]. To control SSP pulmonary TB cases, they suggested investigating the periodic structures of SSP and SSN pulmonary TB cases' temporal patterns individually. Attendants often talked about each of these diseases. Twenty pathogens (Table 2) were described in this seminar. For early diagnosis of DRI, biomarkers' roles were presented, including galectin-9 (Gal-9) in dengue fever (DF) [9], malaria [23], and osteopontin (OPN) in leptospirosis [24]. Neutrophil gelatinase-associated lipocalin (Ngal) and other tubular dysfunction markers were also introduced to diagnose acute kidney injury (AKI) [25,26].

**Table 2.** Pathogens discussed at the seminars.

| Classification (No.) and Pathogens | | |
|---|---|---|
| Virus infection (17) | RNA (14) | *Human Immunodeficiency Virus (HIV); Coronavirus type 1, type 2; Middle east respiratory virus syndrome; Ebola virus; Dengue virus; Zika virus; Severe fever with thrombocytopenia syndrome virus; Rabies; Lyssavirus; Influenza virus; Norovirus; Hepatitis C virus; Measles virus; Rubella virus.* |
| | DNA (3) | *Human papilloma virus; Hepatitis B virus; Varicella zoster virus; Chickenpox virus.* |
| *Bacteria (8)* | *Mycobacterium tuberculosis; Escherichia coli; Clostridium tetani; Legionella; Leptospira* spp.; *Bartonella henselae; Coxiella burnetii; Chlamydia psittaci.* | |
| *Fungi (1)* | *Chytrid fungi* | |
| *Parasite (2)* | *Plasmodium falciparum Malaria; Trypanosoma cruzi;* | |

Table 2 lists the pathogens discussed at the conference. Interestingly, 17 out of 28 (about 60%) are viruses, and 14 out of 17 (82%) are RNA viruses. It is worth mentioning that representative zoonotic pathogens, such as Coronavirus, Influenza virus, Ebola virus, Rabies lyssavirus, and Leptospira, were discussed. Therefore, it is necessary to set human and animal life as countermeasure targets for preventing disaster-related infectious diseases. At the same time, it is necessary to further in vivo research on pathogens such as RNA viruses, as described here.

## 3. Disaster-Related Infectious Diseases

### 3.1. Leptospirosis

Leptospirosis is zoonotic, often occurs after floods, and is mainly endemic to subtropical or tropical countries. It has not been reported since 2009 in the Tohoku region (northern Japan). However, four patients with leptospirosis were found in the region between 2012 and 2014. These cases imply that leptospirosis has reemerged in the region, probably due to global warming [27]. In the Philippines, leptospirosis occurs after floods caused by typhoons or heavy rainfall. The main pathogens consist of numerous serovars (>250). The case fatality rate is 10–20%, and the majority of patients, about 85%, are young males. In addition to rats, its main reservoirs are animals such as wild rodents, herbivores, livestock, and pets, which transmit leptospires through Leptospira-colonized water with urinary excretion in the environment [28,29]. Dominant Leptospira serovars with high virulence include *L. interrogans* serovar Manilae, *L. interrogans* serovar Losbanos, *L. interrogans* serovar Ratnapura, and *L. borgpetersenii*. After a storm surge during the super typhoon Haiyan (Yolanda), pathogenic Leptospira survived in coastal soil in Leyte. Metrological factors showed that leptospirosis occurrence is associated with floods following monsoons in Manila. Besides rainfall, leptospirosis is also associated with relative humidity and temperature in the Philippines. The peak occurrence of leptospirosis preceded DF by only one month, despite occurring 2–3 months later than the peak occurrence of dengue in Thailand [6].

We conducted a biomarker analysis of leptospirosis using two representative matricellular proteins, OPN and Gal-9, in plasma. Both the full-length Gal-9 (FL-Gal9) and OPN (FL-OPN) had increased levels of leptospirosis. Compared to other infectious diseases, pFL-Gal-9 levels showed an inverse correlation with pFL-OPN levels ($r = -0.24$, $p < 0.05$), but no correlation with other markers. By contrast, pFL-OPN levels correlated significantly with other markers of kidney injury, indicating that FL-OPN levels reflect kidney injury in leptospirosis. N-gal was associated with tubular dysfunction in AKI [25].

### 3.2. Tick-Borne Disorders

Scrub typhus or "Tsutsugamushi disease" was recognized in Japan as a Japanese flood fever with high mortality [30]. A recent study in Laos suggested that *O. tsutsugamushi* infection is an important cause of central nervous system infections in Laos [31]. Global warming causes changes to all living things on earth. Tick-borne Lyme disease is increasing annually in the United States and Canada [32], and tick-borne encephalitis (TBE), Lyme borreliosis (LB), and emerging borrelial relapsing fever are widespread in Russia [33,34]. The increased number and distribution of ticks, vulnerability to rain, and increased wild animals, which are sources of blood-sucking for ticks, are involved. Tick and tick-borne pathogen surveillance efforts improve our understanding of geographic variation in risk factors for tick-borne diseases, and efforts to build such programs have increased in recent years [35].

### 3.3. Mosquito-Borne Disorders

Disasters change the behaviors of vectors and increase the incidence of vector-borne diseases, including malaria and DF [36]. Unlike the immediate impacts of flooding, malaria epidemics emerge after the acute phase of the crisis has passed. Heavy precipitation is thought to flush established larval habitats; however, malaria vectors rapidly reestablish, and a surge in disease may occur months after the disaster. Chemo-prevention is useful for reducing the excess disease burden associated with a severe flood [37]. It has also been suggested that DF cases in Manila are influenced by monsoon occurrence, contemporaneous with high temperature, high relative humidity, and heavy rainfall. Heavy rainfall precedes the occurrence of DF cases by two months. This timing can be attributed to the life-cycle of mosquitoes and an adequate number of cases for transmission, which is affected by population density [6]. An epidemic from imported DF occurred in Japan in 2014 and 200 cases were diagnosed. According to the analysis of virus strains, it was found that a single strain may have caused Dengue virus (DENV) cases in Tokyo. It should be noted that the plasma levels of Gal-9 are elevated in both DF and malaria. In malaria, Gal-9 levels were higher at day 0 compared with day 7 and day 28 ($p < 0.0001$). Gal-9 levels were significantly higher in severe malaria (SM) cases than uncomplicated (UM) cases on days 0 and 7. Therefore, Gal-9 is released during acute malaria and reflects its severity in malaria infections [23]. In DENV infection, Gal-9 levels in the critical phase were significantly higher in DENV-infected patients compared with healthy patients or those with non-dengue febrile illness. The highest Gal-9 levels were observed in dengue hemorrhagic fever (DHF) patients. Gal-9 levels significantly declined from peak levels in DF and DHF patients in the recovery phase. Gal-9 levels tracked viral load and reflected the severity of DENV infection [9]. Finally, a dipstick DNA chromatography assay, a single-tag hybridization-printed array strip (STH-PAS), was evaluated for its efficacy in detecting DENV. PCR amplified reverse-transcribed DNA, and the amplified DNA was detected using the STH-PAS system. In clinical studies, the STH-PAS system showed 100% sensitivity with 88.9 and 86.6% specificities compared to Taqman RT-PCR and the SD Dengue Duo NS1 test, respectively. The STH-PAS system was found to have a superior sensitivity to the Taqman system [11].

## 4. COVID-19 Caused a Disaster

The COVID-19 outbreak is primarily a human tragedy, affecting countless people. Thus, many countries have undergone lockdowns, restricting their economic agents from mobilizing from one country to another, even nationally, due to the communicable COVID-19. The virus has had a growing impact on the global economy; unfortunately, the global health crisis has become a global economic crisis due to the cancellation of flights, restriction of labor mobility, volatility in stock markets, and so on. For vulnerable families, loss of income due to the outbreak translates to spikes in poverty, missed meals for children, and reduced access to healthcare beyond COVID-19 [38]. It also affects the education of surgeons in the medical community. Residents and young surgeons have shown a substantial decrease in clinical experience, affecting resident education and practice, and variable access to personal protective equipment (PPE). These wasteful efforts have resulted in emotional problems and burnout [39]. Internationally, governments have been enforcing travel bans, quarantine, isolation, and social distancing. Extended periods spent at home have resulted in reduced physical activity, changes in dietary intake with the potential to accelerate sarcopenia, deterioration of muscle mass and function (especially in older populations), as well as increases in body fat [40]. It was also revealed that SARS-CoV-2 has a lower mutation rate than other RNA viruses because it encodes proofreading enzyme genes. Nevertheless, ongoing rapid transmission between humans increases the genetic diversity of SARS-CoV-2 genomes, especially the Spike gene (or the receptor-binding domain, RBD); the latter is advantageous in virus infectivity, immune escape, and tolerance [41]. Interestingly, these glocally occurring viral genetic changes display a convergent evolution of the SARS-CoV-2 genome worldwide [42]. Therefore, worldwide surveillance of the SARS-CoV-2 genome is important to understanding future epidemics and may help us control COVID-19. The historical background of mRNA-based vaccine development was also introduced during the seminar [43]. Furthermore, immunogenicity and BNT162b2, a lipid nanoparticle-formulated, nucleoside-modified RNA (modRNA) encoding the SARS-CoV-2 full-length spike, modified by two proline mutations that lock it in the prefusion conformation, were proven to be safe and effective [44]. Identifying risk factors for COVID-19 infection is critical to public health importance. Mosaic chromosomal alteration (mCA), a clonal expansion of leukocytes with somatic chromosomal abnormalities, is associated with an increased risk of many infectious diseases, including severe COVID-19 infection [45]. mCA is strongly associated with males and the elderly; however, the association was significant even after controlling for covariates such as age and sex. The presence of cancer enhanced this association. There was also a trend that the higher the patient's fraction of mCA, the higher the infection rate, suggesting that the expansion of cells with large mutations resulted in abnormal immune dysfunction. This mechanism is interesting; targeting abnormally expanded cells may present a new treatment for many infections, including COVID-19. It would be reasonable to stratify people by the presence or absence of mCA, carefully monitor the infections of those with mCA, and provide appropriate advice according to infection risk inferred from the presence or absence of mCA. SARS-CoV-2 RNA in concentrated and purified saliva specimens was detected 37 days after onset, using sugar chain-immobilized gold nanoparticles. It was suggested that early morning saliva specimens are more likely to show positive results than those obtained later in the day [46].

An intravenous administration of the anti-interleukin-6 receptor antibody tocilizumab (TCZ; 400 mg) effectively treated a patient with COVID-19 pneumonia and a kidney injury. An early administration of TCZ was proposed to prevent pneumonia and kidney injury caused by COVID-19 from progressing to hyperinflammatory syndrome [47]. Plasma levels of FL-Gal9 and FL-OPN and their truncated forms (Tr-Gal9, Ud-OPN, respectively) represent inflammatory biomarkers. For COVID-19 infection, Spearman's correlation analysis showed that Tr-Gal9, Ud-OPN, but not FL-Gal9 and FL-OPN, were significantly associated with laboratory markers for lung function, inflammation, coagulopathy, and kidney function in CP patients. It was proposed that the cleaved forms of OPN and Gal-9 can be used to monitor the severity of pathological inflammation and therapeutic effects of TCZ in CP patients [48].

## 5. Discussion

Three times more natural disasters occurred from 2000 to 2009 than 1980 to 1989. Climate-related events have increased, accounting for nearly 80% [49]. It is urgent and critical to anticipate, plan for and reduce disaster risk to protect persons, communities, and countries, their livelihoods, health, cultural heritage, socioeconomic assets, and ecosystems effectively, thus strengthening their resilience [4]. We must initiate measures against Nankai Trough Mega Earthquake [3]. In this manuscript, we summarized 10 consecutive seminars on disaster-related infectious diseases. Various topics, including disaster risk reduction, were discussed. Speakers mentioned various pathogens associated with disasters; about 60% of them (17 out of 28) are viruses, and 14 out of 17 (82%) are RNA viruses. RNA viruses evolve rapidly. The high mutation frequency in RNA virus populations is one source of their ability to rapidly change. A high mutation frequency is a central tenet of the quasi-species theory. Unlike RNA viruses, DNA-based organisms generally have lower mutation frequencies and do not exist near the error threshold [50].

Among the many disaster-related infectious diseases, we proposed that AIDS associated with TB (AIDS/TB) is a disaster because deaths caused by AIDS and tuberculosis (TB) account for 47% of all deaths in South Africa [13]. The encroachment of HIV into TB endemic areas may expand AIDS/TB. We have been researching novel biomarkers to detect AIDS/TB in patients from India [51] and have continued our study as part of a JICA grass-roots project.

The recent COVID-19 pandemic caused by SARS-CoV2 is a global crisis. Genome sequencing early in the pandemic showed that single nucleotide mutations, multi-base insertions and deletions, recombination, and variation in surface glycans all generate the variability that, guided by natural selection, enables both HIV-1′s extraordinary diversity and SARS-CoV-2′s slower pace of mutation accumulation. Although SARS-CoV-2′s diversity is more limited, recently emergent SARS-CoV-2 variants carry Spike mutations with important phenotypic consequences in antibody resistance and enhanced infectivity [52]. This rate of change is about half that of influenza, and one-quarter of HIV owing to the error-correcting enzyme coronaviruses possess, rare among other RNA viruses. There are probably thousands of viral particles in any given infection, each with unique single-letter mutations; however, few if any of these cause the virus to be more infectious. Omicron's rise may be largely due to its ability to infect people immune to Delta through vaccination or previous infection [53].

At the seminar discussed here, we shared our knowledge about the clinical manifestations of various infectious diseases, pathogens, and progress in diagnostic methods. In addition, the significance of matricellular proteins such as OPN and Gal-9, which were reported as markers of severity for tropical infectious diseases, was reconfirmed in COVID-19 infection. Further examination revealed that protease cleaves these proteins, suggesting that cleaved products exert new pathological functions and become new severity markers [54,55]. On the other hand, the countermeasures against COVID-19, which caused the disasters worldwide, have introduced a great deal of knowledge about the pathophysiology and infectious mode of disaster-related infectious diseases. Furthermore, measures against infectious diseases are different for each country. Therefore, it is necessary to conduct such disaster-related infection control seminars on an international scale and share knowledge from each country.

**Author Contributions:** Conceptualization, T.H., S.K., Y.Y. and I.T.; data curation, H.C.-Y.; writing, T.H. and Y.Y.; funding acquisition, T.H. All authors have read and agreed to the published version of the manuscript.

**Funding:** This work was partially supported by the Japan Society for the Promotion of Science (JSPS) Grants-in-Aid for Scientific Research (KAKENHI), Grant Number 23256004, 26257506, JP17H01690.

**Institutional Review Board Statement:** Not applicable.

**Informed Consent Statement:** Not applicable.

**Data Availability Statement:** Not applicable.

**Acknowledgments:** We would like to thank all the speakers listed in Table 1. We would also like to thank the staff of SGH for operating the seminar.

**Conflicts of Interest:** The authors declare no conflict of interest.

## Abbreviations

| | |
|---|---|
| JBCL | Japan Biosciences Co., Ltd.; (Sendai, Miyagi, Japan) |
| U. | University |
| IRIDeS | International Research Institute of Disaster Science; (Tohoku University, Sendai, Miyagi, Japan) |
| SMU | Sapporo Medical University; (Sapporo, Hokkaido, Japan) |
| SGH | Shizuoka General Hospital; (Shizuoka, Shizuoka, Japan) |
| SSH | Saiseikai Shizuoka Hospital; (Shizuoka, Shizuoka, Japan) |
| NCGM | National Center for Global Health and Medicine;(Tokyo, Japan) |
| SCHC | Shizuoka City Health Center; (Shizuoka, Shizuoka, Japan) |
| SSK | Saiseikai Kumamoto Hospital; (Kumamoto, Kumamoto, Japan) |
| TBA | Tohoku Bio-Array Co., Ltd.; (Sendai, Miyagi, Japan) |
| NIID | National Institute for Infectious Disease; (Tokyo, Japan) |
| KIUI | Kibi International University; (Takahashi, Okayama, Japan) |
| CMDS | Crisis Management Department Shizuoka; (Shizuoka, Shizuoka, Japan) |
| NIES | National Institute for Environmental Studies;(Tsukuba, Ibaragi, Japan) |
| KHSU | Kumamoto Health Science University; (Kumamoto, Kumamoto, Japan) |
| ShCH | Shizuoka City Hospital; (Shizuoka, Shizuoka, Japan) |
| IMS | The Institute of Medical Science;(Tokyo, Japan) |
| NMC | Nagoya Medical Center; (Nagoya, Aichi, Japan) |
| OGMC | Osaka General Medical Center; (Osaka, Osaka, Japan) |
| SDCH | Sendai City Hospital; (Sendai, Miyagi, Japan) |
| *E. coli* | *Esherichia coli* |
| DRI | Disaster related infectious diseases |
| DRR | Disaster risk reduction |
| Tropical | Tropical infectious diseases |
| DRHM | Disaster risk health management |
| MTB | Mycobacterium tuberculosis |
| HIV | Human immunodeficiency virus |
| POCT | Point of care test |
| Tick | Tick-borne diseases |
| Pet infection | Pet-derived infectious diseases |
| COVID-19 | Coronavirus Disease in 2019 |

## References


1. Center for Research on the Epidemiology of Disasters, Natural Disaster 2019. Available online: https://landsliderisk.wordpress.com/2020/08/28/cred-report-natural-disasters-2019/ (accessed on 30 December 2021).
2. Hattori, T.; Chagan-Yasutan, H.; Shiratori, B.; Egawa, S.; Izumi, T.; Kubo, T.; Nakajima, C.; Suzuki, Y.; Niki, T.; Alisjahbana, B.; et al. Development of Point-of-Care Testing for Disaster-Related Infectious Diseases. *Tohoku J. Exp. Med.* **2016**, *238*, 287–293. [CrossRef]
3. Ministry of Land, Infrastructure, Transport and Tourism. *Overview of Nankai Trough Mega Earthquake Operation Plan*; MLITT: Tokyo, Japan, 2021.
4. UNDRR. *Sendai Framework for Disaster Risk Reduction 2015–2030*; UNDRR: Geneva, Switzerland, 2016.
5. Torgerson, P.; Hagan, J.; Costa, F.; Calcagno, J.; Kane, M.; Martinez-Silveira, M.S.; Goris, M.G.A.; Stein, C.; Ko, A.; Abela-Ridder, B. Global Burden of Leptospirosis: Estimated in Terms of Disability Adjusted Life Years. *PLoS Negl. Trop. Dis.* **2015**, *9*, e0004122. [CrossRef]
6. Sumi, A.; Telan, E.F.O.; Chagan-Yasutan, H.; Piolo, M.B.; Hattori, T.; Kobayashi, N. Effect of temperature, relative humidity and rainfall on dengue fever and leptospirosis infections in Manila, the Philippines. *Epidemiol. Infect.* **2017**, *145*, 78–86. [CrossRef]
7. Furin, J.; Mathew, T. Tuberculosis Control in Acute Disaster Settings: Case Studies from the 2010 Haiti Earthquake. *Disaster Med. Public Health Prep.* **2013**, *7*, 129–130. [CrossRef]
8. Koenig, S.P.; Rouzier, V.; Vilbrun, S.C.; Morose, W.; Collins, S.E.; Joseph, P.; Decome, D.; Ocheretina, O.; Galbaud, S.; Hashiguchi, L.; et al. Tuberculosis in the aftermath of the 2010 earthquake in Haiti. *Bull. World Health Organ.* **2015**, *93*, 498–502. [CrossRef]
9. Chagan-Yasutan, H.; Ndhlovu, L.; Lacuesta, T.L.; Kubo, T.; Leano, P.S.A.; Niki, T.; Oguma, S.; Morita, K.; Chew, G.M.; Barbour, J.D.; et al. Galectin-9 plasma levels reflect adverse hematological and immunological features in acute dengue virus infection. *J. Clin. Virol.* **2013**, *58*, 635–640. [CrossRef]
10. Phetsuksiri, B.; Rudeeaneksin, J.; Srisungngam, S.; Bunchoo, S.; Roienthong, D.; Mukai, T.; Nakajima, C.; Hamada, S.; Suzuki, Y. Applicability of In-House Loop-Mediated Isothermal Amplification for Rapid Identification of Mycobacterium tuberculosis Complex Grown on Solid Media. *Jpn. J. Infect. Dis.* **2013**, *66*, 249–251. [CrossRef]
11. Liles, V.R.; Pangilinan, L.-A.S.; Daroy, M.L.G.; Dimamay, M.T.A.; Reyes, R.S.; Bulusan, M.K.; Dimamay, M.P.S.; Luna, P.A.S.; Mercado, A.; Bai, G.; et al. Evaluation of a rapid diagnostic test for detection of dengue infection using a single-tag hybridization chromatographic-printed array strip format. *Eur. J. Clin. Microbiol.* **2019**, *38*, 515–521. [CrossRef]
12. Mitsuhashi, S.; Kryukov, K.; Nakagawa, S.; Takeuchi, J.S.; Shiraishi, Y.; Asano, K.; Imanishi, T. A portable system for rapid bacterial composition analysis using a nanopore-based sequencer and laptop computer. *Sci. Rep.* **2017**, *7*, 5657. [CrossRef]
13. *The 2012 National Antenatal Sentinel HIV & Herpes Simplex Type-2 Prevalence Survey in South Africa*; Directorate Epidemiology Cluster, HIMME National Department of Health: Pretoria, South Africa, 2013.
14. Hu, B.; Guo, H.; Zhou, P.; Shi, Z.-L. Characteristics of SARS-CoV-2 and COVID-19. *Nat. Rev. Microbiol.* **2021**, *19*, 141–154. [CrossRef]
15. Nations United. *Human Development Report 1994*; Oxford University Press: Oxford, UK, 1994.
16. Fatehpanah, A.; Jahangiri, K.; Seyedin, S.H.; Kavousi, A.; Malekinezhad, H. Water safety in drought: An indigenous knowledge-based qualitative study. *J. Water Health* **2020**, *18*, 692–703. [CrossRef]
17. McKinnon, J. Community culture: Strengthening persistence to empower resistance. In *Living at the Edge of Thai Society*; Routledge: Oxfordshire, UK, 2003; pp. 64–85.
18. Kato, A.; Nakamura, K.; Hiyama, Y. The 2016 Kumamoto earthquake sequence. *Proc. Jpn. Acad. Ser. B* **2016**, *92*, 358–371. [CrossRef]
19. Yee, E.L.; Palacio, H.; Atmar, R.L.; Shah, U.; Kilborn, C.; Faul, M.; Gavagan, T.E.; Feigin, R.D.; Versalovic, J.; Neill, F.H.; et al. Widespread Outbreak of Norovirus Gastroenteritis among Evacuees of Hurricane Katrina Residing in a Large "Megashelter" in Houston, Texas: Lessons Learned for Prevention. *Clin. Infect. Dis.* **2007**, *44*, 1032–1039. [CrossRef]
20. Harada, T.; Hiroi, M.; Kawamori, F.; Furusawa, A.; Ohata, K.; Sugiyama, K.; Masuda, T. A food poisoning diarrhea outbreak caused by enteroaggregative Escherichia coli serogroup O126:H27 in Shizuoka, Japan. *Jpn. J. Infect. Dis.* **2007**, *60*, 154–155.
21. Pascapurnama, D.N.; Murakami, A.; Chagan-Yasutan, H.; Hattori, T.; Sasaki, H.; Egawa, S. Prevention of Tetanus Outbreak Following Natural Disaster in Indonesia: Lessons Learned from Previous Disasters. *Tohoku J. Exp. Med.* **2016**, *238*, 219–227. [CrossRef]
22. Luo, T.; Sumi, A.; Zhou, D.; Kobayashi, N.; Mise, K.; Yu, B.; Kong, D.; Wang, J.; Duan, Q. Seasonality of reported tuberculosis cases from 2006 to 2010 in Wuhan, China. *Epidemiol. Infect.* **2014**, *142*, 2036–2048. [CrossRef]
23. Dembele, B.P.P.; Chagan-Yasutan, H.; Niki, T.; Ashino, Y.; Tangpukdee, N.; Shinichi, E.; Krudsood, S.; Kano, S.; Hattori, T. Plasma levels of Galectin-9 reflect disease severity in malaria infection. *Malar. J.* **2016**, *15*, 408. [CrossRef]
24. Chagan-Yasutan, H.; Hanan, F.; Niki, T.; Bai, G.; Ashino, Y.; Egawa, S.; Telan, E.F.O.; Hattori, T. Plasma Osteopontin Levels is Associated with Biochemical Markers of Kidney Injury in Patients with Leptospirosis. *Diagnostics* **2020**, *10*, 439. [CrossRef]
25. Mori, K.; Lee, H.T.; Rapoport, D.; Drexler, I.R.; Foster, K.; Yang, J.; Schmidt-Ott, K.M.; Chen, X.; Li, J.Y.; Weiss, S.; et al. Endocytic delivery of lipocalin-siderophore-iron complex rescues the kidney from ischemia-reperfusion injury. *J. Clin. Investig.* **2005**, *115*, 610–621. [CrossRef]

26. Mori, K.; Mori, N. Diagnosis of AKI: Clinical Assessment, Novel Biomarkers, History, and Perspectives. *Acute Kidney Inj. Regen. Med.* **2020**, 47–58. [CrossRef]
27. Saitoh, H.; Koizumi, N.; Seto, J.; Ajitsu, S.; Fujii, A.; Takasaki, S.; Yamakage, S.; Aoki, S.; Nakayama, K.; Ashino, Y.; et al. Leptospirosis in the Tohoku Region: Re-emerging Infectious Disease. *Tohoku J. Exp. Med.* **2015**, *236*, 33–37. [CrossRef] [PubMed]
28. Villanueva, S.Y.A.; Saito, M.; Tsutsumi, Y.; Segawa, T.; Baterna, R.A.; Chakraborty, A.; Asoh, T.; Miyahara, S.; Yanagihara, Y.; Cavinta, L.L.; et al. High virulence in hamsters of four dominant Leptospira serovars isolated from rats in the Philippines. *Microbiology* **2014**, *160*, 418–428. [CrossRef] [PubMed]
29. Saito, M.; Miyahara, S.; Villanueva, S.Y.A.M.; Aramaki, N.; Ikejiri, M.; Kobayashi, Y.; Guevarra, J.P.; Masuzawa, T.; Gloriani, N.G.; Yanagihara, Y.; et al. PCR and Culture Identification of Pathogenic Leptospira spp. from Coastal Soil in Leyte, Philippines, after a Storm Surge during Super Typhoon Haiyan (Yolanda). *Appl. Environ. Microbiol.* **2014**, *80*, 6926–6932. [CrossRef] [PubMed]
30. Kawamura, R. Studies on tsutsugamushi disease (Japanese flood fever). *Med Bull. Coll. Med. Univ. Cincinnati* **1926**, *4*, 217–222.
31. Dittrich, S.; Rattanavong, S.; Lee, S.J.; Panyanivong, P.; Craig, S.B.; Tulsiani, S.M.; Blacksell, S.; Dance, D.; Dubot-Pérès, A.; Sengduangphachanh, A.; et al. Orientia, rickettsia, and leptospira pathogens as causes of CNS infections in Laos: A prospective study. *Lancet Glob. Health* **2015**, *3*, e104–e112. [CrossRef]
32. Marx, G.E.; Spillane, M.; Beck, A.; Stein, Z.; Powell, A.K.; Hinckley, A.F. Emergency Department Visits for Tick Bites–United States, January 2017–December 2019. *MMWR. Morb. Mortal. Wkly. Rep.* **2021**, *70*, 612–616. [CrossRef]
33. Krause, P.; Fish, D.; Narasimhan, S.; Barbour, A. Borrelia miyamotoi infection in nature and in humans. *Clin. Microbiol. Infect.* **2015**, *21*, 631–639. [CrossRef]
34. Platonov, A.E.; Karan, L.S.; Kolyasnikova, N.M.; Makhneva, N.A.; Toporkova, M.G.; Maleev, V.V.; Fish, D.; Krause, P.J. Humans Infected with Relapsing Fever SpirocheteBorrelia miyamotoi, Russia. *Emerg. Infect. Dis.* **2011**, *17*, 1816–1823. [CrossRef]
35. Eisen, R.J.; Paddock, C.D. Tick and Tickborne Pathogen Surveillance as a Public Health Tool in the United States. *J. Med. Entomol.* **2021**, *58*, 1490–1502. [CrossRef]
36. Charnley, G.E.C.; Kelman, I.; Gaythorpe, K.; Murray, K. Understanding the risks for post-disaster infectious disease outbreaks: A systematic review protocol. *BMJ Open* **2020**, *10*, e039608. [CrossRef]
37. Boyce, R.M.; Hollingsworth, B.D.; Baguma, E.; Xu, E.; Goel, V.; Brown-Marusiak, A.; Muhindo, R.; Reyes, R.; Ntaro, M.; Siedner, M.J.; et al. Dihydroartemisinin-Piperaquine Chemoprevention and Malaria Incidence After Severe Flooding: Evaluation of a Pragmatic Intervention in Rural Uganda. *Clin. Infect. Dis.* **2021**. [CrossRef] [PubMed]
38. Singh, M.K.; Neog, Y. Contagion effect ofCOVID-19 outbreak: Another recipe for disaster on Indian economy. *J. Public Aff.* **2020**, 2171. [CrossRef] [PubMed]
39. Ellison, E.C.; Shabahang, M.M. COVID-19 Pandemic and the Need for Disaster Planning in Surgical Education. *J. Am. Coll. Surg.* **2021**, *232*, 135–137. [CrossRef]
40. Kirwan, R.; McCullough, D.; Butler, T.; De Heredia, F.P.; Davies, I.G.; Stewart, C. Sarcopenia during COVID-19 lockdown restrictions: Long-term health effects of short-term muscle loss. *GeroScience* **2020**, *42*, 1547–1578. [CrossRef]
41. Miyasaka, M. COVID-19 and immunity: Quo vadis? *Int. Immunol.* **2021**, *33*, 507–513. [CrossRef]
42. Kamikubo, Y.; Takahashi, A. Epidemic trends of SARS-CoV-2 modulated by economic activity, ethnicity, and vaccination. *Camb. Open Engag.* **2021**. Available online: https://researchmap.jp/read0146204/published_papers/31864267 (accessed on 30 December 2021).
43. Sugiyama, T.; Gursel, M.; Takeshita, F.; Coban, C.; Conover, J.; Kaisho, T.; Akira, S.; Klinman, D.M.; Ishii, K.J. CpG RNA: Identification of Novel Single-Stranded RNA That Stimulates Human CD14+CD11c+Monocytes. *J. Immunol.* **2005**, *174*, 2273–2279. [CrossRef]
44. Polack, F.P.; Thomas, S.J.; Kitchin, N.; Absalon, J.; Gurtman, A.; Lockhart, S.; Perez, J.L.; Pérez Marc, G.; Moreira, E.D.; Zerbini, C.; et al. Safety and efficacy of the BNT162b2 mRNA COVID-19 vaccine. *N. Engl. J. Med.* **2020**, *383*, 2603–2615. [CrossRef]
45. Zekavat, S.M.; Lin, S.-H.; Bick, A.G.; Liu, A.; Paruchuri, K.; Wang, C.; Uddin, M.; Ye, Y.; Yu, Z.; Liu, X.; et al. Hematopoietic mosaic chromosomal alterations increase the risk for diverse types of infection. *Nat. Med.* **2021**, *27*, 1012–1024. [CrossRef]
46. Tajima, Y.; Suda, Y.; Yano, K. A case report of SARS-CoV-2 confirmed in saliva specimens up to 37 days after onset: Proposal of saliva specimens for COVID-19 diagnosis and virus monitoring. *J. Infect. Chemother.* **2020**, *26*, 1086–1089. [CrossRef]
47. Ashino, Y.; Chagan-Yasutan, H.; Hatta, M.; Shirato, Y.; Kyogoku, Y.; Komuro, H.; Hattori, T. Successful Treatment of a COVID-19 Case with Pneumonia and Renal Injury Using Tocilizumab. *Reports* **2020**, *3*, 29. [CrossRef]
48. Bai, G.; Furushima, D.; Niki, T.; Matsuba, T.; Maeda, Y.; Takahashi, A.; Hattori, T.; Ashino, Y. High Levels of the Cleaved Form of Galectin-9 and Osteopontin in the Plasma Are Associated with Inflammatory Markers That Reflect the Severity of COVID-19 Pneumonia. *Int. J. Mol. Sci.* **2021**, *22*, 4978. [CrossRef] [PubMed]
49. Leaning, J.; Guha-Sapir, D. Natural Disasters, Armed Conflict, and Public Health. *N. Engl. J. Med.* **2013**, *369*, 1836–1842. [CrossRef] [PubMed]
50. Crotty, S.; Cameron, C.E.; Andino, R. RNA virus error catastrophe: Direct molecular test by using ribavirin. *Proc. Natl. Acad. Sci. USA* **2001**, *98*, 6895–6900. [CrossRef]
51. Shete, A.; Bichare, S.; Pujari, V.; Virkar, R.; Thakar, M.; Ghate, M.; Patil, S.; Vyakarnam, A.; Gangakhedkar, R.; Bai, G.; et al. Elevated Levels of Galectin-9 but Not Osteopontin in HIV and Tuberculosis Infections Indicate Their Roles in Detecting MTB Infection in HIV Infected Individuals. *Front. Microbiol.* **2020**, *11*, 1685. [CrossRef]
52. Fischer, W.; Giorgi, E.E.; Chakraborty, S.; Nguyen, K.; Bhattarcharya, T.; Theiler, J.; Goloboff, P.A.; Yoon, H.; Abfalterer, W.; Foley, B.T.; et al. HIV-1 and SARS-CoV-2: Patterns in the evolution of two pandemic pathogens. *Cell Host Microbe* **2021**, *29*, 1093–1110. [CrossRef]

53. Callaway, E. Beyond Omicron: What's next for COVID's viral evolution. *Nature* **2021**, *600*, 204–207. [CrossRef]
54. Iwasaki-Hozumi, H.; Chagan-Yasutan, H.; Ashino, Y.; Hattori, T. Blood Levels of Galectin-9, an Immuno-Regulating Molecule, Reflect the Severity for the Acute and Chronic Infectious Diseases. *Biomolecules* **2021**, *11*, 430. [CrossRef]
55. Hattori, T.; Iwasaki-Hozumi, H.; Bai, G.; Chagan-Yasutan, H.; Shete, A.; Telan, E.F.; Takahashi, A.; Ashino, Y.; Matsuba, T. Both Full-Length and Protease-Cleaved Products of Osteopontin Are Elevated in Infectious Diseases. *Biomedicine* **2021**, *9*, 1006. [CrossRef]

reports

MDPI

Article

# COVID-19 Outcomes in a US Cohort of Persons Living with HIV (PLWH)

**Amanda Blair Spence [1,*], Sameer Desale [2], Jennifer Lee [1], Princy Kumar [1], Xu Huang [2], Stanley Evan Cooper [3], Stephen Fernandez [2] and Seble G. Kassaye [1]**

1 Division of Infectious Diseases, Georgetown University Medical Center, Washington, DC 20007, USA
2 MedStar Health Research Institute, Hyattsville, MD 20782, USA
3 Department of Medicine, Georgetown University Medical Center, Washington, DC 20007, USA
* Correspondence: abs132@georgetown.edu

**Abstract:** Reported coronavirus disease 2019 (COVID-19) outcomes in persons living with HIV (PLWH) vary across cohorts. We examined clinical characteristics and outcomes of PLWH with COVID-19 compared with a matched HIV-seronegative cohort in a mid-Atlantic US healthcare system. Multivariate logistic regression was used to explore factors associated with hospitalization and death/mechanical ventilation among PLWH. Among 281 PLWH with COVID-19, the mean age was 51.5 (SD 12.74) years, 63% were male, 86% were Black, and 87% had a HIV viral load <200 copies/mL. Overall, 47% of PLWH versus 24% ($p < 0.001$) of matched HIV-seronegative individuals were hospitalized. Rates of COVID-19 associated cardiovascular and thrombotic events, AKI, and infections were similar between PLWH and HIV-seronegative individuals. Overall mortality was 6% ($n = 18/281$) in PLWH versus 3% ($n = 33/1124$) HIV-seronegative, $p < 0.0001$. Among admitted patients, mortality was 14% ($n = 18/132$) for PLWH and 13% ($n = 33/269$) for HIV-seronegative, $p = 0.75$. Among PLWH, hospitalization associated with older age aOR 1.04 (95% CI 1.01, 1.06), Medicaid insurance aOR 2.61 (95% CI 1.39, 4.97) and multimorbidity aOR 2.98 (95% CI 1.72, 5.23). Death/mechanical ventilation associated with older age aOR 1.06 (95% CI 1.01, 1.11), Medicaid insurance aOR 3.6 (95% CI 1.36, 9.74), and multimorbidity aOR 4.4 (95% CI 1.55, 15.9) in adjusted analyses. PLWH were hospitalized more frequently than the HIV-seronegative group and had a higher overall mortality rate, but once hospitalized had similar mortality rates. Older age, multimorbidity and insurance status associated with more severe outcomes among PLWH suggesting the importance of targeted interventions to mitigate the effects of modifiable inequities.

**Keywords:** HIV; COVID-19; SARS-CoV-2; complications; outcomes



**Citation:** Spence, A.B.; Desale, S.; Lee, J.; Kumar, P.; Huang, X.; Cooper, S.E.; Fernandez, S.; Kassaye, S.G. COVID-19 Outcomes in a US Cohort of Persons Living with HIV (PLWH). *Reports* **2022**, 5, 41. https://doi.org/10.3390/reports5040041

Academic Editors: Toshio Hattori and Yugo Ashino

Received: 13 July 2022
Accepted: 30 September 2022
Published: 9 October 2022



## 1. Introduction

Data are mixed regarding the severity and clinical outcomes of coronavirus disease 2019 (COVID-19) among persons living with HIV (PLWH) and there are reports of both similar and worse clinical outcomes among different populations of PLWH co-infected with SARS-CoV-2. Early studies indicated a similar COVID-19 illness severity among PLWH and HIV-seronegative counterparts, but many of these reports were case series and/or had no matched controls [1–11]. There are also reports of higher rates of death and/or more severe disease among PLWH internationally and domestically [11–15]. Much of the literature describing COVID-19 in PLWH is limited to case series, single-center studies, includes mostly individuals on antiretroviral therapy (ART), and/or does not have matched control cohorts [1,3,9,16]. However, even among population-based or registry studies, there is variability in reported outcomes, with some reporting increased mortality risk or hospitalizations and others not noting this association [14,15,17,18]. Thus, additional data across are needed to describe the impact of COVID-19 on PLWH.

There are consistent reports of higher disease severity or worse outcomes among PLWH with COVID-19 who have medical comorbidities such as diabetes, cardiovascular disease, obesity and/or chronic lung disease [19,20]. COVID-19-associated complications such as acute kidney injury (AKI), cardiac events/myocardial injury, thrombosis, and stroke are well reported in the literature, and risk factors for these events include pre-existing disease and/or other medical comorbidities [21–33]. However, the occurrence of these COVID-associated events have not yet been described in PLWH, a population with high prevalence of medical comorbidities including diabetes, obesity, hypertension, and dyslipidemia [34–37]. These COVID-19-associated events can account for significant morbidity, mortality, and healthcare expenditure among persons affected by COVID-19. Thus, an assessment of COVID-19 related outcomes and infection associated events is needed among PLWH.

We conducted a retrospective analysis of all PLWH diagnosed with COVID-19 seen in the MedStar Healthcare system. The MedStar Healthcare system is the largest healthcare provider in the Maryland and Washington, DC area that includes 10 hospitals and provides ambulatory care services in the hospitals and at free standing sites in the surrounding communities. These facilities serve urban, suburban, and rural populations [38]. The District of Columbia and Maryland have some of the highest rates of HIV in the country with 2360.8 and 652.9 diagnoses per 100,000, respectively [39]. Our sampling provides a representative sample of PLWH in the Mid-Atlantic region who sought clinical care. This allows for a detailed analysis of clinical characteristics of PLWH compared to a matched cohort as well as examination of COVID-19 associated events as we sought to characterize clinical characteristics of PLWH who were infected with COVID-19 as well as outcomes as compared to the HIV-seronegative.

## 2. Methods

***Cohort Population and Data Sources:*** All persons with a diagnosis of HIV, determined either via International Classification of Diseases (ICD-10) coding or laboratory testing with a diagnosis of COVID-19, who received care in the Medstar Healthcare system were included in this analysis. Individuals were considered to have a diagnosis of COVID-19 if an ICD-10 diagnosis code for COVID-19 or positive laboratory testing for SARS-CoV-2 by polymerase chain reaction (PCR) was documented between January 2020 and November 2020. In addition, an age- and sex/gender-frequency-matched control group of HIV-seronegative individuals with a diagnosis of COVID-19 was generated in a 1:4 ratio for comparison. There were no required standardized hospital protocols for hospital admission or COVID treatment and patient care decisions were based on the discretion of individual care providers.

***Variable Selection:*** Demographic and clinical data were extracted from the Electronic Health Data Warehouse (MedStar Analytics Platform). Clinical data for this analysis included laboratory testing, medications/therapeutics, comorbid diagnoses as determined by ICD-10 coding, socio-demographics, oxygen requirements, and hospital length of stay. Individuals were considered to have multimorbidity (e.g., the co-occurrence of two or more chronic conditions) [40] if they had more than one of the following diagnoses: cardiovascular disease, obesity, diabetes, chronic renal disease, malignancy, or transplant. To determine accuracy of ICD-10 coding diagnoses, 25% of participants with each reported comorbid diagnosis were verified by manual chart review and the overall accuracy rate was 79% which is similar to other reports of discharge coding accuracy in the literature [41]. For those hospitalized, all laboratory data during the hospital admission were extracted. HIV viral load and CD4 + T lymphocyte count were obtained from the time most proximal to admission and/or COVID-19 diagnosis and viral loads were obtained until November 2020.

***Analytic Plan:*** Descriptive statistics were used to describe cohort characteristics. Chi-square or Fisher's exact tests were used for categorical variables and t-tests or Kruskal–Wallis tests were used for continuous variables to determine group differences [42] We examined differences in PLWH diagnosed with COVID-19 and PLWH without a diagnosis of COVID-19 as well as PLWH and HIV-seronegative individuals with a diagnosis of COVID-19. Univariate and multivariate logistic regression was used to explore factors associated with hospitalization and incident death/mechanical ventilation requirement among PLWH. Variables with a *p*-value < 0.05 in the univariate analysis or selected based on known effect on SAR-CoV-2 outcomes were included in the multivariate analysis [43]. Data utilized for these analyses are included in the manuscript text and tables. All analyses were completed in R 4.0.0.

## 3. Results

In total, 1632 PLWH were tested for SARS-CoV-2 infection among the 20,662 who received care within the MedStar healthcare system, Figure 1. Characteristics of PLWH who tested for SARS-CoV-2 versus those who did not test for SARS-CoV-2 are outlined in Table S1. A total of 249 PLWH had a SARS-CoV-2 PCR confirmed infection, and an additional 32 had an ICD-10 coded COVID-19 diagnosis for a total of 281 PLWH with COVID-19.

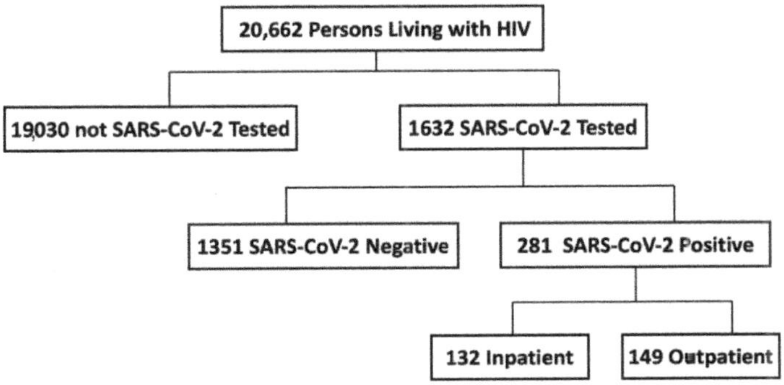


**Figure 1. PLWH seen in the MedStar healthcare system with and without SARS-CoV-2 Testing.** Flow chart of persons living with HIV seen in the MedStar Healthcare system. Abbreviations: HIV, Human Immunodeficiency Virus; PLWH, Persons Living with HIV; SARS-CoV-2, Severe Acute Respiratory Syndrome Coronavirus 2.

The mean age of PLWH with COVID-19 was 51.5 (SD 12.7) years, 63% ($n = 177$) were male, and 86% ($n = 237$) were African American/Black. The median CD4 + T lymphocyte count was 623 cells/mm$^3$ [IQR 383, 938] and 87% had a HIV viral load <200 copies/mL. Characteristics of tested PLWH with COVID-19 versus without COVID-19 are described in Table S2. Among those tested for SARS-CoV-2, PLWH who tested positive had lower rates of chronic renal disease (11% versus 12%, $p = 0.030$), higher rates of obesity (40% versus 33, $p = 0.046$), and higher median nadir CD4 + T lymphocyte counts (533 versus 413, $p = 0.036$). Among those tested, mean age in years, sex at birth, healthcare insurance status, CD4+ T lymphocyte count, and total number with HIV viral load <200 copies/mL were similar between those with and without SARS-CoV-2 infection.

Incident inpatient and outpatient SARS-CoV-2 infections among PLWH and HIV-seronegative individuals are depicted in Figure 2. Compared to age- and sex-matched HIV-negative individuals, more PLWH were hospitalized at 47% ($n = 132$) versus 24% ($n = 269$), $p < 0.001$. Characteristics of PLWH and the matched cohort of HIV-seronegative individuals with COVID-19 are outlined in Table 1. The majority of PLWH, 86% ($n = 237$) were Black/African American versus 44% ($n = 388$) in the matched HIV-negative control group, $p < 0.001$. There were more privately insured persons in the HIV-negative group at 75% ($n = 818$) versus 58% ($n = 161$), $p < 0001$ among PLWH. Comorbid conditions were more common among PLWH including chronic liver disease at 24% ($n = 70$) versus 6% ($n = 62$), $p < 0.001$; hypertension 59% ($n = 165$) versus 36% ($n = 403$), $p < 0.001$; cardiovascular disease 62% ($n = 174$) versus 38% ($n = 423$), $p < 0.001$; malignancy 10% ($n = 28$) versus 2% ($n = 19$), $p < 0.001$; chronic lung disease 31% ($n = 86$) versus 12%($n = 134$), $p < 0.001$; chronic renal disease 25% ($n = 69$) and 10% ($n = 117$), $p < 0.001$; and diabetes 33% ($n = 92$) versus 20%

($n = 226$), $p < 0.001$. However, rates of post-COVID-19 cardiovascular, thrombotic, AKI, and infection events were similar between HIV-seropositive and HIV-seronegative groups overall as well among individuals who required hospitalization.

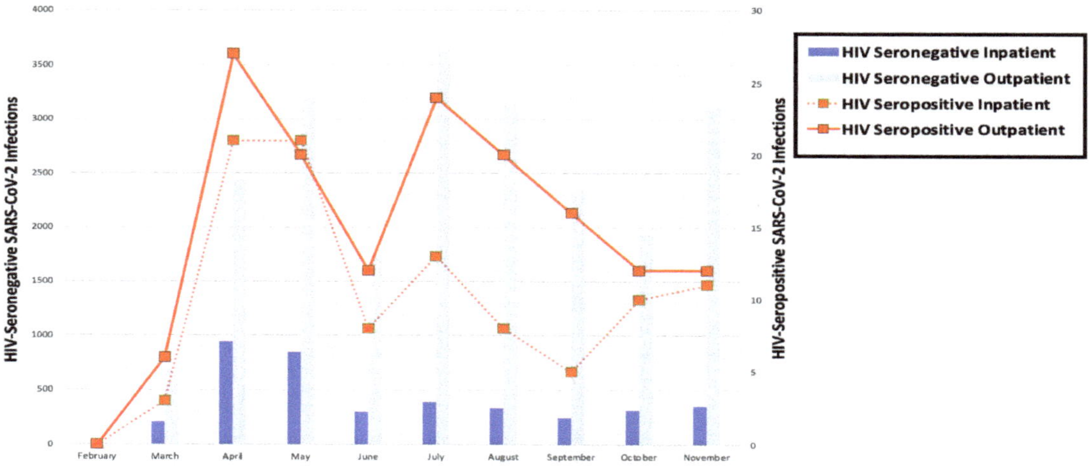


**Figure 2. Persons with COVID-19 seen in the MedStar Healthcare system.** Figure of persons living with HIV and HIV-seronegative individuals seen in the MedStar Healthcare system with COVID-19. Abbreviations: HIV, Human Immunodeficiency Virus; COVID-19, coronavirus disease 2019.

**Table 1.** Comparison of age and sex matched PLWH and age/sex matched HIV-seronegative individuals with COVID-19.

| Characteristic | HIV-Seronegative ($n$ = 1124) | HIV-Seropositive ($n$ = 281) | $p$-Value |
|---|---|---|---|
| Age mean years (SD) | 51.2 (13.7) | 51.5 (12.7) | 1 |
| Sex at Birth, $n$ (%) | | | |
| Male | 708 (63) | 177 (63) | 1 |
| Female | 416 (37) | 104 (37) | |
| Race, $n$ (%) | | | |
| African American/Black | 388 (44) | 237 (86) | <0.001 |
| White | 341 (39) | 20 (7) | |
| Other | 157 (18) | 18 (7) | |
| Ethnicity | | | |
| Non-Hispanic | 813 (92) | 258 (98) | 0.001 |
| Hispanic | 69 (8) | 6 (2) | |
| Insurance, $n$ (%) | | | |
| Private | 818 (75) | 161 (58) | <0.001 |
| Medicaid | 79 (7) | 67 (24) | |
| Medicare | 146 (13) | 45 (16) | |
| Non-Insured | 46 (4) | 6 (2) | |

**Table 1.** *Cont.*

| Characteristic | HIV-Seronegative (*n* = 1124) | HIV-Seropositive (*n* = 281) | *p*-Value |
|---|---|---|---|
| Co-Morbid Conditions, *n* (%) | | | |
| Cardiovascular Disease | 423 (38) | 174 (62) | <0.001 |
| Hypertension | 403 (36) | 165 (59) | <0.001 |
| Obesity | 280 (25) | 111 (40) | <0.001 |
| Diabetes Mellitus | 226 (20) | 92 (33) | <0.001 |
| Chronic Renal Disease | 117 (10) | 31 (11) | <0.001 |
| Chronic Liver Disease | 62 (6) | 70 (25) | <0.001 |
| Malignancy | 19 (2) | 28 (10) | <0.001 |
| Transplant | 14 (1) | 8 (3) | 0.062 |
| Post-Infection Events, *n* (%) | | | |
| Thrombotic | 2 (1) | 1 (0.4) | 0.489 |
| Infections | 14 (1) | 7 (2) | 0.206 |
| Cardiovascular | 22 (2) | 9 (3) | 0.253 |
| Acute Kidney Injury | 6 (1) | 4 (1) | 0.120 |
| INPATIENT | N = 269 | N = 132 | |
| Median Length of Stay, days (IQR) | 6 (3, 11) | 5.5 (3, 11) | 0.889 |
| ICU Median Length of Stay, days (IQR) | 7 (3, 15) | 3 (1, 7.25) | 0.008 |
| Deceased, *n* (%) | 33 (13) | 18 (14) | 0.750 |
| Comorbid Conditions, *n* (%) | | | |
| Diabetes Mellitus | 110 (41) | 50 (38) | 0.589 |
| Cardiovascular Disease | 67 (35) | 35 (27) | 0.716 |
| Chronic Renal Disease | 30 (11) | 22 (17) | 0.154 |
| Chronic Liver Disease | 10 (4) | 21 (16) | <0.001 |
| Malignancy | 19 (7) | 25 (18) | <0.001 |
| Post-Infection Events, *n* (%) | | | |
| Thrombotic | 1 (0.4) | 1 (0.4) | 0.551 |
| Infections | 12 (5) | 3 (2) | 0.421 |
| Cardiovascular | 20 (7) | 5 (4) | 0.190 |
| Acute Kidney Injury | 4 (2) | 1 (1) | 1 |
| COVID Treatments [a], *n* (%) | | | |
| Remdesivir | 39 (15) | 18 (14) | 0.880 |
| Dexamethasone | 65 (24) | 32 (24) | 1 |
| Azithromycin | 120 (45) | 58 (44) | 0.915 |
| Hydroxychloroquine | 49 (18) | 22 (17) | 0.781 |
| Tocilizumab | 18 (7) | 6 (5) | 0.504 |

**Table 1.** *Cont.*

| Characteristic | HIV-Seronegative ($n$ = 1124) | HIV-Seropositive ($n$ = 281) | $p$-Value |
|---|---|---|---|
| Supplemental Oxygen, $n$ (%) | | | |
| Room Air | 38 (18) | 27 (25) | |
| Nasal Cannula | 82 (39) | 33 (30) | 0.097 |
| Non-Rebreather/HFNC | 29 (14) | 25 (23) | |
| Ventilator | 53 (25) | 21 (19) | |
| Laboratory Data (Admission [b]), (IQR) | | | |
| Median WBC ($\times 10^3$ cells/µL) | 7 (5.3, 9.6) | 6.80 (4.60, 9.20) | 0.060 |
| Median Absolute Lymphocyte count ($\times 10^3$ cells/µL) | 1.05 (0.80, 1.50) | 1.30 (0.80, 1.80) | 0.032 |
| Mean Hemoglobin (gm/dL) | 12.98 (12.98) | 12.23 (2.40) | 0.006 |
| Mean Platelets ($\times 10^3$ cells/µL) | 233 (95.52) | 211.07 (91.78) | 0.036 |
| Median Creatinine (mg/dL) | 1.11 (0.83, 1.71) | 1.17 (0.89, 2.48) | 0.175 |
| Mean eGFR (mL/min/1.73 $m^2$) | 50.07 (17.96) | 46.10 (20.67) | 0.062 |
| Median ALT (IU/L) | 37.00 (23, 58.50) | 33.00 (22, 49.50) | 0.224 |
| Median CPK (units/L) | 148.50 (78.25, 326) | 142 (75, 394) | 0.834 |
| Median Troponin (ng/mL) | 0.02 (0.01, 0.03) | 0.02 (0.01, 0.04) | 0.248 |
| Median Procalcitonin (ng/mL) | 0.19 (0.10, 0.73) | 0.34 (0.10, 0.86) | 0.398 |
| Median Ferritin (ng/mL) | 592 (300, 1330.40) | 565.15 (262.40, 1367.22) | 0.573 |
| Median Lactate Dehydrogenase (units/L) | 343.50 (264.50, 460.50) | 312.50 (238.5, 161.5) | 0.477 |
| Median D-Dimer (mcg/mL FEU) | 1.66 (0.78, 3.06) | 1.44 (0.78, 3.46) | 0.902 |
| Median C-Reactive Protein (mg/L) | 82.80 (35.05, 127.50) | 93.70 (53.50, 161.50) | 0.285 |
| Laboratory Data (Peak), (IQR) | | | |
| Median WBC ($\times 10^3$ cells/µL) | 10.20 (6.93, 14.97) | 8.90 (6, 12.70) | 0.010 |
| Median Platelets ($\times 10^3$ cells/µL) | 307 (236.75, 417.75) | 263 (194, 371) | 0.008 |
| Median Procalcitonin (ng/mL) | 0.22 (0.10, 2.30) | 0.39 (0.10, 1.70) | 0.498 |
| Median Ferritin (ng/mL) | 896.1 (373.45, 1817.15) | 707.40 (345, 1798.20) | 0.420 |

**Table 1.** *Cont.*

| Characteristic | HIV-Seronegative ($n$ = 1124) | HIV-Seropositive ($n$ = 281) | $p$-Value |
|---|---|---|---|
| Median Lactate Dehydrogenase (units/L) | 400.50 (284.50, 574) | 355.5 (271, 576.75) | 0.615 |
| Median D-Dimer (mcg/mL FEU) | 1.88 (1.09, 5.07) | 1.94 (0.93, 3.83) | 0.655 |
| Mean C-Reactive Protein (mg/L) | 109 (47.40) | 121.50 (61.70, 172.25) | 0.573 |
| Median Interleukin-6 (pg/mL) | 12.10 (5, 43.50) | 9 (5, 18.60) | 0.412 |

Abbreviations: PLWH, persons living with HIV; N, number; SD, standard deviation; IQR, interquartile range; HFNC, high-flow nasal cannula; WBC, white blood cell count; mcL, microliters; gm, gram; dL, deciliter; eGFR, estimated glomerular filtration rate; mg, milligrams; mL, milliliter; min, minute; m, meter; IU, CPK, creatinine phosphokinase; international units, L, liter; ng, nanogram; mcg, micrograms; pg, picogramss. [a] Other investigational treatments/treatments included vagepant ($n$ = 0, HIV-seronegative; $n$ = 1, HIV-seropositive) and extracorporeal membrane oxygenation (ECMO) ($n$ = 0, HIV-seronegative; $n$ = 1, HIV-seropositive). [b] Laboratory data are from admission or first available.

Among those hospitalized, the PLWH had higher prevalence of liver disease at 16% ($n$ = 21) versus 4% ($n$ = 10), $p < 0.001$) and malignancy 19% ($n$ = 25) versus 7% ($n$ = 19), $p = 0.001$. The oxygen requirements and treatments were similar between the HIV-seropositive and HIV-seronegative groups. A total of 33% ($n$ = 44) PLWH versus 31% ($n$ = 83), $p = 0.648$, of HIV-seronegative individuals were admitted to the ICU. Among those admitted to the ICU, median length of stay was shorter among PLWH at 3 [IQR 1, 7.25] days versus 7 [IQR 3, 15] days. A total of 33% ($n$ = 44) PLWH versus 31% ($n$ = 83), $p = 0.648$, of HIV-seronegative individuals were admitted to the ICU. Inpatient mortality was similar for PLWH ($n$ = 18/132) and HIV-seronegative individuals ($n$ = 33/269) at 14% versus 13%, respectively, $p = 0.750$. The median length of hospital stay was 6 days [IQR 3, 11] for PLWH and 5.5 days [IQR 3, 11] for HIV-seronegative individuals, $p = 0.889$. Overall mortality was 6% ($n$ = 18/281) in PLWH versus 3% ($n$ = 33/1124) in HIV-seronegative individuals, $p < 0.0001$.

In analyses adjusted for age, sex, insurance status and multimorbidity, hospitalization among PLWH associated with older age aOR 1.04 (95% CI 1.01, 1.06), Medicaid insurance aOR 2.61 (95% CI 1.39, 4.97) and multimorbidity aOR 2.98 (95% CI 1.72, 5.23) (Table 2). Death/mechanical ventilation requirement was associated with older age aOR 1.06 (95% CI 1.01, 1.11), Medicaid insurance aOR 3.6 (95% CI 1.36, 9.74), and multimorbidity aOR 4.4 (95% CI 1.55, 15.9) in analyses adjusted for age, sex, insurance status and multimorbidity (Table 3).

**Table 2.** Factors associated with hospitalization among persons living with HIV with COVID-19.

| Characteristic | OR | $p$-Value | aOR * | $p$-Value |
|---|---|---|---|---|
| Age, years | 1.05 (1.03, 1.07) | <0.001 | 1.04 (1.01, 1.06) | 0.002 |
| Sex at Birth | | | | |
| Female (reference) | — | — | — | — |
| Male | 1.12 (0.69, 1.83) | 0.646 | 1.5 (0.87, 2.62) | 0.152 |
| Race | | | | |
| White (reference) | — | — | — | — |
| African American/Black | 0.6 (0.23, 1.5) | 0.278 | — | — |
| Other | 0.26 (0.06, 0.96) | 0.051 | — | — |

**Table 2.** *Cont.*

| Characteristic | OR | *p*-Value | aOR * | *p*-Value |
|---|---|---|---|---|
| Ethnicity | | | | |
| Non-Hispanic (reference) | – | – | – | – |
| Hispanic | 1.13 (0.21, 6.22) | 0.88 | – | – |
| HIV Viral Load | | | | |
| <200 (reference) | – | – | – | – |
| >200 | 1 (1, 1) | 0.34 | | |
| CD4 + T Lymphocyte | | | | |
| >200 (reference) | – | – | – | – |
| <200 | 0.98 (0.91, 1.06) | 0.624 | – | – |
| Insurance | | | | |
| Private (reference) | – | – | – | – |
| Medicaid | 2.22 (1.25, 4) | 0.007 | 2.61 (1.39, 4.97) | 0.003 |
| Medicare | 2.4 (1.23, 4.77) | 0.011 | 1.41 (0.67, 3.01) | 0.362 |
| Uninsured/Self-Pay | 0.8 (0.11, 4.22) | 0.798 | 0.78 (0.09, 5.39) | 0.803 |
| Multimorbidity ** | 3.74 (2.29, 6.21) | <0.001 | 2.98 (1.72, 5.23) | <0.001 |

Abbreviations: SARS CoV-2, severe acute respiratory syndrome coronavirus 2; OR, odds ratio; aOR, adjusted odds ratio. * Multivariable model adjusted for age, sex, insurance status, and multimorbidity, ** Multimorbidity = two or more comorbidities including cardiovascular disease, obesity, diabetes mellitus, chronic renal disease, or malignancy.

**Table 3.** Factors associated with death/mechanical ventilation among hospitalized PLWH with COVID-19.

| Characteristic | OR (CI 95%) | *p*-Value | aOR * | *p*-Value |
|---|---|---|---|---|
| Age, years | 1.06 (1.03, 1.1) | <0.0001 | 1.06 (1.01, 1.11) | 0.013 |
| Sex at Birth | | | | |
| Female (reference) | – | – | – | – |
| Male | 0.87 (0.4, 1.93) | 0.72 | 0.97 (0.42, 2.34) | 0.94 |
| Race | | | | |
| White (reference) | – | – | – | – |
| African American/Black | 2.34 (0.46, 42.92) | 0.416 | – | – |
| Other | 0 (0, $2.44 \times 10^{15}$) | 0.987 | – | – |
| Ethnicity | | | | |
| Non-Hispanic (reference) | – | – | – | – |
| Hispanic | 1.95 (0.1, 12.76) | 0.55 | – | – |
| HIV Viral Load | | | | |
| <200 (reference) | – | – | – | – |
| >200 | 0.97 (0.84, 1) | 0.592 | – | – |
| CD4 + T Lymphocyte | | | | |
| >200 (reference) | – | – | – | – |
| <200 | 1.05 (0.86, 1.31) | 0.64 | – | – |
| Insurance | | | | |
| Private (reference) | – | – | – | – |
| Medicaid | 2.97 (1.19, 7.49) | 0.019 | 3.6 (1.36, 9.74) | 0.01 |
| Medicare | 2.78 (0.95, 7.73) | 0.051 | 1.33 (0.42, 3.99) | 0.614 |
| Uninsured/Self-Pay | 7.55 (0.97, 43.98) | 0.029 | 12.09 (1.17, $1.26 \times 10^2$) | 0.027 |
| Multimorbidity ** | 6.55 (2.47, 22.68) | <0.001 | 4.4 (1.55, 15.9) | 0.011 |

Abbreviations: OR, odds ratio; aOR, adjusted odds ratio. * Multivariable model adjusted for age, sex, insurance status, and multimorbidity, ** Multimorbidity = two or more comorbidities including cardiovascular disease, obesity, diabetes mellitus, chronic renal disease, or malignancy.

## 4. Discussion

In a clinical cohort of PLWH seeking healthcare in the mid-Atlantic US, 281 were diagnosed with COVID-19 between March 2020 and November 2020. Patients were seen in a variety of care settings including ambulatory and inpatient. This group was predominantly African American/Black, carried a heavy burden of prevalent medical comorbidities, and had mostly virologically well controlled HIV. PLWH were admitted to the inpatient setting more frequently than an age- and sex-matched cohort and had a higher overall mortality rate, but once admitted, had similar mortality to their HIV-seronegative counterparts. Despite more frequent hospital admissions, more comorbid illnesses, and higher overall mortality COVID-19 associated complications including AKI, thrombosis, cardiovascular events, and other infections were similar between PLWH and the matched HIV-seronegative control group. As in the general population, older age and multimorbidity are associated with more severe outcomes. Differences in outcomes were also noted by insurance status, some of which may be attributed to age but may also reflect social determinants of health. This study adds to the existing studies that suggest that older age, multiple medical comorbidities, and social determinants of health influence on COVID-19 outcomes.

COVID-19-associated complications such as cardiovascular events, AKI, and thrombotic events are frequently noted in the literature. AKI frequently complicates SARS-CoV-2 infection, and incidence rates are variable, but rates of up to 57% are reported among those hospitalized and/or admitted to an intensive care unit [21] AKI in the setting of COVID-19 is associated with Black/African American or Hispanic race, male sex, older age and other comorbidities such as diabetes, cardiovascular disease, hypertension, or baseline chronic kidney disease [21–24]. Further, myocardial injury is commonly reported among hospitalized patient with COVID-19, with risk factors being older age and a history of cardiovascular disease [25]. Thrombotic events are also common in persons with COVID-19 and pulmonary emboli and deep venous thrombosis have been reported in 20 to 30% of persons with COVID-19 with risk factors of older age and cardiovascular disease [30,31,44]. Persons with deep venous thrombosis and COVID-19 were older, had higher rates of cardiac injury, and oxygenation index [45]. HIV is a known risk factor for chronic kidney disease, cardiovascular disease, and venous thrombosis [46–49]. PLWH also have known higher rates of medical comorbidities, which was reflected in our cohort [34–37]. Thus, we initially hypothesized higher rates of COVID-19 associated complications. Studies are limited regarding COVID-19-associated complications among PLWH, but Durstenfeld et al. reported that hospitalized PLWH did not have elevated risk of major adverse cardiac events, mortality, or severity of disease.[18] Although the methodology was different, these findings, combined with our study findings of similar rates of COVID-19-related complications, suggest the need for additional study. Potential insights may be gained by further examining the immunologic response to disease among both PLWH as immune dysregulation is thought to contribute to SARS-CoV-2 pathogenesis including end organ disease such as myocardial injury, other cardiovascular dysfunction, or kidney dysfunction [50].

As other studies have reported, hospitalization rates were higher among PLWH in our cohort [14,51,52]. As more PLWH were admitted to the inpatient setting, overall mortality among all COVID-19 positive individuals, hospitalized and non-hospitalized was higher among PLWH versus the HIV-seronegative cohort. However, inpatient mortality was similar between PLWH and the HIV seronegative cohort. Differential hospitalization rates between the two groups may be reflective of differential admission practices and burden of comorbid disorders among PLWH. Our study corroborates the excess morbidity related to COVID-19 among PLWH found in other studies; however, our analysis may overestimate the mortality differences between PLWH and the HIV-seronegative group as we assume patients not admitted to our healthcare system survived infection and there may be unaccounted deaths in the outpatient group. Our study adds to the existing literature exploring the effect of COVID-19 on mortality among PLWH, yet additional work is needed to determine the effect of COVID-19 in PLWH as studies in various populations show differing outcomes [8,12,15,17,18,52–56].

We determined risk factors related to hospitalization for SARS-CoV-2 or death/mechanical ventilation and found they were associated with age, insurance status, and multimorbidity. These findings are similar to those noted in the general HIV-seronegative population where known risk factors for hospitalization or severe disease include older age, or the presence of other comorbid disorders [57–59]. This is corroborated in other studies of PLWH with COVID-19 older PLWH or those with multiple comorbidities have more severe disease/worse outcomes [19,20,54,60–62]. However, we did not observe more severe disease among ethnic/racial minorities as previously reported [14,60,63]. Our population was skewed with a majority of African American PLWH; thus, the assessment of the influence of race/ethnicity on COVID-19 severity is limited in our analysis. To our knowledge, the association of insurance type with hospitalization for COVID-19 or death/mechanical ventilation among PLWH has not been reported in the literature. However, those that are uninsured/self-pay and Medicaid recipients are socially and economically vulnerable populations [64,65], and the higher rates of severe COVID-19 disease may be reflective of differences in health seeking behavior, health service delivery, or other social determinants of health that are confounders in the relationship. The association of social determinants of health and COVID-19 outcomes has been described in the literature and access and delivery of care may be targets for intervention [66,67].

## 5. Limitations

Our study utilized the data available in the Medstar Health electronic medical registry, so we are unable to account for care sought outside this healthcare system, HIV treatment history, or duration of HIV infection. Additionally, all comorbid diagnoses were determined by ICD-10 codes. These codes were developed for administrative use and have their own inherent bias, but they are used by public health organizations to conduct surveillance and have also successfully been used by researchers including in large studies of COVID-19 [52,68–70]. To ensure the data accuracy we conducted manual abstraction of a subset of the population and the data accuracy was consistent with that of the published literature [41]. The majority of the participants in this study were virologically suppressed and sought healthcare. Thus, our findings may not be representative of persons with advanced HIV or not receiving care. Additionally, the therapeutic approaches to treatment and prevention of COVID-19 changed over the duration of the study which likely impacted outcomes and ability to compare our results with that of studies performed early in the pandemic. We utilized electronic health records that do not capture genomic surveillance data, but the data analyzed for this study included individuals diagnosed with COVID-19 between March 2020 and November 2020. The alpha (B.1.1.7.) variant was first reported in the United Kingdom in December of 2020. Thus, individuals in our cohort likely were likely infected with the original COVID-19 strain. The emergence of the alpha, delta, and omicron variants likely affected disease severity and outcomes and our findings may not be generalizable to those infected with other variants. Our cohort was predominantly African American/Black, and although representative of the HIV-epidemic in the area, this may have affected our outcomes as other studies have noted differences in outcomes by race. Other studies noted differences by race and COVID-19 outcomes, our population was predominantly African American and this may have influenced outcomes [71–73]. We were not able to fully assess difference by race given the unequal racial population distribution Additional studies are needed to identify emerging trends in hospitalizations, morbidity, and mortality among PLWH with more recent SARS-CoV-2 variants, and contemporary SARS-CoV-2 prevention and treatment modalities.

## 6. Conclusions

Our findings suggest disparities in COVID-19 morbidity among PLWH in the form of excess hospitalizations and higher mortality when including both inpatients and outpatient COVID-19 diagnoses. Despite higher burdens of baseline comorbid illness, PLWH did not experience more cardiovascular, acute kidney injury, or thrombotic events. Similar to other studies, older age, multimorbidity, and Medicaid insurance were associated with more severe outcomes among PLWH. Ongoing assessments of these findings and COVID-19 prevention efforts are needed among PLWH, especially socially or economically vulnerable populations, those with advanced age, or multiple comorbidities.

**Supplementary Materials:** The following are available online at https://www.mdpi.com/article/10.3390/reports5040041/s1, Table S1: Characteristics of PLWH and SARS-CoV-2 testing status; Table S2: Characteristics of persons living with HIV who completed SARS-CoV-2 testing with and without infection.

**Author Contributions:** Conceptualization, A.B.S. and S.G.K.; formal analysis, S.D.; data curation, X.H., S.F., J.L. and S.E.C.; writing—original draft preparation, A.B.S.; writing—review and editing, S.G.K., P.K., J.L., S.E.C. and S.D. All authors have read and agreed to the published version of the manuscript.

**Funding:** This research has been supported by the services and resources provided by the District of Columbia Center for AIDS Research, a National Institutes of Health funded program (P30 AI117970). S.E.C is supported under T32 AI007613 by the National Institute of Allergy and Infectious Diseases.

**Institutional Review Board Statement:** This study was approved by the Georgetown University Intuitional Review Board (STUDY00001455).

**Informed Consent Statement:** Not Applicable.

**Data Availability Statement:** Data is contained within the article and Supplement Material.

**Conflicts of Interest:** P.K. reports research grants from Eli Lilly, G.S.K , Merck, Gilead, Regeneron, and American Gene Technologies and financial interest in Merck, Johnson & Johnson, G.S.K., Gilead, and Pfizer.

## References

1. Inciarte, A.; Gonzalez-Cordon, A.; Rojas, J.; Torres, B.; de Lazzari, E.; de la Mora, L.; Martinez-Rebollar, M.; Laguno, M.; Callau, P.; Gonzalez-Navarro, A.; et al. Clinical characteristics, risk factors, and incidence of symptomatic coronavirus disease 2019 in a large cohort of adults living with HIV: A single-center, prospective observational study. *AIDS* **2020**, *34*, 1775–1780. [CrossRef]
2. Huang, J.; Xie, N.; Hu, X.; Yan, H.; Ding, J.; Liu, P.; Ma, H.; Ruan, L.; Li, G.; He, N.; et al. Epidemiological, Virological and Serological Features of Coronavirus Disease 2019 (COVID-19) Cases in People Living with Human Immunodeficiency Virus in Wuhan: A Population-based Cohort Study. *Clin. Infect. Dis.* **2020**, *73*, e2086–e2094. [CrossRef]
3. Gervasoni, C.; Meraviglia, P.; Riva, A.; Giacomelli, A.; Oreni, L.; Minisci, D.; Atzori, C.; Ridolfo, A.; Cattaneo, D. Clinical features and outcomes of HIV patients with coronavirus disease 2019. *Clin. Infect. Dis.* **2020**, *71*, 2276–2278. [CrossRef]
4. Byrd, K.M.; Beckwith, C.G.; Garland, J.M.; Johnson, J.E.; Aung, S.; Cu-Uvin, S.; Farmakiotis, D.; Flanigan, T.; Gillani, F.S.; Macias-Gil, R.; et al. SARS-CoV-2 and HIV coinfection: Clinical experience from Rhode Island, United States. *J. Int. AIDS Soc.* **2020**, *23*, e25573. [CrossRef]
5. Calza, L.; Bon, I.; Tadolini, M.; Borderi, M.; Colangeli, V.; Badia, L.; Verucchi, G.; Rossini, G.; Vocale, C.; Gaibani, P.; et al. COVID-19 in patients with HIV-1 infection: A single-centre experience in northern Italy. *Infection* **2021**, *49*, 333–337. [CrossRef]
6. Okoh, A.K.; Bishburg, E.; Grinberg, S.; Nagarakanti, S. COVID-19 pneumonia in patients with HIV—A Case Series. *J. Acquir. Immune Defic. Syndr.* **2020**, *85*, e4–e5. [CrossRef]
7. Shalev, N.; Scherer, M.; LaSota, E.D.; Antoniou, P.; Yin, M.T.; Zucker, J.; Sobieszczyk, M.E. Clinical Characteristics and Outcomes in People Living with Human Immunodeficiency Virus Hospitalized for Coronavirus Disease 2019. *Clin. Infect. Dis.* **2020**, *71*, 2294–2297. [CrossRef] [PubMed]
8. Sigel, K.; Swartz, T.; Golden, E.; Paranjpe, I.; Somani, S.; Richter, F.; De Freitas, J.K.; Miotto, R.; Zhao, S.; Polak, P.; et al. Covid-19 and People with HIV Infection: Outcomes for Hospitalized Patients in New York City. *Clin. Infect. Dis.* **2020**, *71*, 2933–2938. [CrossRef]
9. Collins, L.F.; Moran, C.A.; Oliver, N.T.; Moanna, A.; Lahiri, C.D.; Colasanti, J.A.; Kelley, C.F.; Nguyen, M.L.; Marconi, V.C.; Armstrong, W.S.; et al. Clinical characteristics, comorbidities and outcomes among persons with HIV hospitalized with coronavirus disease 2019 in Atlanta, Georgia. *AIDS* **2020**, *34*, 1789–1794. [CrossRef]
10. Ridgway, J.P.; Farley, B.; Benoit, J.-L.; Frohne, C.; Hazra, A.; Pettit, N.; Pho, M.; Pursell, K.; Saltzman, J.; Schmitt, J.; et al. A Case Series of Five People Living with HIV Hospitalized with COVID-19 in Chicago, Illinois. *AIDS Patient Care STDS* **2020**, *34*, 331–335. [CrossRef] [PubMed]
11. Guo, W.; Ming, F.; Feng, Y.; Zhang, Q.; Mo, P.; Liu, L.; Gao, M.; Tang, W.; Liang, K. Patterns of HIV and SARS-CoV-2 co-infection in Wuhan, China. *J. Int. AIDS Soc.* **2020**, *23*, e25568. [CrossRef]
12. Boulle, A.; Davies, M.-A.; Hussey, H.; Ismail, M.; Morden, E.; Vundle, Z.; Zweigenthal, V.; Mahomed, H.; Paleker, M.; Pienaar, D.; et al. Risk factors for COVID-19 death in a population cohort study from the Western Cape Province, South Africa. *Clin. Infect. Dis.* **2020**, *73*, e2005–e2015. [CrossRef]
13. Miyashita, H.; Kuno, T. Prognosis of coronavirus disease 2019 (COVID-19) in patients with HIV infection in New York City. *HIV Med.* **2021**, *22*, e1–e2. [CrossRef]

14. Tesoriero, J.M.; Swain, C.-A.E.; Pierce, J.L.; Zamboni, L.; Wu, M.; Holtgrave, D.R.; Gonzalez, C.J.; Udo, T.; Morne, J.E.; Hart-Malloy, R.; et al. COVID-19 Outcomes Among Persons Living with or without Diagnosed HIV Infection in New York State. *JAMA Netw. Open* **2021**, *4*, e2037069. [CrossRef]
15. Geretti, A.M.; Stockdale, A.J.; Kelly, S.H.; Cevik, M.; Collins, S.; Waters, L.; Villa, G.; Docherty, A.; Harrison, E.M.; Turtle, L.; et al. Outcomes of Coronavirus Disease 2019 (COVID-19) Related Hospitalization among People with Human Immunodeficiency Virus (HIV) in the ISARIC World Health Organization (WHO) Clinical Characterization Protocol (UK): A Prospective Observational Study. *Clin. Infect. Dis.* **2021**, *73*, e2095–e2106. [CrossRef]
16. Vizcarra, P.; Pérez-Elías, M.J.; Quereda, C.; Moreno, A.; Vivancos, M.J.; Dronda, F.; Casado, J.L.; COVID-19 ID Team. Description of COVID-19 in HIV-infected individuals: A single-centre, prospective cohort. *Lancet HIV* **2020**, *7*, e554–e564. [CrossRef]
17. Durstenfeld, M.S.; Sun, K.; Ma, Y.; Rodriguez, F.; Secemsky, E.A.; Parikh, R.V.; Hsue, P.Y. Association of HIV infection with outcomes among adults hospitalized with COVID-19. *AIDS* **2022**, *36*, 391–398. [CrossRef] [PubMed]
18. Bhaskaran, K.; Rentsch, C.T.; MacKenna, B.; Schultze, A.; Mehrkar, A.; Bates, C.J.; Eggo, R.M.; Morton, C.E.; Bacon, S.C.J.; Inglesby, P.; et al. HIV infection and COVID-19 death: A population-based cohort analysis of UK primary care data and linked national death registrations within the OpenSAFELY platform. *Lancet HIV* **2021**, *8*, e24–e32. [CrossRef]
19. Dandachi, D.; Geiger, G.; Montgomery, M.W.; Karmen-Tuohy, S.; Golzy, M.; Antar, A.A.R.; Llibre, J.M.; Camazine, M.; Díaz-De Santiago, A.; Carlucci, P.M.; et al. Characteristics, Comorbidities, and Outcomes in a Multicenter Registry of Patients with HIV and Coronavirus Disease-19. *Clin. Infect. Dis.* **2021**, *73*, e1964–e1972. [CrossRef] [PubMed]
20. Ambrosioni, J.; Blanco, J.L.; Reyes-Urueña, J.M.; Davies, M.-A.; Sued, O.; Marcos, M.A.; Martínez, E.; Bertagnolio, S.; Alcamí, J.; Miro, J.M.; et al. Overview of SARS-CoV-2 infection in adults living with HIV. *Lancet HIV* **2021**, *8*, e294–e305. [CrossRef]
21. Nugent, J.; Aklilu, A.; Yamamoto, Y.; Simonov, M.; Li, F.; Biswas, A.; Ghazi, L.; Greenberg, J.; Mansour, S.; Moledina, D.; et al. Assessment of Acute Kidney Injury and Longitudinal Kidney Function after Hospital Discharge Among Patients with and without COVID-19. *JAMA Netw. Open* **2021**, *4*, e211095. [CrossRef] [PubMed]
22. Fisher, M.; Neugarten, J.; Bellin, E.; Yunes, M.; Stahl, L.; Johns, T.S.; Abramowitz, M.K.; Levy, R.; Kumar, N.; Mokrzycki, M.H.; et al. AKI in Hospitalized Patients with and without COVID-19: A Comparison Study. *J. Am. Soc. Nephrol.* **2020**, *31*, 2145–2157. [CrossRef] [PubMed]
23. Hirsch, J.S.; Ng, J.H.; Ross, D.W.; Sharma, P.; Shah, H.H.; Barnett, R.L.; Hazzan, A.D.; Fishbane, S.; Jhaveri, K.D.; Northwell COVID-19 Research Consortium; et al. Acute kidney injury in patients hospitalized with COVID-19. *Kidney Int.* **2020**, *98*, 209–218. [CrossRef] [PubMed]
24. Chan, L.; Chaudhary, K.; Saha, A.; Chauhan, K.; Vaid, A.; Zhao, S.; Paranjpe, I.; Somani, S.; Richter, F.; Miotto, R.; et al. AKI in Hospitalized Patients with COVID-19. *J. Am. Soc. Nephrol.* **2021**, *32*, 151–160. [CrossRef]
25. Lala, A.; Johnson, K.W.; Januzzi, J.L.; Russak, A.J.; Paranjpe, I.; Richter, F.; Zhao, S.; Somani, S.; Van Vleck, T.; Vaid, A.; et al. Prevalence and Impact of Myocardial Injury in Patients Hospitalized With COVID-19 Infection. *J. Am. Coll. Cardiol.* **2020**, *76*, 533–546. [CrossRef]
26. Kotecha, T.; Knight, D.S.; Razvi, Y.; Kumar, K.; Vimalesvaran, K.; Thornton, G.; Patel, R.; Chacko, L.; Brown, J.T.; Coyle, C.; et al. Patterns of myocardial injury in recovered troponin-positive COVID-19 patients assessed by cardiovascular magnetic resonance. *Eur. Heart J.* **2021**, *42*, 1866–1878. [CrossRef]
27. Huang, L.; Zhao, P.; Tang, D.; Zhu, T.; Han, R.; Zhan, C.; Liu, W.; Zeng, H.; Tao, Q.; Xia, L. Cardiac Involvement in Patients Recovered From COVID-2019 Identified Using Magnetic Resonance Imaging. *JACC Cardiovasc. Imaging* **2020**, *13*, 2330–2339. [CrossRef]
28. Ojha, V.; Verma, M.; Pandey, N.N.; Mani, A.; Malhi, A.S.; Kumar, S.; Jagia, P.; Roy, A.; Sharma, S. Cardiac Magnetic Resonance Imaging in Coronavirus Disease 2019 (COVID-19): A Systematic Review of Cardiac Magnetic Resonance Imaging Findings in 199 Patients. *J. Thorac. Imaging* **2021**, *36*, 73–83. [CrossRef]
29. Puntmann, V.O.; Carerj, M.L.; Wieters, I.; Fahim, M.; Arendt, C.; Hoffmann, J.; Shchendrygina, A.; Escher, F.; Vasa-Nicotera, M.; Zeiher, A.M.; et al. Outcomes of Cardiovascular Magnetic Resonance Imaging in Patients Recently Recovered from Coronavirus Disease 2019 (COVID-19). *JAMA Cardiol.* **2020**, *5*, 1265–1273. [CrossRef]
30. Hanff, T.C.; Mohareb, A.M.; Giri, J.; Cohen, J.B.; Chirinos, J.A. Thrombosis in COVID-19. *Am. J. Hematol.* **2020**, *95*, 1578–1589. [CrossRef]
31. Malas, M.B.; Naazie, I.N.; Elsayed, N.; Mathlouthi, A.; Marmor, R.; Clary, B. Thromboembolism risk of COVID-19 is high and associated with a higher risk of mortality: A systematic review and meta-analysis. *EClinicalMedicine* **2020**, *29*, 100639. [CrossRef] [PubMed]
32. Qureshi, A.I.; Baskett, W.I.; Huang, W.; Shyu, D.; Myers, D.; Raju, M.; Lobanova, I.; Suri, M.F.K.; Naqvi, S.H.; French, B.R.; et al. Acute Ischemic Stroke and COVID-19: An Analysis of 27 676 Patients. *Stroke* **2021**, *52*, 905–912. [CrossRef] [PubMed]
33. Merkler, A.E.; Parikh, N.S.; Mir, S.; Gupta, A.; Kamel, H.; Lin, E.; Lantos, J.; Schenck, E.J.; Goyal, P.; Bruce, S.S.; et al. Risk of Ischemic Stroke in Patients with Coronavirus Disease 2019 (COVID-19) vs Patients with Influenza. *JAMA Neurol.* **2020**, *77*, 1366. [CrossRef]
34. Palella, F.J.; Hart, R.; Armon, C.; Tedaldi, E.; Yangco, B.; Novak, R.; Battalora, L.; Ward, D.; Li, J.; Buchacz, K.; et al. Non-AIDS comorbidity burden differs by sex, race, and insurance type in aging adults in HIV care. *AIDS* **2019**, *33*, 2327–2335. [CrossRef] [PubMed]

35. Collins, L.F.; Sheth, A.N.; Mehta, C.C.; Naggie, S.; Golub, E.T.; Anastos, K.; French, A.L.; Kassaye, S.; Taylor, T.; Fischl, M.A.; et al. The Prevalence and Burden of Non-AIDS Comorbidities Among Women Living with or at Risk for Human Immunodeficiency Virus Infection in the United States. *Clin. Infect. Dis.* **2021**, *72*, 1301–1311. [CrossRef]
36. Schouten, J.; Wit, F.W.; Stolte, I.G.; Kootstra, N.A.; van der Valk, M.; Geerlings, S.E.; Prins, M.; Reiss, P.; AGEhIV Cohort Study Group. Cross-sectional comparison of the prevalence of age-associated comorbidities and their risk factors between HIV-infected and uninfected individuals: The AGEhIV cohort study. *Clin. Infect. Dis.* **2014**, *59*, 1787–1797. [CrossRef] [PubMed]
37. Ronit, A.; Gerstoft, J.; Nielsen, L.; Mohey, R.; Wiese, L.; Kvinesdal, B.; Obel, N.; Ahlströhm, M.G. Non-AIDS Comorbid Conditions in Persons Living with Human Immunodeficiency Virus (HIV) Compared With Uninfected Individuals 10 Years Before HIV Diagnosis. *Clin. Infect. Dis.* **2018**, *67*, 1291–1293. [CrossRef]
38. Facts and Figures. Available online: https://www.medstarhealth.org/mhs/about-medstar/facts-and-figures/ (accessed on 12 July 2021).
39. Centers for Disease Control and Prevention. Monitoring selected national HIV prevention and care objectives by using HIV surveillance data—United States and 6 dependent areas, 2018. *HIV Surveill. Suppl. Rep.* **2020**, *25*. Available online: https://www.cdc.gov/hiv/pdf/library/reports/surveillance/cdc-hiv-surveillance-supplemental-report-vol-25-2.pdf (accessed on 12 July 2021).
40. Navickas, R.; Petric, V.-K.; Feigl, A.B.; Seychell, M. Multimorbidity: What do we know? What should we do? *J. Comorb.* **2016**, *6*, 4–11. [CrossRef] [PubMed]
41. Burns, E.M.; Rigby, E.; Mamidanna, R.; Bottle, A.; Aylin, P.; Ziprin, P.; Faiz, O.D. Systematic review of discharge coding accuracy. *J. Public Health* **2012**, *34*, 138–148. [CrossRef] [PubMed]
42. Peck, R.; Olsen, C.; Devore, J.L. *Introduction to Statistics and Data Analysis*; Cengage Learning: Boston, MA, USA, 2015.
43. Schriger, D.L. Book and media review. *Ann. Emerg. Med.* **2008**, *52*, 480. [CrossRef]
44. Bilaloglu, S.; Aphinyanaphongs, Y.; Jones, S.; Iturrate, E.; Hochman, J.; Berger, J.S. Thrombosis in Hospitalized Patients with COVID-19 in a New York City Health System. *JAMA* **2020**, *324*, 799–801. [CrossRef]
45. Zhang, L.; Feng, X.; Zhang, D.; Jiang, C.; Mei, H.; Wang, J.; Zhang, C.; Li, H.; Xia, X.; Kong, S.; et al. Deep Vein Thrombosis in Hospitalized Patients with COVID-19 in Wuhan, China: Prevalence, Risk Factors, and Outcome. *Circulation* **2020**, *142*, 114–128. [CrossRef]
46. Naicker, S.; Rahmanian, S.; Kopp, J.B. HIV and chronic kidney disease. *Clin. Nephrol.* **2015**, *83*, 32–38. [CrossRef]
47. So-Armah, K.; Benjamin, L.A.; Bloomfield, G.S.; Feinstein, M.J.; Hsue, P.; Njuguna, B.; Freiberg, M.S. HIV and cardiovascular disease. *Lancet HIV* **2020**, *7*, e279–e293. [CrossRef]
48. Losina, E.; Hyle, E.P.; Borre, E.D.; Linas, B.P.; Sax, P.E.; Weinstein, M.C.; Rusu, C.; Ciaranello, A.L.; Walensky, R.P.; Freedberg, K.A. Projecting 10-year, 20-year, and Lifetime Risks of Cardiovascular Disease in Persons Living With Human Immunodeficiency Virus in the United States. *Clin. Infect. Dis.* **2017**, *65*, 1266–1271. [CrossRef]
49. Bibas, M.; Biava, G.; Antinori, A. HIV-Associated Venous Thromboembolism. *Mediterr. J. Hematol. Infect. Dis.* **2011**, *3*, e2011030. [CrossRef] [PubMed]
50. Jamal, M.; Bangash, H.I.; Habiba, M.; Lei, Y.; Xie, T.; Sun, J.; Wei, Z.; Hong, Z.; Shao, L.; Zhang, Q. Immune dysregulation and system pathology in COVID-19. *Virulence* **2021**, *12*, 918–936. [CrossRef]
51. Braunstein, S.L.; Lazar, R.; Wahnich, A.; Daskalakis, D.C.; Blackstock, O.J. COVID-19 Infection Among People with HIV in New York City: A Population-Level Analysis of Matched Surveillance Data. *SSRN Electron. J.* **2020**. [CrossRef]
52. Yendewa, G.A.; Perez, J.A.; Schlick, K.; Tribout, H.; McComsey, G.A. Clinical Features and Outcomes of Coronavirus Disease 2019 Among People with Human Immunodeficiency Virus in the United States: A Multicenter Study from a Large Global Health Research Network (TriNetX). *Open Forum Infect. Dis.* **2021**, *8*, ofab272. [CrossRef] [PubMed]
53. Hadi, Y.B.; Naqvi SF, Z.; Kupec, J.T.; Sarwari, A.R. Characteristics and outcomes of COVID-19 in patients with HIV: A multicentre research network study. *AIDS* **2020**, *34*, F3–F8. [CrossRef] [PubMed]
54. Del Amo, J.; Polo, R.; Moreno, S.; Díaz, A.; Martínez, E.; Arribas, J.R.; Jarrín, I.; Hernán, M.A.; The Spanish HIV/COVID-19 Collaboration. Incidence and Severity of COVID-19 in HIV-Positive Persons Receiving Antiretroviral Therapy: A Cohort Study. *Ann. Intern. Med.* **2020**, *173*, 536–541. [CrossRef]
55. Jassat, W.; Cohen, C.; Masha, M.; Goldstein, S.; Kufa-Chakezha, T.; Savulescu, D.; Walaza, S.; Bam, J.-L.; Davies, M.-A.; Prozesky, H.W.; et al. A national cohort study of COVID-19 in-Hospital Mortality in South Africa: The Intersection of Communicable and Non-Communicable Chronic Diseases in a High HIV Prevalence Setting. *medRxiv* **2020**. [CrossRef]
56. Rosenthal, E.M.; Rosenberg, E.S.; Patterson, W.; Ferguson, W.P.; Gonzalez, C.; DeHovitz, J.; Udo, T.; Rajulu, D.T.; Hart-Malloy, R.; Tesoriero, J. Factors associated with SARS-CoV-2-related hospital outcomes among and between persons living with and without diagnosed HIV infection in New York State. *PLoS ONE* **2022**, *17*, e0268978. [CrossRef]
57. Ioannou, G.N.; Locke, E.; Green, P.; Berry, K.; O'Hare, A.M.; Shah, J.A.; Crothers, K.; Eastment, M.C.; Dominitz, J.A.; Fan, V.S. Risk Factors for Hospitalization, Mechanical Ventilation, or Death Among 10 131 US Veterans with SARS-CoV-2 Infection. *JAMA Netw. Open* **2020**, *3*, e2022310. [CrossRef]
58. Panagiotou, O.A.; Kosar, C.M.; White, E.M.; Bantis, L.E.; Yang, X.; Santostefano, C.M.; Feifer, R.A.; Blackman, C.; Rudolph, J.L.; Gravenstein, S.; et al. Risk Factors Associated With All-Cause 30-Day Mortality in Nursing Home Residents with COVID-19. *JAMA Intern. Med.* **2021**, *181*, 439–448. [CrossRef]

59. Booth, A.; Reed, A.B.; Ponzo, S.; Yassaee, A.; Aral, M.; Plans, D.; Labrique, A.; Mohan, D. Population risk factors for severe disease and mortality in COVID-19: A global systematic review and meta-analysis. *PLoS ONE* **2021**, *16*, e0247461. [CrossRef] [PubMed]
60. Yang, X.; Sun, J.; Patel, R.C.; Zhang, J.; Guo, S.; Zheng, Q.; Olex, A.L.; Olatosi, B.; Weissman, S.B.; Islam, J.Y.; et al. Associations between HIV infection and clinical spectrum of COVID-19: A population level analysis based on US National COVID Cohort Collaborative (N3C) data. *Lancet HIV* **2021**, *8*, e690–e700. [CrossRef]
61. Brown, L.B.; Spinelli, M.A.; Gandhi, M. The interplay between HIV and COVID-19: Summary of the data and responses to date. *Curr. Opin. HIV AIDS* **2021**, *16*, 63. [CrossRef]
62. Nomah, D.K.; Reyes-Urueña, J.; Díaz, Y.; Moreno, S.; Aceiton, J.; Bruguera, A.; Vivanco-Hidalgo, R.M.; Llibre, J.M.; Domingo, P.; Falcó, V.; et al. Sociodemographic, clinical, and immunological factors associated with SARS-CoV-2 diagnosis and severe COVID-19 outcomes in people living with HIV: A retrospective cohort study. *Lancet HIV* **2021**, *8*, e701–e710. [CrossRef]
63. Meyerowitz, E.A.; Kim, A.Y.; Ard, K.L.; Basgoz, N.; Chu, J.T.; Hurtado, R.M.; Lee, C.K.; He, W.; Minukas, T.; Nelson, S.; et al. Disproportionate burden of coronavirus disease 2019 among racial minorities and those in congregate settings among a large cohort of people with HIV. *AIDS* **2020**, *34*, 1781–1787. [CrossRef] [PubMed]
64. Bhanja, A.; Lee, D.; Gordon, S.H.; Allen, H.; Sommers, B.D. Comparison of Income Eligibility for Medicaid vs. Marketplace Coverage for Insurance Enrollment Among Low-Income US Adults. *JAMA Health Forum* **2021**, *2*, e210771. [CrossRef]
65. Shafer, P.R.; Anderson, D.M.; Whitaker, R.; Wong, C.A.; Wright, B. Association of Unemployment with Medicaid Enrollment By Social Vulnerability In North Carolina During COVID-19. *Health Aff.* **2021**, *40*, 1491–1500. [CrossRef] [PubMed]
66. Ingraham, N.E.; Purcell, L.N.; Karam, B.S.; Dudley, R.A.; Usher, M.G.; Warlick, C.A.; Allen, M.L.; Melton, G.B.; Charles, A.; Tignanelli, C.J. Racial and Ethnic Disparities in Hospital Admissions from COVID-19: Determining the Impact of Neighborhood Deprivation and Primary Language. *J. Gen. Intern. Med.* **2021**, *36*, 3462–3470. [CrossRef]
67. Dalsania, A.K.; Fastiggi, M.J.; Kahlam, A.; Shah, R.; Patel, K.; Shiau, S.; Rokicki, S.; DallaPiazza, M. The Relationship Between Social Determinants of Health and Racial Disparities in COVID-19 Mortality. *J. Racial Ethn. Health Disparities* **2021**, *9*, 288–295. [CrossRef]
68. Liebovitz, D.M.; Fahrenbach, J. COUNTERPOINT: Is ICD-10 Diagnosis Coding Important in the Era of Big Data? No. *Chest* **2018**, *153*, 1095–1098. [CrossRef]
69. Weiner, M.G. POINT: Is ICD-10 Diagnosis Coding Important in the Era of Big Data? Yes. *Chest* **2018**, *153*, 1093–1095. [CrossRef]
70. ICD-ICD-10-CM-International Classification of Diseases, (ICD-10-CM/PCS) Transition. 2019. Available online: https://www.cdc.gov/nchs/icd/icd10cm_pcs_background.htm (accessed on 14 July 2021).
71. Wiley, Z.; Kubes, J.N.; Cobb, J.; Jacob, J.T.; Franks, N.; Plantinga, L.; Lea, J. Age, Comorbid Conditions, and Racial Disparities in COVID-19 Outcomes. *J. Racial Ethn. Health Disparities* **2022**, *9*, 117–123. [CrossRef]
72. Fu, J.; Reid, S.A.; French, B.; Hennessy, C.; Hwang, C.; Gatson, N.T.; Duma, N.; Mishra, S.; Nguyen, R.; Hawley, J.E.; et al. Racial Disparities in COVID-19 Outcomes Among Black and White Patients with Cancer. *JAMA Netw. Open* **2022**, *5*, e224304. [CrossRef]
73. Shortreed, S.M.; Gray, R.; Akosile, M.A.; Walker, R.L.; Fuller, S.; Temposky, L.; Fortmann, S.P.; Albertson-Junkans, L.; Floyd, J.S.; Bayliss, E.A.; et al. Increased COVID-19 Infection Risk Drives Racial and Ethnic Disparities in Severe COVID-19 Outcomes. *J. Racial Ethn. Health Disparities* **2022**. [CrossRef]

reports

MDPI

*Communication*

# Management of the COVID-19 Pandemic in Singapore from 2020 to 2021: A Revisit

**Zehuan Liao [1,2,*], Devika Menon [1], Le Zhang [3], Ye-Joon Lim [1], Wenhan Li [4], Xuexin Li [5,*] and Yan Zhao [1,*]**

1 School of Biological Sciences, Nanyang Technological University, Singapore 637551, Singapore
2 Department of Microbiology, Tumor and Cell Biology (MTC), Karolinska Institutet, 17177 Stockholm, Sweden
3 Department of Medical Epidemiology and Biostatistics, Karolinska Institutet, 17165 Solna, Sweden
4 School of Physical and Mathematical Sciences, Nanyang Technological University, Singapore 637551, Singapore
5 Department of Medical Biochemistry and Biophysics, Karolinska Institutet, 17165 Solna, Sweden
* Correspondence: liao0058@e.ntu.edu.sg (Z.L.); xuexin.li@ki.se (X.L.); zhaoyan@ntu.edu.sg (Y.Z.)

**Abstract:** The first coronavirus disease 2019 (COVID-19) case was detected in Singapore on 23 January 2020. Over the two years, Singapore witnessed tightening and easing of policies in response to and in anticipation of new variants, stress on the healthcare sector, and new waves of infection. Upon confirming the reliability of the data using Benford's analysis, the collated COVID-19 data and trends were analyzed alongside the policies between 2020 and 2021 in Singapore. Due to the proactive nature of these policies, Singapore was largely successful in reducing the imported cases that would spill over and result in community waves of infection and death. The government has taken necessary steps to support the citizens and reduce the impact of the pandemic on the economy of the country. Furthermore, there were policies that were more responsive and there are lessons to be learned from neighboring countries on their management of the pandemic. Given the endemic approach the government has adopted, the efficacy of these policies comes down to its sustainability. Since the pandemic requires frequent revisiting of these policies, Singapore's long-term management of the pandemic (or endemic) and its impact comes down to the ability of the government to introduce sustainable policies and update these according to new developments in treatments, variants, and vaccines, bearing in mind the socioeconomic condition of the country.

**Keywords:** SARS-CoV-2; COVID-19; Benford's Law; Singapore; pandemic management

check for updates

**Citation:** Liao, Z.; Menon, D.; Zhang, L.; Lim, Y.-J.; Li, W.; Li, X.; Zhao, Y. Management of the COVID-19 Pandemic in Singapore from 2020 to 2021: A Revisit. *Reports* **2022**, 5, 35. https://doi.org/10.3390/reports5030035

Academic Editors: Toshio Hattori and Yugo Ashino

Received: 15 July 2022
Accepted: 11 August 2022
Published: 22 August 2022



## 1. Introduction

In December 2019, a novel coronavirus named severe acute respiratory syndrome coronavirus 2 (SARS-CoV-2) causing serious pneumonia was first reported in Wuhan, China. Coronavirus disease 2019 (COVID-19) was a novel disease with major respiratory symptoms with no effective treatment schemes then. Singapore reported its first COVID-19 case on 23 January 2020 [1]. The Singapore government swiftly implemented various policies to combat COVID-19 while maintaining the economic competitiveness of Singapore. One such example is the Disease Outbreak Response System Condition (DORSCON) framework which serves as a simple way to communicate the level of severity of the current disease situation [2]. The efficient and immediate updates ensured credibility and timeliness of information, which supports the country in recovering from the pandemic crisis. In addition, the COVID-19 multi-ministry taskforce of Singapore also reacted swiftly to the situation and commenced tracking of the global situation from 2 January 2020.

The following months witnessed a rise and fall of cases that were imported, prevalent in the community and within the migrant worker dormitories. This resulted in an all-time peak of cases in May 2020 leading to circuit breaker measures being implemented on 7th April and extended until early June 2020 [3]. This period of increasing cases was met with stricter restrictions imposed by the government. These measures included travel restrictions, compulsory mask mandate, and digital contact tracing systems like Trace Together. Travel restrictions were imposed in February 2020 and became stricter as the cases increased. With increasing community cases, compulsory mask mandate was established in April 2020. To facilitate better contact tracing and early detection of cases, Trace Together was also implemented first in March 2020 [4].

As the number of cases stabilized and the economic repercussions of tighter restrictions were considered, safe and progressive reopening was carried out gradually in three phases. Phase I—Safe Re-opening was implemented on 2 June 2020, and Phase II—Safe Transition was initiated on 19 June 2020. Phase III—Safe Nation started from 28 December 2020 onwards [5]. This approach was designed considering the impact of COVID-19 on the national economy while also being cautious of community spread.

However, following these phases, Singapore witnessed an oscillation between restricting and easing of policies, either in response to or in anticipation of latest developments regarding the pandemic. These developments were often in the form of new variants or sub-variants, new clusters, rise in imported cases or scientific developments such as vaccinations. The situation stabilized by the second half of 2021 as the government adopted an endemic approach when dealing with the pandemic. Recognizing that COVID-19 will continue to exist in the society, the focus was on stabilizing the cases with minimum restrictions using vaccination differentiated measures (VDM) [6].

Throughout the circuit breaker period and the subsequent phases, the cases have displayed interesting patterns that were influenced by policies and reveal how three components of the total cases—imported, community, and dormitory cases—changed over time. This paper revisits the COVID-19 policies over the course of 2020 and 2021 and discusses the consequences of these policies in Singapore.

## 2. Materials and Methods

### 2.1. Data Collation

For this study, data were collected from a combination of the situation reports from Ministry of Health (MOH) News Highlights and the Interactive Situation Report with the epidemic split curve. The situation reports with data from the most recent 14 days was utilized for collating the linked and unlinked cases. However, since the published reports cannot be updated in the same table, the interactive situation report was used. This situation report, updated daily, allowed collection of updated data for imported, community, and dormitory cases as well as the cases that were isolated before detection and detected through surveillance. Additionally, this facilitated cross-checking of the situation report data which may have been later altered due to contact tracing developments (www.moh.gov.sg/covid-19, accessed on 10 July 2022) [6].

### 2.2. Benford's Law Analysis

To determine the accuracy and reliability of our COVID-19 data collated from MOH, we need to show if the dataset obeys Benford's Law, and if there is anomaly in our readings. Benford's Law, also known as the Newcomb-Benford Law or the First-digit Law, was first observed by Newcomb and popularized by Benford. After extensive research about this distribution phenomenon, Benford's law remains an interesting methodology for finding anomalies in data. The law is considered an empirical gem of statistical folklore used for fraud detection in many naturally occurring datasets such as financial reports, election data, macroeconomics data, and scientific data [7]. The same technique has also been deployed in the modeling of behavioral features for social network users. Research conducted by Anran Wei et al. in September 2020 studied the application of Benford's Law to COVID-19 datasets where they targeted data readings of total confirmed cases, total deaths, and daily confirmed cases. They obtained numbers from nineteen countries and the general results showed that COVID-19 data readings follow Benford's Law [8]. The idea behind Benford's Law is that the leading digits $1, 2, \ldots, 9$ of any naturally occurring data follow a certain probability distribution where the probability of digit 1 occurring is approximately 30% of the time and decreases monotonically to less than 5% for digit 9. More precisely, the exact law is given by:

$$P(d) = log_{10}\,(d+1) - log_{10}\,(d) = log_{10}\,(1 + 1/d), for\ all\ (d = 1, \ldots, 9)$$

Here, $d$ denotes the first significant of the decimal digit, e.g.,

$$P(d=1) = log_{10}\,(2/1) = 0.3010, P(d=2) = log_{10}\,(3/2) = 0.1760, \ldots,$$
$$P(d=9) = log_{10}\,(10/9) = 0.04575$$

### *2.3. Policy Evaluation*

The policies were collected from the MOH website (www.moh.gov.sg/covid-19, accessed on 10 July 2022), where daily updates are posted since 2 January 2020 [6]. The updates include the daily new cases, grants given out by the government, trade agreements with other countries other updates on the COVID-19 situation in Singapore. There are multiple updates per day, hence, multiple hyperlinks will be shown under the same date. A table was created to facilitate referencing of the policies updated. These policies were analyzed alongside the COVID-19 data to understand the impact of the pandemic on these policies and vice versa.

## 3. Results

### *3.1. Benford's Law Analysis*

In our study, we superimpose our readings onto the Benford's Law curve and determine whether it will yield a good fit. If the datasets match closely to the Benford's Law curve, then the COVID-19 dataset can be considered reliable for our subsequent analysis. The graph of the first digit of daily cases from 2020–2021 plotted against frequency (in %) seems to follow Benford's distribution closely. The frequency of the first digits obeys the law, more accurately among the higher digits than the lower digits. The shape of the graph matches the expected shape of Benford's distribution. Given that no anomaly was detected (Figure 1), the variation of empirical measurements from the expected values may not be statistically significant.

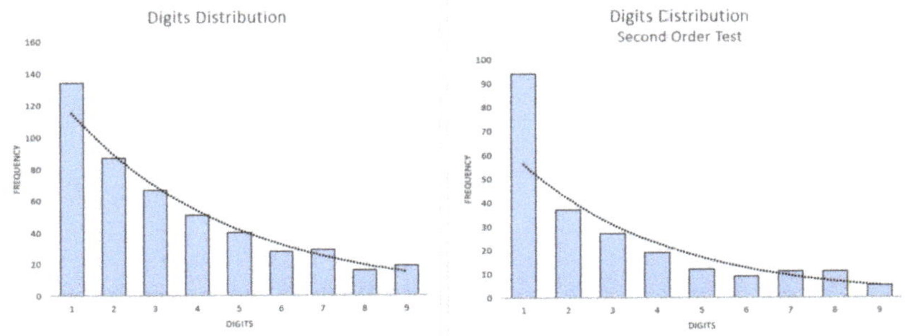


**Figure 1.** First digit distribution and second order test for COVID-19 data from 2020–2021 in Singapore (Benford's test).

Slight deviations in data are acceptable since the Benford's distribution is an ideal case scenario and the real-world examples deviate slightly from the ideal model [3]. Given that Benford's law has been used widely to detect fraudulent reporting and the data largely follow the distribution, it can thus be concluded that the data for COVID-19 cases in Singapore are largely accurate and reliable for further analysis [9].

The digit distribution second order test in Figure 1, related to Benford's Law, could also be used to detect if there are any inconsistencies in the internal pattern of our COVID-19 data. A formal definition of the second order Benford test is as follows: Let $x_1, \ldots, x_N$ be a data set comprising observations drawn from a continuous distribution, and let $y_1, \ldots, y_N$ be the $x_i$'s in increasing order. Then, for many natural data sets, for large N, the digits of the differences between adjacent observations ($y_{i+1} - y_i$) are close to Benford's Law. Therefore, this test helps to detect the relationship and anomaly in our data based on the digits of the difference between the largest number of cases and the smallest number of cases after sorting. As observed in Figure 1, these digit patterns also seem to be closely approximated by the digit frequencies of Benford's Law using the second-order digit distribution test [10].

### 3.2. COVID-19 Trends in Singapore

Singapore reported its first imported case of COVID-19 on 23 January 2020 and continued to report imported cases until March. Imported cases peaked by end March when there was a significant increase in cases. However, this decreased toward the second half of March and April. Ever since travel restrictions were eased by mid-June, imported cases resurfaced and gradually increased until the end of December 2020. Furthermore, the first community case was detected in Singapore during February and steadily increased until April, peaking during the second week of April. With two periods of circuit breaker measures, community cases gradually decreased by June 2020. However, Singapore witnessed what was possibly a second wave of much weaker intensity in July. This could be attributed to the easing of circuit breaker measures in June, which increased community transmission. However, most of the dormitories were only cleared in August, while the second wave is seemed to have started as early as July. Another possible explanation is from an immunological standpoint. In his paper on the second wave of COVID-19, O Hossein argues that the second wave of the pandemic in several countries is likely a cause of pathogen–host interaction pattern rather than relaxed social distancing measures [11]. Healthy individuals infected with the virus possibly cleared the viral load before adaptive immune response could be initiated. Thus, making them more susceptible to a second round of infection due to a lack of memory cells. Eventually the community cases tapered out and was negligible by November of 2020 (Figure 2).

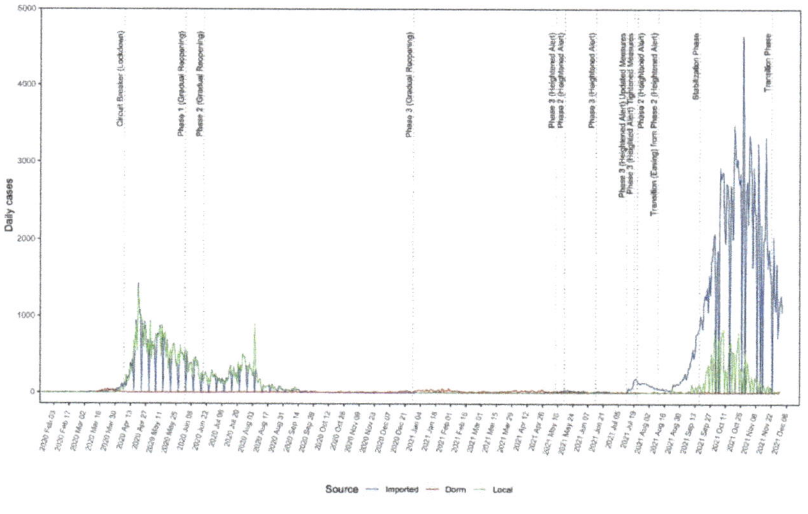


**Figure 2.** COVID-19 cases and phases in Singapore (2020–2021).

Meanwhile, the dormitory cases, first detected in March 2020, experienced a dramatic rise in cases, peaking in April 2020. This could be attributed to two reasons. First, the significant number of community cases that were prevalent at the time and infected dormitory workers. Second and possibly of greater importance is the high density of dorm workers living within small spaces under poor living conditions that favored rapid transmission within the dormitories [12]. With frequent testing and isolation, the number of dorm cases decreased subsequently. However, there was still a significant number of cases resurfacing in September owing to a second peak that emerged in August. When the dorms were intended to be cleared on 7 August, the number of cases leading to this day reached a three-month high [13]. Eventually, all dormitories were cleared and there were practically no dorm cases reported by December 2020.

Taken together, the data for imported, community, and dormitory cases together make it evident that a spike in imported cases was followed by community cases within two weeks during the first half of the year. The first wave of community cases seemed to follow Farr's Law, tapering off owing to circuit breaker measures [10]. The second wave of community cases is about a month after phase 1 was initiated and was possibly due to a lax in restrictions. Once travel restrictions and quarantine were imposed, while the imported cases started increasing, community cases remained low. This is because most of the imported cases became isolated before detection, decreasing the chances of it spilling into the community, thereby decreasing the percentage of imported cases that turned into community cases. However, this did not prevent community cases from spilling into dorm once again in July/August 2020—a week after the community peak of the second wave since most dorms were open by then. By the end of December 2020, both community and dormitory cases were close to zero and only newly imported cases were prevalent.

However, in 2021, Singapore witnessed several new challenges in management of the pandemic. More COVID-19 cases started to resurface, and Singapore reverted to a heightened alert in Phase 3 during May. This was followed by several rounds of tightening and subsequent easing of measures. In July 2021, the government announced several measures tightening the restrictions within Phase 3 (heightened alert). Following this announcement, Singapore witnessed the largest wave it had seen since the beginning of the pandemic.

To understand the evolution of pandemic management from 2020 to 2021, these policies enforced during this period are sufficient. The government clearly adopted an endemic approach to managing the pandemic—accepting that COVID-19 will remain in the society and measures must focus on gradual reopening without placing a burden on the healthcare system rather than complete restrictions on activities. Recognizing the impact that COVID-19 has had on the economy of Singapore, it was crucial to strike a balance between the cost of the infections, its impact on the healthcare system, and the economic consequences of a zero-COVID strategy.

As Singapore's largest COVID-19 wave placed an immense burden on healthcare workers, the stabilization phase was announced on 27 September 2021 when Singapore reported 1641 daily cases. The aim of this phase was to stabilize the cases and ease the burden on the healthcare system. Hence, this period was further extended until November 2021. In November 2021, when cases were still high, Singapore exited the stabilization phase and entered the transition phase. This period was characterized by lifting of several restrictions that were imposed for stabilization. A significant difference between this wave and the COVID-19 wave in 2020 was the nature of the cases. Most of these reported cases were imported cases and unlike 2020, the government managed to contain these cases without spilling over into the community. Hence, community transmission was less severe compared to 2020 and is further a testament to the success of pandemic management in Singapore.

## 4. Discussion

### *4.1. What Has Singapore Done Well?*

#### 4.1.1. Information Transparency

As a role model to some countries, the Singapore government tackled the pandemic effectively, be it reducing the economic impacts as much as possible or slowing down community spread. Singapore's success in effectively managing the pandemic can be largely attributed to the public willingness to cooperate and adherence to the policies that were enforced. This can be attributed to the transparency from the government regarding the COVID-19 situation in Singapore as well as the rationale behind all of the policies enforced [14]. The Singapore government communicated daily developments and situation updates through press releases and situation reports. The Gov.sg WhatsApp channel was a medium to disseminate important announcements to the public in an accessible manner daily [15]. This was done to disseminate information, reduce panic, and debunk misinformation that was spreading throughout the Internet [16]. This level of transparency has been crucial in solidifying the public trust in the government, contributing to their role in pandemic management.

#### 4.1.2. Efficient Screening

To curb the spread of cases, liberal testing was conducted on the population, with Singapore being one the countries with one of the greatest numbers of swab tests done [17]. On top of the testing done, contact tracing and the SafeEntry were implemented to break the chain of transmission, with the contact tracing being widely commended for its efficiency [18]. The Public Health Preparedness Clinic (PHPC) was also activated. The PHPCs are clinics across the country that are activated during public health emergencies which dispense medications, administer vaccinations, and provide subsidized treatments. The PHPCs are adequately prepared since they have been receiving constant training before the pandemic [19]. By serving as the intermediary between the community and hospitals, these PHPCs help to increase the efficiency and reduce the stress on hospitals by supplementing manpower to screen for patients and categorize them into low-risk and high-risk groups [20].

#### 4.1.3. Vaccination

One of the most important factors that shaped Singapore's response to the pandemic in 2021 has been its vaccination campaign. With an aggressive campaign, the Singapore government aimed to ease restrictions largely allowing vaccinated individuals to return to almost pre-COVID-19 levels of activity while protecting the unvaccinated population. Singapore initiated the vaccination rollout on 30 December 2020, prioritizing health care workers who are most at risk. The subsequent phases of the campaign targeted senior citizens and the vulnerable before reaching the young adult population and children. As of 29 December 2021, 87% of the population had been fully vaccinated. To attain this, the government mobilized several clinics as centers where walking vaccinations were encouraged. As a result, vaccination-differentiated measures were introduced in 2021 wherein vaccinated individuals could carry out activities to greater level of freedom in comparison to non-vaccinated individuals allowing easing of restrictions while protecting the unvaccinated [21].

This campaign is frequently updated based on latest scientific developments and expert advice on the types of vaccines and doses required as the pandemic progresses and variants like Delta are identified. Booster vaccine doses were encouraged and were determined as necessary to be considered fully vaccinated. The Singapore government has been largely transparent regarding the vaccination situation in Singapore and even prepared the public for a possibility of taking booster shots periodically to maintain their fully vaccinated status according to the vaccinated differentiated measures [22]. Vaccination has been crucial in the stabilization that was achieved in 2021 while avoiding a strain on the health care system as well as protecting the vulnerable senior citizens in Singapore.

#### 4.1.4. Providing Grants

To protect the economy from the consequences of the COVID-19 pandemic, different grants and packages were distributed. For instance, the Unity Budget, Resilience and Solidarity Budget, and the Fortitude Budget were approved to help offset the costs and protect the livelihood of many [23]. These budgets were targeted toward employment-related issues, sectors that were affected by COVID-19, and stimulating the economy. For example, the SGUnited Jobs and Skills package aids jobseekers in looking for a job and grants such as the self-employed person income relief scheme (SIRS) help to ease the costs for the self-employed. Industries such as the Arts & Culture sector and the tourism sector received $55 million and $90 million respectively as they were hit hard by the impact of COVID-19 [24]. Besides the different subsidies for businesses and industries, the government also provided subsidies to offset the costs of healthcare. This is important, especially in times when healthcare is most needed by the people. Through the one-off COVID-19 subsidy and additional support to the lower and middle income, as well as the elderly of the Merdeka and Pioneer generation, Singaporeans can now receive healthcare without worrying about the costs [25]. As a country that is heavily reliant on imported products, Singapore has been constantly stockpiling its supplies and is well-prepared for a disruption in the supply chain. Even though production and exports were reduced by many countries during the pandemic, the Singapore government had months' worth of essential items and food for the country. These stockpiles allowed more time for the government to source for alternative productions [26].

### 4.2. *What Could Have Been Done Better?*

#### 4.2.1. Electronic Tracking

To date, there are different ways of tracking the places a person has visited in Singapore. This includes the SafeEntry, Trace together application, and the Trace Together token. The SafeEntry was implemented on 12 May 2020, the Trace together application was launched on 20 March 2020, and the Trace together token was distributed from 14 September 2020 onwards [27–29]. Prior to the implementation of electronic tracking, contact tracing was done manually and involved greater time and manpower. This process included monitoring the movement of the patient for the past 14 days, investigation and identification of close contacts, and notifying the close contacts [30]. Interviewing the patient was also the most crucial process in identifying potential clusters and hence, a patient's memory and integrity are vital to identifying close contacts. While the contact tracing methods in Singapore has been commended for its high accuracy and persistence in tracking, some lapse in contact tracing is inevitable as patients could lie about their history or suffer from recall biases especially when these patients are already unwell [18,19,31]. Therefore, the use of electronic tracking in the earlier phase could have been implemented to a greater extent to prevent such lapses.

While SafeEntry is compulsory, downloading of the Trace together application is voluntary. The Trace together application acts like the Trace together token where it tracks whether a person had been in close proximity to an infected individual. Short-distance Bluetooth signals that are exchanged between the application or the token mean that these individuals are near each other [32]. Therefore, the Trace together application is much more accurate in determining whether a person is in close contact with the patient compared to SafeEntry, which only tracks whether a person has entered a certain premise. Furthermore, SafeEntry could be less accessible to elderly who are not proficient in technology since it requires the use of smartphones [4]. Even though the National Registration Identity Card (NRIC) could replace our smart phones for SafeEntry, not all places are equipped with the NRIC scanner. Thus, the Trace Together token, which tracks the location more accurately and is simpler in terms of usage, would be more convenient and appropriate for contact tracing. However, owing to the lack of time, the tokens could not be manufactured in time. Thus, earlier implementation of the SafeEntry could have made the contact tracing process more efficient.

#### 4.2.2. Mask Mandate

Policies regarding mask wearing are a crucial element of the pandemic, which if managed more closely, could have prevented the outbreak from spreading within the community in Singapore. Singapore confirmed the first case of COVID-19 on 23 January 2020. At that time, only sick persons (with obvious symptoms) were required to wear masks and the public was specifically instructed by the government to not wear masks unless they were sick. This was to prevent any shortage of mask supply due to excessive use. Until 5 June, the World Health Organization (WHO) did not encourage the public to wear masks at all times. However, as of now, WHO announced that mask wearing may become a part of normal life. [33]

The Singapore Government only enforced compulsory mask wearing from 15 April 2020 onwards. According to the policies, individuals who did not wear a mask could be fined $300 the first time and $1000 the second time. Based on medical recommendation, children below two years of age and adults doing strenuous exercise were exempted from mask wearing [34]. For evidence that the decrease in community spread was due to compulsory mask enforcements, Singapore has to look no further than Vietnam. The first case of COVID-19 was detected in Vietnam on 17 January 2020. The government made wearing masks on public transport and all public places compulsory on 21 February and 16 March respectively [35]. Vietnam's limited community spread and well-controlled second wave is likely due to these policies [36].

Furthermore, Taiwan's success in managing COVID-19 has been attributed to its compulsory mask wearing policies and medical care [37]. M. T Leffler et al. found that the per capacity mortality of countries where mask wearing was practiced diligently was significantly lower than other countries that did not strictly enforce mask wearing [38]. Scientifically, this is attributed to masks acting a barrier, preventing almost all droplets from an infected person being suspended in the atmosphere [39]. Epidemiologically, the impact of mask wearing of daily COVID-19 cases has been established. A Health Affairs study on the COVID-19 spread in 15 U.S. states has found that there was a significant decline in the growth of daily COVID-19 cases in states with strict mask mandates [40]. These evidence illustrate that an early intervention to make masks compulsory while securing mask supplies could have significantly decreased community cases in Singapore.

#### 4.2.3. Travel Restrictions

Since the outbreak of COVID-19 in Wuhan, Singapore has consistently been monitoring its epidemiological spread and imposing travel advisories and restrictions to Wuhan. All inbound flights from Wuhan, China were ceased when the first COVID-19 case in Singapore was confirmed [41]. By February 2020, all travel to Hubei province in mainland China, and non-essential travel to the rest of mainland China, Iran, Japan, and the Republic of Korea were issued travel advisories. Thereafter, Singapore continued to impose travel restrictions and advisories on countries with very high numbers of cases such as Italy, France, Spain and Germany [42]. On 23 March 2020, all short-term visitors were not allowed entry or transit through Singapore [43].

In the early stages of a pandemic outbreak, mobility plays a significant role in the spread of a disease [44]. This was demonstrated in a recent study on the outbreak of COVID-19 which showed that mobility is indeed a strong contributor to the global spread of the virus [44]. As a country that is highly connected to the rest of the world, there would naturally be visitors from many countries. Inevitably, there were imported cases which led to a few clusters. Two clusters were linked to tourists from China while another was the Grand Hyatt cluster which involved several overseas cases [45]. Although the clusters were closed, there were other unlinked cases which emerged. These could be linked to undetected imported cases since air travel was still active in March, when Singapore received the greatest number of visitors from Indonesia, UK and Australia [46]. In these three countries, COVID-19 cases started increasing since the start of March [47–49]. Since some travelers could be asymptomatic or pre-symptomatic, those that were in Singapore before 23 March 2020 might have already been infected with the virus. Furthermore, there were cases in Indonesia that went unreported due to low testing rate [50,51]. Hence, cases in Indonesia could be higher than recorded. Moreover, European countries and the USA had high number of cases as well [52]. Even though Singapore received fewer visitors from these countries, there could be higher chance of having an infected visitor from these countries. This was especially so in Europe, where cases in Italy multiplied more than nine times in ten days within the period when Singapore was still receiving travelers from Europe [46]. Cases also escalated in USA and was as high as that in China in mid-March [52]. Hence, the Singapore government could have prevented the sudden spike in the number of cases if stricter travel restrictions were implemented earlier.

## 5. Conclusions

In summary, Singapore has tackled the pandemic effectively, balancing restrictions with economic impact. The government has constantly updated the public on the COVID-19 situations through different platforms. To curb the spread of cases, extensive testing was conducted. To protect the economy from the consequences of the COVID-19 pandemic, different grants and packages were distributed as well. However, there were several policies and measures that could have been more effectively established. For instance, the late establishment of a compulsory mask mandate due to limited mask supply may have contributed to the spread during the early months of the pandemic. Furthermore, restricting travelers earlier could have decreased the imported cases that enter the community. However, with emerging nature of the pandemic, the success of these policies eventually comes down to the government's ability to be flexible and responsive to latest developments, whether regarding new variants or vaccines.

**Author Contributions:** Conceptualization, Z.L.; methodology, Z.L., D.M., L.Z., Y.-J.L. and W.L.; formal analysis, Z.L., D.M., L.Z., Y.-J.L. and W.L.; investigation, Z.L., D.M., L.Z., Y.-J.L. and W.L.; resources, Y.Z.; writing—original draft preparation, Z.L., D.M., Y.-J.L. and W.L.; writing—review and editing, Z.L., X.L. and Y.Z.; supervision, Z.L., X.L. and Y.Z.; funding acquisition, Y.Z. All authors have read and agreed to the published version of the manuscript.

**Funding:** We would like to acknowledge the funding support from Nanyang Technological University —URECA Undergraduate Research Programme for this research project (Funding No: SBS21033).

**Institutional Review Board Statement:** Not applicable.

**Informed Consent Statement:** Not applicable.

**Data Availability Statement:** Data used in this paper is published by MOH and is available publicly (www.moh.gov.sg/covid-19) as accessed from 2 January 2020 to 1 July 2022.

**Conflicts of Interest:** The authors declare no conflict of interest.

## References

1. Abdullah, A.Z.; Salamat, H. Singapore Confirms First Case of Wuhan Virus. CNA. 23 January 2020. Available online: https://www.channelnewsasia.com/singapore/wuhan-virus-pneumonia-singapore-confirms-first-case-786446 (accessed on 1 January 2022).
2. What Do the Different DORSCON Levels Mean. Gov.SG. 6 February 2020. Available online: https://www.gov.sg/article/what-do-the-different-dorscon-levels-mean (accessed on 1 January 2022).
3. Baker, J.A. Singapore's Circuit Breaker and Beyond: Timeline of the COVID-19 Reality. CNA. 2 June 2020. Available online: https://www.channelnewsasia.com/singapore/covid-19-circuit-breaker-chronicles-charting-evolution-645586 (accessed on 1 January 2022).
4. Asher, S. TraceTogether: Singapore Turns to Wearable Contact-Tracing COVID Tech. 2020. Available online: https://www.bbc.com/news/technology-53146360 (accessed on 1 January 2022).
5. Post-Circuit Breaker–When Can We Move on to Phases 2 and 3? Gov.SG. 28 May 2020. Available online: https://www.gov.sg/article/post-circuit-breaker-when-can-we-move-on-to-phases-2-and-3 (accessed on 1 January 2022).
6. Updates on Singapore's COVID-19 Situation. Ministry of Health. Available online: https://www.moh.gov.sg/covid-19 (accessed on 1 January 2022).
7. Berger, A.; Hill, T.P. *An Introduction to Benford's Law*; Princeton University Press: Princeton, NJ, USA, 2015.
8. Anran Wei, A.E.V. Is COVID-19 Data Reliable? A Statistical Analysis with Benford's Law. *Preprint* **2020**. [CrossRef]
9. Diekmann, A. Not the first digit! using Benford's law to detect fraudulent scientif ic data. *J. Appl. Stat.* **2007**, *34*, 321–329. [CrossRef]

10. Nigrini, M.J.; Miller, S.J. Data Diagnostics using second-order tests of Benford's law. *Audit. A J. Pract. Theory* **2009**, *28*, 305–324. [CrossRef]
11. Hussein, O. Second wave of COVID-19 is determined by immune mechanism. *Med. Hypotheses* **2020**, *144*, 110238. [CrossRef] [PubMed]
12. Tan Eugene, K.B. Tan Eugene, K.B. Time for Singapore to Address Some Uncomfortable Questions on Its Migrant Workers. TODAY. 24 April 2020. Available online: https://www.todayonline.com/commentary/time-singapore-address-uncomfortable-questions-migrant-workers-covid-19-dormitories (accessed on 1 January 2022).
13. Wei, T.T. All Migrant Worker Dormitories to be Cleared of Coronavirus by Aug 7, Says Lawrence Wong. *The Straits Times*. 24 July 2020. Available online: https://www.straitstimes.com/singapore/health/all-migrant-worker-dormitories-to-be-cleared-of-coronavirus-by-aug-7-says-lawrence (accessed on 1 January 2022).
14. MOH–News Highlights. Available online: https://www.moh.gov.sg/news-highlights (accessed on 1 July 2022).
15. Gov.sg Launches New Channels to Keep the Public Informed about COVID-19. MCI. 2020. Available online: https://www.mci.gov.sg/pressroom/news-and-stories/pressroom/2020/4/gov-sg-launches-new-channels-to-keep-the-public-informed-about-covid-19 (accessed on 1 January 2022).
16. Lim, J. How Singapore Is Taking On COVID-19. 2020. Available online: https://www.asianscientist.com/2020/04/features/singapore-covid-19-response/ (accessed on 1 January 2022).
17. Goh, T. Coronavirus: Singapore's Testing Rate is Tops in Asean, with over 1m Swabs Done. 2020. Available online: https://www.straitstimes.com/singapore/health/spores-testing-rate-is-tops-in-asean-with-over-1m-swabs-done (accessed on 1 January 2022).
18. The Importance of Contact Tracing in Singapore and the Role Technology Plays. 2020. Available online: https://opengovasia.com/the-importance-of-contact-tracing-in-singapore-and-the-role-technology-plays/ (accessed on 1 January 2022).
19. MOH National Schemes. 2020. Available online: https://www.primarycarepages.sg/practice-management/moh-national-schemes/public-health-preparedness-clinic-(phpc) (accessed on 1 January 2022).
20. Oppah Kuguyo, A.P.K.; Dandara, C. Singapore COVID-19 Pandemic Response as a Successful Model Framework for Low-Resource Health Care Settings in Africa? *A J. Integr. Biol.* **2020**, *24*, 470–478. [CrossRef] [PubMed]
21. Rebecca, P.; Stephanie, A. Tracking Singapore's COVID-19 Vaccination Progress. *The Straits Times*. 26 June 2021. Available online: https://www.straitstimes.com/multimedia/graphics/2021/06/singapore-covid-vaccination-tracker/index.html (accessed on 1 January 2022).
22. Chong, C. Boosters Needed for Extension of Full Vaccination Status as COVID-19 Variants Emerge. *The Straits Times*. 16 December 2021. Available online: https://www.straitstimes.com/singapore/exception-to-enter-vaccination-differentiated-places-for-recovered-covid-19-patients (accessed on 1 January 2022).
23. Budget 2020. 2020. Available online: https://www.gov.sg/features/budget2020 (accessed on 1 January 2022).
24. Singapore. (n.d.). KPMG. Available online: https://home.kpmg/xx/en/home/insights/2020/04/singapore-government-and-institution-measures-in-response-to-covid.html (accessed on 1 January 2022).
25. Government to Provide about $2.2 Billion to Help Singaporeans with MediShield Life Premium Adjustments. Report.sg | The Singapore Report. 29 September 2020. Available online: https://report.sg/government-to-provide-about-2-2-billion-to-help-singaporeans-with-medishield-life-premium-adjustments/ (accessed on 1 January 2022).
26. Lam, L. Singapore has Months' Worth of Stockpiles, Planned for Disruption of Supplies Online Malaysia for Years: Chan Chun Sing. 2020. Available online: https://www.channelnewsasia.com/news/singapore/coronavirus-covid-19-chan-chun-sing-food-supply-12545326 (accessed on 1 January 2022).
27. Implementing Safe Entry and Safe Management Practices. Ministry of Health. 9 May 2020. Available online: https://www.moh.gov.sg/news-highlights/details/implementing-safeentry-and-safe-management-practices (accessed on 1 January 2022).
28. Koh, D. Singapore Government Launches New App for Contact Tracing to Combat Spread of COVID-19. 2020. Available online: https://www.mobihealthnews.com/news/asia-pacific/singapore-government-launches-new-app-contact-tracing-combat-spread-covid-19 (accessed on 1 January 2022).
29. Distribution of TraceTogether Tokens Starts; Aim is for 70% Participation in Contact Tracing Scheme. 2020. Available online: https://www.straitstimes.com/singapore/government-aiming-for-70-participation-in-tracetogether-programme-says-vivian-on-first-day (accessed on 1 January 2022).
30. 9 in 10 Coronavirus Patients in Singapore are Linked to Worker Dormitories. 2020. Available online: https://www.straitstimes.com/singapore/health/novel-coronavirus-cases-in-singapore (accessed on 1 January 2022).
31. Alkhatib, S. Coronavirus: Couple Online China Charged with Giving False Info to MOH Officials. 2020. Available online: https://www.straitstimes.com/singapore/courts-crime/coronavirus-china-couple-charged-after-allegedly-giving-false-info-to-moh#:~{}:text=SINGAPORE%20%2D%20A%20couple%20Online%20China,the%20process%20of%20contact%20tracing (accessed on 1 January 2022).
32. Lai, S.H.S.; Tang, C.Q.Y.; Kurup, A.; Thevendran, G. The experience of contact tracing in Singapore in the control of COVID-19: Highlighting the use of digital technology. *Int. Orthop.* **2021**, *45*, 65–69. [CrossRef] [PubMed]
33. Ellis, R. WHO Changes Stance, Says Public Should Wear Masks. 2020. Available online: https://www.webmd.com/lung/news/20200608/who-changes-stance-says-public-should-wear-masks (accessed on 1 January 2022).

34. Ang Hwee Min, R.P. COVID-19: Compulsory to Wear Mask When Leaving the House, Says Lawrence Wong. 2020. Available online: https://www.channelnewsasia.com/news/singapore/covid19-wearing-masks-compulsory-lawrence-wong-12640828 (accessed on 1 January 2022).
35. Which Countries Have Made Wearing Face Masks Compulsory? 2020. Available online: https://www.aljazeera.com/news/2020/8/17/which-countries-have-made-wearing-face-masks-compulsory (accessed on 1 January 2022).
36. Duong, M.C. Commentary: Masks Could Be Secret behind Vietnam's COVID-19 Success. Minh Cuong Duong. 2020. Available online: https://www.channelnewsasia.com/news/commentary/coronavirus-covid-19-vietnam-case-mask-who-symptom-spread-travel-13471616 (accessed on 1 January 2022).
37. Su, V.Y.F.; Yen, Y.F.; Yang, K.Y.; Su, W.J.; Chou, K.T.; Chen, Y.M.; Perng, D.W. Masks and Medical Care: Two Keys to Taiwan's Success in Preventing COVID-19 Spread. *Travel. Med. Infect. Dis.* **2020**, *38*, 101780.
38. Christopher, T.; Leffler, E.B.I.; Joseph, D.; Lykins, V.; Matthew, C.; Hogan, C.; McKeown, A.; Grzybowski, A. Association of country-wide coronavirus mortality with demographics, testing, lockdowns, and public wearing of masks. *Am. J. Trop. Med. Hyg.* **2020**, *103*, 2400.
39. Philip Anfinrud, V.S.; Christina, E. Bax, Adriaan Bax, Visualizing Speech-Generated Oral Fluid Droplets with Laser Light Scattering. *N. Engl. J. Med.* **2020**, *382*, 2061–2063. [CrossRef] [PubMed]
40. Lyu, W.; Wehby, G.L. Community Use Of Face Masks And COVID-19: Evidence Online A Natural Experiment of State Mandates In The US. *Health Aff.* **2020**, *39*, 1419–1425. [CrossRef] [PubMed]
41. How is Singapore Limiting the Spread of Coronavirus Disease 2019? 2020. Available online: https://www.gov.sg/article/how-is-singapore-limiting-the-spread-of-covid-19 (accessed on 1 January 2022).
42. Additional Precautionary Measures To Prevent Further Importation and Spread of COVID-19 Cases. 2020. Available online: https://www.moh.gov.sg/news-highlights/details/additional-precautionary-measures-to-prevent-further-importation-and-spread-of-covid-19-cases (accessed on 1 January 2022).
43. Additional Border Control Measures To Reduce Further Importation of COVID-19 Cases. Ministry of Health. 22 March 2020. Available online: https://www.moh.gov.sg/news-highlights/details/additional-border-control-measures-to-reduce-further-importation-of-covid-19-cases (accessed on 1 January 2022).
44. Linka, K.; Peirlinck, M.; Sahli Costabal, F.; Kuhl, E. Outbreak dynamics of COVID-19 in Europe and the effect of travel restrictions. *Comput. Methods Biomech. Biomed. Eng.* **2020**, *23*, 710–717. [CrossRef] [PubMed]
45. Heng, M. Yong Thai Hang Medical Shop and Grand Hyatt COVID-19 Clusters no Longer Active. *The Straits Times*. 11 March 2020. Available online: https://www.straitstimes.com/singapore/yong-thai-hang-medical-shop-and-grand-hyatt-covid-19-clusters-no-longer-active (accessed on 1 January 2022).
46. Board, S.T. Monthly Visitor 2020. Arrivals. Available online: https://stan.stb.gov.sg/public/sense/app/254dd6c2-eaf7-46c4-bf7a-39b5df6ff847/sheet/3101ecdd-af88-4d5d-be49-6c7f90277948/state/analysis (accessed on 1 January 2022).
47. Worldometer. Australia. 2020. Available online: https://www.worldometers.info/coronavirus/country/australia/ (accessed on 1 January 2022).
48. Worldometer. Indonesia. 2020. Available online: https://www.worldometers.info/coronavirus/country/indonesia/ (accessed on 1 January 2022).
49. Worldometer. UK. 2020. Available online: https://www.worldometers.info/coronavirus/country/uk/ (accessed on 1 January 2022).
50. Grace Sihombing, A.A. Virus Deaths May Be Three Times Official Tally in Indonesia. 2020. Available online: https://www.bloomberg.com/news/articles/2020-05-29/virus-deaths-may-be-three-times-the-official-tally-in-indonesia (accessed on 1 January 2022).
51. Soeriaatmadja, W. Coronavirus: Indonesia Estimates More Than 500,000 Had Contact with Virus Suspects. *The Straits Times*. 22 March 2020. Available online: https://www.straitstimes.com/asia/se-asia/coronavirus-indonesian-president-vows-to-use-all-powers-to-tackle-health-economic-woes (accessed on 1 January 2022).
52. Analysis April 2, & GlobalData. COVID-19 Coronavirus: Top Ten Most-Affected Countries. Pharmaceutical Technology. 7 September 2020. Available online: https://www.pharmaceutical-technology.com/analysis/covid-19-coronavirus-top-ten-most-affected-countries/ (accessed on 1 January 2022).

reports

Systematic Review

# Clinical Outcomes after Immunotherapies in Cancer Setting during COVID-19 Era: A Systematic Review and Meta-Regression

**Mona Kamal [1,2,*], Massimo Baudo [3], Jacinth Joseph [4,5], Yimin Geng [6] and Aiham Qdaisat [7]**

1. Department of Symptom Research, Unit 1450, The University of Texas MD Anderson Cancer Center, 1515 Holcombe Boulevard, Houston, TX 77030, USA
2. Clinical Oncology, Faculty of Medicine, Ain Shams University, Cairo 11591, Egypt
3. Department of Cardiac Surgery, Spedali Civili di Brescia, 25123 Brescia, Italy; massimo.baudo@icloud.com
4. Department of Stem Cell Transplantation, The University of Texas MD Anderson Cancer Center, Houston, TX 77030, USA; drjacinthjoy@yahoo.com
5. Blood and Marrow Transplant Center, Methodist Le Bonheur, Memphis, TN 38104, USA
6. Research Medical Library, The University of Texas MD Anderson Cancer Center, Houston, TX 77030, USA; ygeng@mdanderson.org
7. Department of Emergency Medicine, The University of Texas MD Anderson Cancer Center, Houston, TX 77030, USA; aqdaisat@mdanderson.org

* Correspondence: mkjomaa@mdanderson.org; Tel.: +1-(832)-873-0163

**Abstract:** Background: This study aims to describe COVID-19–related clinical outcomes after immunotherapies (ICIs) for cancer patients. Methods: In this meta-analysis, we searched databases to collect data that addressed outcomes after immunotherapies (ICIs) during the COVID-19 pandemic. The primary endpoint was COVID-19–related mortality. Secondary endpoints included COVID-related hospital readmission, emergency room (ER) visits, opportunistic infections, respiratory complications, need for ventilation, and thrombo-embolic events. Pooled event rates (PERs) were calculated and a meta-regression analysis was performed. Results: A total of 262 studies were identified. Twenty-two studies with a total of forty-four patients were eligible. The PER of COVID-19–related mortality was 39.73%, while PERs of COVID-19–related ER visits, COVID-19–related pulmonary complications, and COVID-19–related ventilator needs were 40.75%, 40.41%, and 34.92%, respectively. The PER of opportunistic infections was 34.92%. The PERs of the use of antivirals, antibiotics, steroids, prophylactic anticoagulants, and convalescent plasma were 62.12%, 57.12%, 51.36%, 41.90%, and 26.48%, respectively. There was a trend toward an association between previous respiratory diseases and COVID-19–related mortality. Conclusion: The rates of COVID-19–related mortality, ER visits, pulmonary complications, need for a ventilator, and opportunistic infections are still high after ICIs during the COVID-19 pandemic. There was a trend toward an association between previous respiratory diseases and COVID-19–related mortality.

**Keywords:** ICIs; COVID-19; cancer; mortality; meta-analysis



**Citation:** Kamal, M.; Baudo, M.; Joseph, J.; Geng, Y.; Qdaisat, A. Clinical Outcomes after Immunotherapies in Cancer Setting during COVID-19 Era: A Systematic Review and Meta-Regression. *Reports* **2022**, *5*, 31. https://doi.org/10.3390/reports5030031

Academic Editors: Toshio Hattori and Yugo Ashino

Received: 29 June 2022
Accepted: 19 July 2022
Published: 25 July 2022



## 1. Introduction

Cancer patients could be more susceptible to COVID-19 infection because of their vulnerable immunity status due to the cancer itself, as well as the cancer treatment [1]. Administering immune checkpoint inhibitors (ICIs) during the COVID-19 era comes with challenges [2,3]. However, the data addressing the impact of ICIs on COVID-19–related outcomes are unclear [4,5], considering the known fact that ICIs restore immune competency [6]. Some data showed that receipt of ICIs does not negatively impact the outcomes after COVID-19 infection [5]. Thus, such challenges, debatable outcomes, and limited existing data necessitate a systematic review.

The challenges of administering ICIs during the COVID-19 era include the potential overlap between COVID-19–related interstitial pneumonia and possible ICI-induced lung injury [2,3,7]. The overall incidence rate of ICI-induced pneumonitis ranges from 2.5% to 10%; yet, it could be fatal, accounting for 35% of ICI-related mortality [2,8]. This challenge is greater in lung cancer patients receiving ICIs with or without local radiotherapy who are at risk for COVID-19 infection [9]. The immune hyperactivation induced by ICIs initiates cytokine release syndrome (CRS) (elevated interleukins and cytokines with subsequent organ failure and death). Similar cytokine storms have been observed after COVID-19 infection with similarly fatal outcomes of organ failure and death [10,11]. Given the similarity of the presentations of underlying COVID-19–induced and ICI-induced lung injury, diagnostic difficulty or delay and the synergistic effect of ICI- and COVID-19–induced lung injury could add to the fatality of the outcomes [12]. Fortunately, ICI-induced CRS is quite rare, and a COVID-19–induced cytokine storm is not an early event in the COVID-19 trajectory [7]. Such observations leave space for early intervention and careful patient screening/selection and monitoring to allow cancer patients in need of ICIs to receive their treatment safely and effectively during the COVID-19 era.

Given that the duration of the pandemic and the trajectory of COVID-19 infections are still unknown and unpredictable, we undertook a systematic review to obtain solid data showing patient characteristics and COVID-19–related outcomes after ICIs during the COVID-19 era. Care providers need these data to create effective, tolerable ICI treatment plans without compromising safety or outcomes. The objective of this systematic review was to address the clinical outcomes after ICIs for cancer patients during the COVID-19 era. The primary endpoint was COVID-19–related mortality and the secondary endpoints included COVID-19–related therapy, readmission to the hospital, ER visits, opportunistic infections, respiratory complications, need for ventilation, need for tracheostomy, and thrombo-embolic events.

## 2. Methodology

This study was conducted according to the Preferred Reporting Items for Systematic Reviews and Meta-Analyses (PRISMA) guidelines. The Newcastle–Ottawa Quality Assessment Scale for cohort studies was used [13].

### 2.1. Literature Search

We searched the Ovid MEDLINE, Ovid Embase, Clarivate Analytics Web of Science, PubMed, and Wiley-Blackwell Cochrane Library databases for publications in the English language from 1 December 2019 to 15 October 2020. The following concepts were searched for using subject headings and keywords as needed: "COVID-19", "severe acute respiratory syndrome coronavirus 2", "SARS-CoV-2", "coronavirus infections", "novel coronavirus", "cancer", "neoplasms", "tumor", "leukemia", "lymphoma", "melanoma", "carcinoma", "sarcoma", "oncology", "checkpoint inhibitors", "programmed cell death 1", "programmed death ligand 1", "PD-1", "PD-L1", "cytotoxic T lymphocyte associated antigen 4", "CTLA 4", "ipilimumab", "pembrolizumab", "nivolumab", "atezolizumab", "durvalumab", "avelumab", "cemiplimab", "chimeric antigen receptor t-cell therapy", "adoptive immunotherapy", etc. The search terms were combined by "or" if they represented similar concepts and combined by "and" if they represented different concepts. The complete search strategies are detailed in Tables S1–S4.

### 2.2. Study Selection

Eligible studies were required to evaluate measurable outcomes related to COVID-19 infection in cancer patients on ICIs during the COVID-19 pandemic. Owing to limited publications in this unique cohort, we included case presentations and case studies. To ensure inclusion of all available data, all bibliographies were searched for potential eligible studies (i.e., backward snowballing). Nevertheless, abstracts, reviews, and expert opinions were excluded, as were studies that were not exclusively of ICI-treated patients and studies with insufficient information about the characteristics or outcomes (listed below).

### 2.3. Data Extraction and Endpoints

Two reviewers (M.K. and A.Q.) independently assessed the eligibility. Then M.K., A.Q., and J.J. extracted the data from the eligible studies and tabulated the data using Excel software (Microsoft Corporation, Redmond, WA, USA).

Data on study period, study center, country, type of cancer, type of study, and sample size were retrieved. We abstracted age, gender, presence of hypertension, diabetes mellitus, renal insufficiency, smoking history, pre-existing chronic obstructive pulmonary disease, cerebrovascular accident, and dyslipidemia.

We also collected information about previous and current cancer treatments, type of cancer and ICI(s), cancer status, in-hospital COVID-19 infection, onset of COVID-19 infection in relation to receipt of ICIs, and laboratory and pulmonary findings at diagnosis of COVID-19 infection and their follow-up data if presented. To assess COVID-19–related therapy use, we recorded use of steroids (yes/no, dosage, and duration), use of antivirals, antibiotics, convalescent plasma, prophylactic coagulations, and antibodies. Finally, we assessed the following outcomes when they occurred because of COVID-19 infection: rates of readmission, emergency room (ER) visits, intensive care unit (ICU) admission, need for tracheostomy, need for ventilation, mortality, and complications, for instance pulmonary problems, thrombo-embolic events, and fungal and other opportunistic infections.

The primary endpoint of the analysis was COVID-19–related mortality. Secondary endpoints included COVID-19–related therapy, readmission to the hospital, ER visits, opportunistic infections, respiratory complications, need for ventilation, need for tracheostomy, and thrombo-embolic events.

### 2.4. Statistical Analysis

Pooled event rates (PERs) with 95% confidence intervals (CIs) were calculated for the study outcomes. Meta-regression was performed to explore the relationship between COVID-19–related mortality and clinical characteristics. These results were reported as a regression coefficient (i.e., beta). In all analyses, studies were weighted by the inverse of the variance of the estimate for that study, and between-study variance was estimated with the DerSimonian–Laird method with a random-effects model. Studies with zeros were included in the meta-analysis, and treatment arm continuity correction was applied in studies with zero cell frequencies.

Heterogeneity was based on the Cochran Q test, with I2 values. In the case of heterogeneity I2 > 50%, individual study inference analysis was performed through a "leave-one-out" sensitivity analysis. Funnel plots by graphical inspection and Egger regression test were used for assessment of publication bias. In the case of asymmetry positivity, visual assessment and Duval and Tweedie's "trim and fill" method were used for further assessment.

Hypothesis testing for equivalence was set at the two-tailed 0.05 level. All analyses were performed using R version 4.1.0 (R Project for Statistical Computing) and RStudio version 1.4.1717, using the "meta" and "metafor" packages.

## 3. Results

A total of 262 studies were identified in the databases. After exclusion of duplicates, 162 studies were screened. Then, we excluded 122 non-eligible studies. Forty full-text articles were assessed for eligibility. Finally, 22 studies with a total of 44 patients met the eligibility criteria. Supplementary Figure S1 shows the PRISMA flow diagram. Table 1 shows the studies' characteristics and patient demographics. Supplementary Table S5 shows the overall baseline patient demographics. Patients' average age was 57.2 ± 17.4 years. A total of 66% were men, and 53% were current/former smokers. Totals of 61%, 36%, 30%, and 15% had hypertension, pre-existing chronic obstructive pulmonary disease, diabetes mellitus, and cerebrovascular accident, respectively. A total of 58% of patients had previous cancer therapy before receipt of ICIs. The top presenting COVID-19 symptoms were fever (74%), cough (57%), and dyspnea (52%), while ground glass opacity (64%), infiltrate (27%), and consolidation (27%) were the top radiologic findings. The Newcastle–Ottawa Quality Assessment Scale for cohort studies is shown in Supplementary Table S6 [13].

The PER of COVID-19–related mortality was 39.73% (95% CI: 26.32–54.87%) (Figure 1), while the PER of COVID-19–related ER visits, pulmonary complications, and need for ventilation were 40.75% (95% CI: 19.63–65.95%), 40.41% (95% CI: 21.81–62.25%), and 34.92% (95% CI: 17.34–57.86%), respectively (Figures 2 and 3, Supplementary Figure S2). The PER of opportunistic infections was 34.92% (95% CI: 17.34–57.86%) (Supplementary Figure S3). Table 2 and Supplementary Figures S4–S8 show the PERs of the use of antivirals (62.12%), antibiotics (57.12%), steroids (51.36%), prophylactic anticoagulants (41.90%), and convalescent plasma (26.48%). As shown in Table 2, none of the patients in the included studies received antibodies, needed readmission, needed tracheostomy, or developed thrombo-embolic events due to COVID-19 infection. Nevertheless, 27% of patients had airway problems after COVID-19 infection in the nine included studies that assessed this outcome.

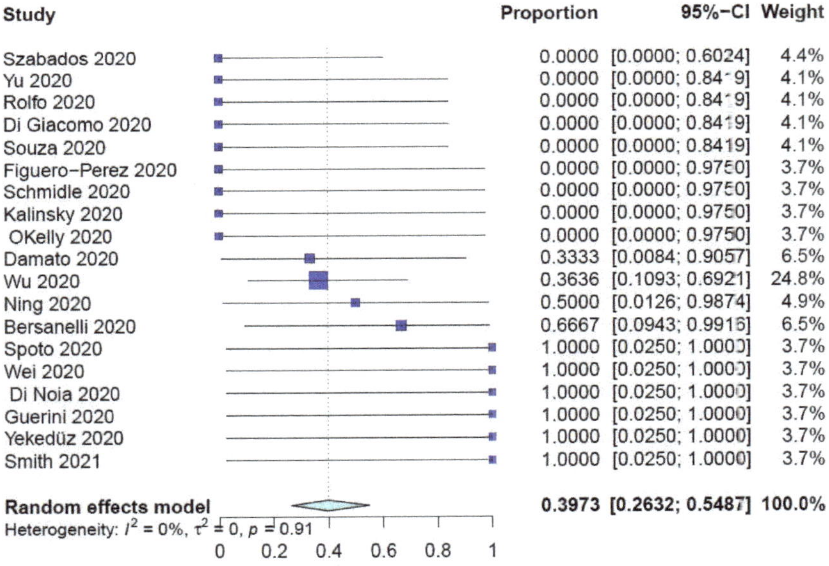


**Figure 1.** Forest plot of the primary endpoint of COVID-19–related mortality.

**Table 1.** Characteristics of the eligible studies and demographics of the patients in the included studies.

| Author | Year | Institution | Country | Study Type | N | Mean Age | Male | Smoking History | HTN | DM | Dyslipidemia | CKD | Respiratory Conditions | CVA |
|---|---|---|---|---|---|---|---|---|---|---|---|---|---|---|
| Yu | 2020 | Zhongnan Hospital of Wuhan University | China | Case series | 2 | NA | 2 | NA | NA | NA | NA | NA | NA | NA |
| Figuero-Perez | 2020 | University of Salamanca | Spain | Case report | 1 | 76 | 1 | NA | NA | NA | NA | NA | 1 | NA |
| Damato | 2020 | Oncologico e Tecnologie Avanzate, Azienda USL—IRCCS Reggio Emilia | Italy | Case series | 3 | 60.3 | 2 | 2 | NA | NA | NA | NA | NA | NA |
| Schmidle | 2020 | Technical University of Munich | Germany | Case report | 1 | 47 | 0 | NA | NA | NA | NA | NA | NA | NA |
| Kalinsky | 2020 | Columbia University Irving Medical Center | USA | Case report | 1 | 32 | 0 | 0 | NA | NA | NA | NA | NA | NA |
| Shaverdian | 2020 | Memorial Sloan Kettering Cancer Center | USA | Case series | 1 | 73 | 0 | NA | NA | NA | NA | NA | NA | NA |
| Ning | 2020 | The University of Texas MD Anderson Cancer Center | USA | Case series | 2 | 61.5 | 1 | NA | NA | NA | NA | NA | NA | NA |
| Rolfo | 2020 | Marlene and Stewart Comprehensive Cancer Center | USA | Case series | 2 | 65 | 1 | 2 | NA | NA | NA | NA | NA | NA |
| Spoto | 2020 | University Campus Bio-Medico of Rome | Italy | Case report | 1 | 55 | 0 | 0 | 0 | 1 | 0 | 0 | 0 | 0 |
| Di Giacomo | 2020 | University Hospital of Siena | Italy | Case series | 2 | 62.5 | 1 | 0 | 0 | 0 | 0 | 0 | 0 | 0 |
| Wei | 2020 | Huazhong University of Science and Technology | China | Case series | 1 | 30 | 1 | NA | NA | NA | NA | NA | NA | NA |
| OKelly | 2020 | Mater Misericordiae University Hospital | Ireland | Case report | 1 | 22 | 0 | 0 | 0 | 0 | 0 | 0 | 0 | 0 |
| Souza | 2020 | Hospital Israelita Albert Einstein | Brazil | Case series | 2 | 78.5 | 1 | NA | NA | NA | NA | NA | NA | NA |
| Di Noia | 2020 | Cliniche Humanitas Gavazzeni | Italy | Case report | 1 | 53 | 1 | NA | NA | NA | NA | NA | NA | NA |
| Guerini | 2020 | Università degli Studi di Brescia | Italy | Case report | 1 | 75 | 1 | 1 | 1 | 0 | 0 | 0 | 1 | 0 |
| da Costa | 2020 | | Brazil | Case report | 1 | 66 | 1 | 1 | NA | NA | NA | NA | NA | NA |
| Yekedüz | 2020 | | Turkey | Case report | 1 | 75 | 1 | NA | 1 | 1 | 0 | 0 | 1 | 1 |
| Szabados | 2020 | | UK | Case series | 4 | 64.5 | 4 | 2 | 4 | 1 | 0 | 0 | 0 | 0 |
| Bersanelli | 2020 | 82 Italian centers | Italy | Case series | 3 | 71.7 | 3 | 3 | 2 | NA | NA | NA | 2 | 1 |
| Grover | 2020 | | USA | Case report | 1 | 54 | 0 | NA | NA | NA | NA | NA | NA | NA |
| Wu | 2020 | Zhongnan Hospital of Wuhan University and the Tongji Hospital of Huazhong University of Science and Technology | China | Case series | 11 | 56 | 8 | 5 | NA | NA | NA | NA | NA | NA |
| Smith | 2021 | Baylor College of Medicine | USA | Case report | 1 | 23 | 0 | NA | NA | NA | NA | NA | NA | NA |

HTN = hypertension; DM = diabetes; CKD = chronic kidney disease; CVA = cerebrovascular accident.

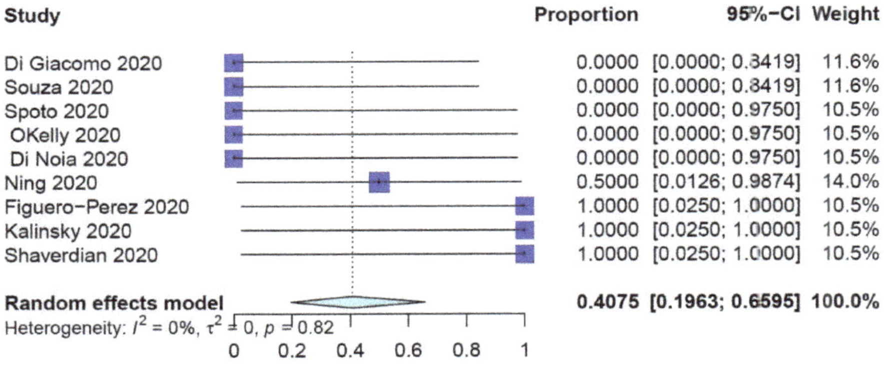


**Figure 2.** Forest plot of COVID-19–related ER visits.

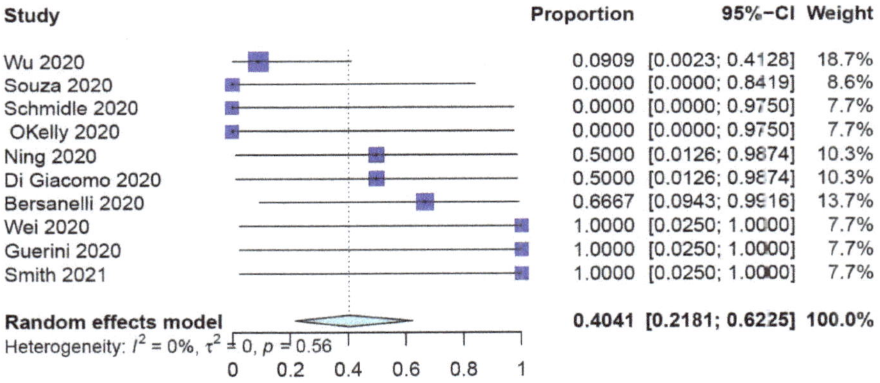


**Figure 3.** Forest plots of pulmonary complications due to COVID-19 infection.

**Table 2.** Outcomes summary.

| Outcome | No. of Studies | Estimate | 95% CI | Heterogeneity: $I^2$, $p$-Value | Egger Test ($p$-Value) |
|---|---|---|---|---|---|
| Steroid use | 14 | 51.36% | 34.99–67.44 | 0%, $p$ = 0.757 | $p$ = 0.6754 |
| Antiviral use | 10 | 62.10% | 41.04–79.41 | 0%, $p$ = 0.5457 | $p$ = 0.1625 |
| Antibiotics use | 13 | 57.12% | 37.03–75.10 | 0%, $p$ = 0.9824 | $p$ = 0.0017 |
| Convalescent plasma use | 8 | 26.48% | 10.59–52.28 | 0%, $p$ = 0.9470 | NA |
| Prophylactic anticoagulant use | 10 | 41.90% | 21.35–65.72 | 0%, $p$ = 0.7297 | $p$ = 0.6215 |
| Antibody treatment | 6 | 0% | NA | NA | NA |
| Readmission to hospital | 5 | 0% | NA | NA | NA |
| ER visit | 9 | 40.75% | 19.16–65.95 | 0%, $p$ = 0.8221 | NA |
| COVID-19–related mortality | 19 | 39.73 | 26.32–54.87 | 0%, $p$ = 0.9077 | $p$ = 0.7214 |
| Airway problem | 9 | 27.28% | 11.79–51.30 | 0%, $p$ = 0.8272 | NA |
| Pulmonary complication | 10 | 40.41% | 21.81–62.25 | 0%, $p$ = 0.5596 | |
| Need for ventilator | 11 | 34.92% | 17.34–57.86 | 0%, $p$ = 0.7252 | $p$ = 0.0030 |
| Need for tracheostomy | 9 | 0% | NA | NA | NA |
| Thrombo-embolic event | 8 | 0% | NA | NA | NA |
| Opportunistic infection | 9 | 29.45% | 12.84–54.18 | 0%, $p$ = 0.8681 | NA |

The meta-regression (Table 3) indicated a trend toward association between previous respiratory diseases and COVID-19–related mortality ($p$ = 0.0861). No other characteristic showed a significant association with COVID-19–related mortality in the meta-regression analysis.

**Table 3.** Meta-regression of COVID-related mortality.

| Variable | No. of Studies | Beta ± SE | *p*-Value |
|---|---|---|---|
| Mean age | 18 | −0.0073 ± 0.0211 | 0.7300 |
| Male sex | 19 | 0.0034 ± 0.0089 | 0.7009 |
| Respiratory disease | 7 | 0.0220 ± 0.0128 | *0.0861* |
| History of smoking | 10 | 0.0078 ± 0.0114 | 0.4917 |
| Diabetes | 5 | 0.0166 ± 0.0189 | 0.3813 |
| Hypertension | 6 | 0.0131 ± 0.0144 | 0.3634 |
| Dyslipidemia | 5 | −0.6263 ± 0.7086 | 0.3768 |
| Chronic kidney disease | 5 | −0.6263 ± 0.7086 | 0.3768 |
| Cerebrovascular accident | 6 | 0.0236 ± 0.0178 | 0.1858 |
| Previous cancer treatment | 8 | 0.0043 ± 0.0121 | 0.7194 |

Results are expressed as β ± standard error, *p*-value. Positive beta reflects an increase in the event when the frequency of the variable increases, while negative beta reflects a decrease in the event with the increase in the frequency of the variable. SE = standard error.

## 4. Discussion

Our systematic review of COVID-19–related outcomes after ICIs reported the rates of COVID-19–related mortality, ER visits, pulmonary complications, need for a ventilator, and opportunistic infections in cancer patients on ICIs during the COVID-19 pandemic. While there was a trend toward association between previous respiratory diseases and COVID-19-related mortality, no other characteristic was associated with COVID-19-related mortality in the meta-regression analysis.

Immunotherapies have revolutionized cancer care. Nevertheless, immunotherapies modulate the immune system, induce unique adverse events, and are usually administered for long durations. Further, managing the resultant, potentially fatal morbidities after immunotherapies is a clinical challenge, especially during the pandemic [1,14]. However, the exact impact of COVID-19 infection on the risk of mortality and morbidities after immunotherapies is still uncertain. Our data showed that the PER of COVID-19–related mortality was 39.73% in cancer patients treated with ICIs during the pandemic. Similarly high COVID-19–related mortality rates in patients on ICI therapy during the pandemic were reported by Dai et al. (33%) [1] and Robilotti et al. (36%). Yet, Robilotti et al. [15] highlighted that receiving ICIs did not impact the death rate during the COVID-19 era.

While patients on ICIs have a certain level of risk for developing infectious diseases [16], the risk of COVID-19 infection after ICIs increased only after the use of corticosteroids and/or TNF-α inhibitors [17]. However, other studies reported that COVID-19 infection rates are low after ICIs and that receipt of ICIs did not increase the risk of COVID-19 infection [18]. These low rates have been attributed in part to the high compliance with social distancing and mask-wearing in cancer-setting care. Additionally, the immunosuppressive effect of ICIs modulates the cytokine release syndrome associated with severe COVID-19 infection [19–22]. For these reasons, some ICI-treated patients with COVID-19 infection are asymptomatic and subsequently do not seek to be tested for COVID-19. Further, at certain stages of the treatment course, ICIs restore cellular immunocompetence, which makes patients on ICIs less prone to infection [6,23]. However, close monitoring is still needed.

Based on the data from this meta-analysis, the top presenting COVID-19 symptoms were fever (74%), cough (57%), and dyspnea (52%), while ground glass opacity (64%), infiltrate (27%), and consolidation (27%) were the most common imaging findings. Considering the high rate of pulmonary complications and need for ventilators (40% and 35%), close and cautious monitoring is warranted [24], with particular focus on excluding bacterial co-infection, which has been found to increase the risk of poor outcomes. The similarities in presentation, response to steroids/antibodies, chest imaging findings, and pathological characterization between the lung injury induced by COVID-19 and ICIs are clinical challenges in the management of cases treated with ICIs during the COVID-19 era [2,11,12]. The massive amount of activated immune cells after ICI therapy may delay the diagnosis of COVID-19 infection, as these cells are very hypermetabolic on fluorodeoxyglucose positron emission tomography [25]. Further, steroids could relieve both COVID-19– and ICI-induced lung injury. On the basis of pathological findings after COVID-19 infection (hyaline membrane formation and pulmonary edema), steroids could resolve COVID-19–induced lung injury. However, steroid use should be timely optimized to treat severe respiratory stress after COVID-19 infection [11]. Additionally, monoclonal antibodies showed improvement in levels of organ toxicity induced by either ICIs or COVID-19 [26,27]. Yet, the efficacy of monoclonal antibodies in treating COVID-19–induced injury is still under investigation. Further, the granulocyte colony-stimulating factor and erythropoietin play important roles whenever indicated [28,29].

Managing COVID-19–related complications in patients on ICIs is another challenge. We found that the PER of opportunistic infections was 34.92% Nevertheless, none of the patients in the included studies needed readmission, needed tracheostomy, or developed thrombo-embolic events due to COVID-19 infection. However, 27% of the patients in nine included studies had airway problems after COVID-19 infection. We also presented PERs of the use of antivirals (62.12%), antibiotics (57.12%), steroids (51.36%), prophylactic anticoagulants (41.90%), and convalescent plasma (26.48%) after COVID-19 infection. Most cancer care centers agree on continuing ICIs after COVID-19 infection [4,30], and Amin et al. advised continuing the standard management of immunotherapy-induced adverse events in these patients as long as protective measures are closely adhered to [21]. Nevertheless, timing is key; since most patients experience immunotherapy-induced adverse events within the first 6 months of treatment [7], patients who are going to start ICIs during the pandemic must be carefully selected and monitored. Furthermore, pathological activation of immune response usually occurs during the late stage of COVID-19 infection [11].

Some authors have explored the effect of treatment frequency and time elapsed after ICIs on COVID-19 infection severity. Robilotti et al. [15] mentioned that ICIs were one of the predictors of the need for hospitalization and developing severe COVID-19 infection, while others did not observe any statistically significant association between receipt of ICIs and the severity of COVID-19 infection [18,31]. We may better explain these findings when we have a better understanding of the crosstalk between the respective immune activation pathways that are secondary to ICI treatment and COVID-19–induced cytokine release syndrome. Nevertheless, modulating the dosage and schedule of ICIs may benefit individual patients [32]. On the other hand, the severity of COVID-19 infection has been observed to be high in patients with lung cancer [33,34], especially after ICIs, as reported by Robilotti et al. [15]. However, Robilotti et al. [15] mentioned that the severity of COVID-19 infection was similarly high in non-lung-cancer patients who had ICIs. Nevertheless, other studies did not find an association between receipt of ICIs and poor outcomes of COVID-19 infection [4,18,33]. Of note, Robilotti et al. attributed the difference between their findings and other studies to their inclusion of more patients and their assessment of infection severity in terms of significant oxygen need rather than death, which was the outcome evaluated by studies that did not show any association between severity and outcomes.

We found a trend toward the association between previous respiratory diseases and COVID-19–related mortality. No other characteristic showed a significant association with COVID-19–related mortality in the meta-regression analysis. Our systematic review provides essential information to guide the care after ICIs during the COVID-19 era. Yet, we acknowledge that the existing data are still limited. Global, harmonized data collection is exceptionally needed to support solid guidelines. We believe that further understanding of the COVID-19- and ICI-induced lung injury will improve our management of patients during the COVID-19 era.

**Supplementary Materials:** The following supporting information can be downloaded at: https://www.mdpi.com/article/10.3390/reports5030031/s1, Figure S1: Preferred reporting items for systematic reviews and meta-analyses diagram of the included studies; Figure S2: Forest plots of the need for ventilation due to COVID-19 infection; Figure S3: Forest plot of opportunistic infections; Figure S4: Forest plot of the use of antivirals for COVID-19 infection; Figure S5: Forest plot of the use of antibiotics for COVID-19 infection; Figure S6: Forest plot of the use of steroids due to COVID-19 infection; Figure S7: Forest plot of the use of prophylactic anticoagulants due to COVID-19 infection; Figure S8: Forest plot of the use of prophylactic convalescent plasma due to COVID-19 infection; Table S1: Ovid MEDLINE search strategy; Table S2: Ovid Embase search strategy; Table S3: Web of Science search strategy; Table S4: Cochrane Library search strategy; Table S5: Overall baseline patient demographics; Table S6: Newcastle–Ottawa Scale of included studies.

**Author Contributions:** Conceptualization, M.K. and Y.G.; methodology, M.K., Y.G. and M.B.; software, M.B.; validation, M.K., Y.G., M.B., A.Q. and J.J.; formal analysis, M.B.; investigation, M.K., Y.G., M.B., A.Q. and J.J.; data curation, M.K., Y.G., M.B., A.Q. and J.J.; writing—original draft preparation, M.K., Y.G. and M.B.; writing—review and editing, M.K., Y.G., M.B., A.Q. and J.J.; visualization, M.B. and M.K.; supervision, M.K.; project administration, M.K. All authors have read and agreed to the published version of the manuscript.

**Funding:** This research received no external funding.

**Institutional Review Board Statement:** Not applicable.

**Informed Consent Statement:** Not applicable.

**Data Availability Statement:** Not applicable.

**Acknowledgments:** The authors appreciate the support from the Research Medical Library at The University of Texas MD Anderson Cancer Center, especially the great help from Sarah Bronson for editing the draft.

**Conflicts of Interest:** The authors declare no conflict of interest.

## References

1. Dai, M.; Liu, D.; Liu, M.; Zhou, F.; Li, G.; Chen, Z.; Zhang, Z.; You, H.; Wu, M.; Zheng, Q.; et al. Patients with Cancer Appear More Vulnerable to SARS-CoV-2: A Multicenter Study during the COVID-19 Outbreak. *Cancer Discov.* **2020**, *10*, 783–791. [CrossRef] [PubMed]
2. Kalisz, K.R.; Ramaiya, N.H.; Laukamp, K.R.; Gupta, A. Immune Checkpoint Inhibitor Therapy–related Pneumonitis: Patterns and Management. *RadioGraphics* **2019**, *39*, 1923–1937. [CrossRef] [PubMed]
3. Bersanelli, M. Controversies about COVID-19 and anticancer treatment with immune checkpoint inhibitors. *Immunotherapy* **2020**, *12*, 269–273. [CrossRef] [PubMed]
4. Lee, L.Y.; Cazier, J.B.; Angelis, V.; Arnold, R.; Bisht, V.; Campton, N.A.; Chackathayil, J.; Cheng, V.W.; Curley, H.M.; Fittall, M.W.; et al. COVID-19 mortality in patients with cancer on chemotherapy or other anticancer treatments: A prospective cohort study. *Lancet* **2020**, *395*, 1919–1926. [CrossRef]
5. Szabados, B.; Abu-Ghanem, Y.; Grant, M.; Choy, J.; Bex, A.; Powles, T. Clinical Characteristics and Outcome for Four SARS-CoV-2-infected Cancer Patients Treated with Immune Checkpoint Inhibitors. *Eur. Urol.* **2020**, *78*, 276–280. [CrossRef]
6. Bersanelli, M.; Scala, S.; Affanni, P.; Veronesi, L.; Colucci, M.E.; Banna, G.L.; Cortellini, A.; Liotta, F. Immunological insights on influenza infection and vaccination during immune checkpoint blockade in cancer patients. *Immunotherapy* **2020**, *12*, 105–110. [CrossRef] [PubMed]
7. Choi, J.; Lee, S.Y. Clinical Characteristics and Treatment of Immune-Related Adverse Events of Immune Checkpoint Inhibitors. *Immune Netw.* **2020**, *20*, e9. [CrossRef]
8. Wang, D.Y.; Salem, J.E.; Cohen, J.V.; Chandra, S.; Menzer, C.; Ye, F.; Zhao, S.; Das, S.; Beckermann, K.E.; Ha, L.; et al. Fatal Toxic Effects Associated with Immune Checkpoint Inhibitors: A Systematic Review and Meta-analysis. *JAMA Oncol.* **2018**, *4*, 1721–1728. [CrossRef]
9. Zhang, L.; Zhu, F.; Xie, L.; Wang, C.; Wang, J.; Chen, R.; Jia, P.; Guan, H.Q.; Peng, L.; Chen, Y.; et al. Clinical characteristics of COVID-19-infected cancer patients: A retrospective case study in three hospitals within Wuhan, China. *Ann. Oncol.* **2020**, *31*, 894–901. [CrossRef]
10. Chen, C.; Zhang, X.R.; Ju, Z.Y.; He, W.F. Advances in the research of mechanism and related immunotherapy on the cytokine storm induced by coronavirus disease 2019. *Zhonghua Shao Shang Za Zhi* **2020**, *36*, 471–475.
11. Xu, Z.; Shi, L.; Wang, Y.; Zhang, J.; Huang, L.; Zhang, C.; Liu, S.; Zhao, P.; Liu, H.; Zhu, L.; et al. Pathological findings of COVID-19 associated with acute respiratory distress syndrome. *Lancet Respir. Med.* **2020**, *8*, 420–422. [CrossRef]

12. Artigas, C.; Lemort, M.; Mestrez, F.; Gil, T.; Flamen, P. COVID-19 Pneumonia Mimicking Immunotherapy-Induced Pneumonitis on 18F-FDG PET/CT in a Patient Under Treatment with Nivolumab. *Clin. Nucl. Med.* **2020**, *45*, e381–e382. [CrossRef] [PubMed]
13. Wells, G.A.; Shea, B.; O'Connell, D.; Peterson, J.; Welch, V.; Losos, M.; Tugwell, P. The Newcastle-Ottawa Scale (NOS) for Assessing the Quality of Nonrandomised Studies in Meta-Analyses. Available online: http://www.ohri.ca/programs/clinical_epidemiology/oxford.asp (accessed on 1 March 2022).
14. Brahmer, J.R.; Lacchetti, C.; Schneider, B.J.; Atkins, M.B.; Brassil, K.J.; Caterino, J.M.; Chau, I.; Ernstoff, M.S.; Gardner, J.M.; Ginex, P.; et al. Management of Immune-Related Adverse Events in Patients Treated with Immune Checkpoint Inhibitor Therapy: American Society of Clinical Oncology Clinical Practice Guideline. *J. Clin. Oncol.* **2018**, *36*, 1714–1768. [CrossRef] [PubMed]
15. Robilotti, E.V.; Babady, N.E.; Mead, P.A.; Rolling, T.; Perez-Johnston, R.; Bernardes, M.; Bogler, Y.; Caldararo, M.; Figueroa, C.J.; Glickman, M.S.; et al. Determinants of COVID-19 disease severity in patients with cancer. *Nat. Med.* **2020**, *26*, 1218–1223. [CrossRef] [PubMed]
16. Fujita, K.; Kim, Y.H.; Kanai, O.; Yoshida, H.; Mio, T.; Hirai, T. Emerging concerns of infectious diseases in lung cancer patients receiving immune checkpoint inhibitor therapy. *Respir. Med.* **2019**, *146*, 66–70. [CrossRef] [PubMed]
17. Del Castillo, M.; Romero, F.A.; Argüello, E.; Kyi, C.; Postow, M.A.; Redelman-Sidi, G. The Spectrum of Serious Infections Among Patients Receiving Immune Checkpoint Blockade for the Treatment of Melanoma. *Clin. Infect. Dis.* **2016**, *63*, 1490–1493. [CrossRef] [PubMed]
18. Luo, J.; Rizvi, H.; Egger, J.V.; Preeshagul, I.R.; Wolchok, J.D.; Hellmann, M.D. Impact of PD-1 Blockade on Severity of COVID-19 in Patients with Lung Cancers. *Cancer Discov.* **2020**, *10*, 1121–1128. [CrossRef] [PubMed]
19. Matrajt, L.; Leung, T. Evaluating the effectiveness of social distancing interventions to delay or flatten the epidemic curve of coronavirus disease. *Emerg. Infect. Dis.* **2020**, *26*, 1740. [CrossRef]
20. Veronese, N.; Demurtas, J.; Yang, L.; Tonelli, R.; Barbagallo, M.; Lopalco, P.; Lagolio, E.; Celotto, S.; Pizzol, D.; Zou, L.; et al. Use of Corticosteroids in Coronavirus Disease 2019 Pneumonia: A Systematic Review of the Literature. *Front. Med.* **2020**, *7*, 170. [CrossRef]
21. Amin, R.; Thomas, A.S.; Khurana, S.; Panneerselvam, K.; Zou, F.; Ma, W.; Chari, S.T.; Wang, Y. Management of Immune-Related Colitis During the COVID-19 Pandemic. *Inflamm. Bowel Dis.* **2020**, *26*, e110–e111. [CrossRef]
22. Rotz, S.J.; Leino, D.; Szabo, S.; Mangino, J.L.; Turpin, B.K.; Pressey, J.G. Severe cytokine release syndrome in a patient receiving PD-1-directed therapy. *Pediatr. Blood Cancer* **2017**, *64*, e26642. [CrossRef] [PubMed]
23. Bersanelli, M.; Giannarelli, D.; Castrignanò, P.; Fornarini, G.; Panni, S.; Mazzoni, F.; Tiseo, M.; Rossetti, S.; Gambale, E.; Rossi, E.; et al. Influenza vaccine indication during therapy with immune checkpoint inhibitors: A transversal challenge. The INVIDIa Study. *Immunotherapy* **2018**, *10*, 1229–1239. [CrossRef] [PubMed]
24. Souza, I.L.; Fernandes, Í.; Taranto, P.; Buzaid, A.C.; Schvartsman, G. Immune-related pneumonitis with nivolumab and ipilimumab during the coronavirus disease 2019 (COVID-19) pandemic. *Eur. J. Cancer* **2020**, *135*, 147–149. [CrossRef] [PubMed]
25. Ding, Y.; Wang, H.; Shen, H.; Li, Z.; Geng, J.; Han, H.; Cai, J.; Li, X.; Kang, W.; Weng, D.; et al. The clinical pathology of severe acute respiratory syndrome (SARS): A report from China. *J. Pathol. A J. Pathol. Soc. Great Br. Irel.* **2003**, *200*, 282–289. [CrossRef] [PubMed]
26. Stroud, C.R.; Hegde, A.; Cherry, C.; Naqash, A.R.; Sharma, N.; Addepalli, S.; Cherukuri, S.; Parent, T.; Hardin, J.; Walker, P. Tocilizumab for the management of immune mediated adverse events secondary to PD-1 blockade. *J. Oncol. Pharm. Pract.* **2019**, *25*, 551–557. [CrossRef]
27. Horisberger, A.; La Rosa, S.; Zurcher, J.P.; Zimmermann, S.; Spertini, F.; Coukos, G.; Obeid, M. A severe case of refractory esophageal stenosis induced by nivolumab and responding to tocilizumab therapy. *J. Immunother. Cancer* **2018**, *6*, 156. [CrossRef] [PubMed]
28. Hadadi, A.; Mortezazadeh, M.; Kolahdouzan, K.; Alavian, G. Does recombinant human erythropoietin administration in critically ill COVID-19 patients have miraculous therapeutic effects? *J. Med. Virol.* **2020**, *92*, 915–918. [CrossRef]
29. Sereno, M.; Gutiérrez-Gutiérrez, G.; Sandoval, C.; Falagan, S.; Jimenez-Gordo, A.M.; Merino, M.; López-Menchaca, R.; Martínez-Martin, P.; Roa, S.; Casado, E.; et al. A favorable outcome of pneumonia COVID 19 in an advanced lung cancer patient with severe neutropenia: Is immunosuppression a risk factor for SARS-CoV2 infection? *Lung Cancer* **2020**, *145*, 213–215. [CrossRef]
30. Vivarelli, S.; Falzone, L.; Grillo, C.M.; Scandurra, G.; Torino, F.; Libra, M. Cancer Management during COVID-19 Pandemic: Is Immune Checkpoint Inhibitors-Based Immunotherapy Harmful or Beneficial? *Cancers* **2020**, *12*, 2237. [CrossRef]
31. Wu, Q.; Chu, Q.; Zhang, H.; Yang, B.; He, X.; Zhong, Y.; Yuan, X.; Chua, M.L.; Xie, C. Clinical outcomes of coronavirus disease 2019 (COVID-19) in cancer patients with prior exposure to immune checkpoint inhibitors. *Cancer Commun.* **2020**, *40*, 374–379. [CrossRef]
32. Goldstein, D.A.; Ratain, M.J.; Saltz, L.B. Weight-Based Dosing of Pembrolizumab Every 6 Weeks in the Time of COVID-19. *JAMA Oncol.* **2020**, *6*, 1694–1695. [CrossRef] [PubMed]
33. Mehta, V.; Goel, S.; Kabarriti, R.; Cole, D.; Goldfinger, M.; Acuna-Villaorduna, A.; Pradhan, K.; Thota, R.; Reissman, S.; Sparano, J.A.; et al. Case Fatality Rate of Cancer Patients with COVID-19 in a New York Hospital System. *Cancer Discov.* **2020**, *10*, 935–941. [CrossRef] [PubMed]
34. Luo, J.; Rizvi, H.; Preeshagul, I.R.; Egger, J.V.; Hoyos, D.; Bandlamudi, C.; McCarthy, C.G.; Falcon, C.J.; Schoenfeld, A.J.; Arbour, K.C.; et al. COVID-19 in patients with lung cancer. *Ann. Oncol.* **2020**, *31*, 1386–1396. [CrossRef] [PubMed]

reports

MDPI

*Article*

# COVID-19 Signs and Symptom Clusters in Long-Term Care Facility Residents: Data from the GeroCovid Observational Study

**Alba Malara [1,*], Marianna Noale [2], Angela Marie Abbatecola [3], Gilda Borselli [4], Carmine Cafariello [5], Stefano Fumagalli [6], Pietro Gareri [7], Enrico Mossello [6], Caterina Trevisan [8,9], Stefano Volpato [9], Fabio Monzani [10], Alessandra Coin [8], Giuseppe Bellelli [11], Chukwuma Okoye [10], Stefania Del Signore [12], Gianluca Zia [12], Raffaele Antonelli Incalzi [13] and on behalf of the GeroCovid LTCFs Working Group †**

1 ANASTE-Humanitas Foundation, Via dei Gracchi 137, 00192 Rome, Italy
2 Aging Branch, Neuroscience Institute, National Research Council, Via Giustiniani 2, 35128 Padua, Italy; marianna.noale@in.cnr.it
3 Alzheimer's Disease Clinic Department, Azienda Sanitaria Locale (ASL), Via Colle Melfa 75, 03042 Atina, Italy; angela_abbatecola@yahoo.com
4 Italian Society of Gerontology and Geriatrics (SIGG), Via G.C. Vanini 5, 50129 Florence, Italy; gilda.borselli@sigg.it
5 Geriatrics Outpatient Clinic and Territorial Residences, Italian Hospital Group, Via Tiburtina 188, 00012 Guidonia, Italy; ccafariello@italianhospitalgroup.com
6 Department of Experimental, Clinical Medicine, Division of Geriatric and Intensive Care Medicine, University of Florence and AOU, Largo Brambilla 3, 50134 Florence, Italy; stefano.fumagalli@unifi.it (S.F.); enrico.mossello@unifi.it (E.M.)
7 Center for Cognitive Disorders and Dementia (CDCD) Catanzaro Lido–ASP Catanzaro 214, 88100 Catanzaro Lido, Italy; pietro.gareri@me.com
8 Geriatric Division, Department of Medicine (DIMED), University of Padua, Via Giustiniani 2, 35128 Padua, Italy; caterina.trevisan.5@studenti.unipd.it (C.T.); alessandra.coin@unipd.it (A.C.)
9 Geriatric and Orthogeriatric Division, Department of Medical Science, University of Ferrara, Via Aldo Moro 2, 44124 Cona, Italy; vlt@unife.it
10 Geriatrics Unit, Department of Clinical and Experimental Medicine, University of Pisa, Via Paradisa 2, 56124 Pisa, Italy; fabio.monzani@unipi.it (F.M.); chuma@hotmail.it (C.O.)
11 Acute Geriatric Unit, School of Medicine and Surgery, University of Milano-Bicocca, San Gerardo Hospital, Via G. B. Pergolesi 33, 20900 Monza, Italy; giuseppe.bellelli@unimib.it
12 Bluecompanion Ltd., 237 Vauxhall Bridge Rd, Pimlico, London SW1V 1EJ, UK; susanna.ds@bluecompanion.eu (S.D.S.); gianluca.zia@bluecompanion.eu (G.Z.)
13 Department of Internal Medicine and Geriatrics, Campus Bio-Medico University, Via Alvaro del Portillo 200, 00128 Rome, Italy; r.antonelli@unicampus.it
* Correspondence: albamalara@gmail.com
† The GeroCovid LTCFs Working Group members list is shown in the Acknowledgements.



**Citation:** Malara, A.; Noale, M.; Abbatecola, A.M.; Borselli, G.; Cafariello, C.; Fumagalli, S.; Gareri, P.; Mossello, E.; Trevisan, C.; Volpato, S.; et al. COVID-19 Signs and Symptom Clusters in Long-Term Care Facility Residents: Data from the GeroCovid Observational Study. *Reports* **2022**, *5*, 30. https://doi.org/10.3390/reports5030030

Academic Editors: Toshio Hattori and Yugo Ashino

Received: 24 June 2022
Accepted: 18 July 2022
Published: 21 July 2022



**Abstract:** Background: Long-term care facility (LTCF) residents often present asymptomatic or paucisymptomatic features of SARS-CoV-2 infection. We aimed at investigating signs/symptoms, including their clustering on SARS-CoV-2 infection and mortality rates associated with SARS-CoV-2 infection in LTCF residents. Methods: This is a cohort study of 586 aged $\geq$ 60 year-old residents at risk of or affected with COVID-19 enrolled in the GeroCovid LTCF network. COVID-19 signs/symptom clusters were identified using cluster analysis. Cluster analyses associated with SARS-CoV-2 infection and mortality were evaluated using logistic regression and Cox proportional hazard models. Results: Cluster 1 symptoms (delirium, fever, low-grade fever, diarrhea, anorexia, cough, increased respiratory rate, sudden deterioration in health conditions, dyspnea, oxygen saturation, and weakness) affected 39.6% of residents and were associated with PCR swab positivity (OR = 7.21, 95%CI 4.78–10.80; $p < 0.001$). Cluster 1 symptoms were present in deceased COVID-19 residents. Cluster 2 (increased blood pressure, sphincter incontinence) and cluster 3 (new-onset cognitive impairment) affected 20% and 19.8% of residents, respectively. Cluster 3 symptoms were associated with increased mortality (HR = 5.41, 95%CI 1.56–18.8; $p = 0.008$), while those of Cluster 2 were not associated with mortality (HR = 0.82, 95%CI 0.26–2.56; $p = 730$). Conclusions: Our study highlights that delirium, fever, and low-grade fever, alone or in clusters should be considered in identifying and predicting the prognosis of SARS-CoV-2 infection in older LTCF patients.

**Keywords:** COVID-19; long term care facilities; gerocovid observational study; symptoms cluster

---

## 1. Introduction

Clinical presentations of coronavirus disease-19 (COVID-19) can significantly vary from asymptomatic infection to severe respiratory failure [1]. In adults, common clinical manifestations of COVID-19 include nasal secretions, cough, dyspnea, fever, myalgia, and occasionally diarrhea. Approximately 15% have developed acute respiratory distress syndrome that may last from 5 to 14 days [2]. Reflecting that COVID-19 infection symptoms particularly vary in older LTCF adults, numerous atypical manifestations including delirium, falls, muscle wasting, anorexia, and cachexia have been shown to be associated with COVID-19 infection [3]. Therefore, the need to quickly recognize COVID-19 infection in these residents in order to protect against negative prognostic outcomes as well as rapidly reduce the spread of the infection in this setting remains crucial. Indeed, older residents commonly suffer from multiple comorbidities that may mimic SARS-CoV-2 infection, thus underlining clinical difficulties related to identifying COVID-19 in this setting. Recent literature has underlined that older residents with three or more chronic diseases, such as dementia or cognitive impairment, malnutrition, or central and peripheral arterial disease have a higher risk of an infection from SARS-CoV-2 [4]. Interestingly, these authors also found that mortality was significantly higher in SARS-CoV-2-positive residents than in SARS-CoV-2-negative residents with suspicious symptoms (21.6% vs. 10.8%, respectively) [4]. At the moment, implications and clinical relevance of asymptomatic and paucisymptomatic COVID-19 residents remain unclear as well as specific treatment options and type of clinical monitoring in LTCF residents [5]. The prevalence of asymptomatic cases greatly varies, from 16% to 69.7% in populations worldwide [6].

Even though anti-SARS-CoV-2 vaccines have shown to significantly lower mortality rates, infection rates in LTCFs remain high. It also is still unclear why clinical presentations of COVID-19 infection in older patients largely vary (asymptomatic, typical clinical symptoms or atypical symptoms), thus underlining an urgent need to identify which presentations may be significantly related to negative clinical outcomes. In this study, we aimed at identifying signs or symptoms, as well as the clustering of signs/symptoms, associated with a SARS-CoV-2 infection and evaluate the related risk on negative outcomes including mortality.

## 2. Materials and Methods

GeroCovid LTCFs is a part of the GeroCovid Observational Study, a multi-center and multi-setting study evaluating the impact of the COVID-19 pandemic on the health outcomes of older patients in numerous clinical settings of acute and long-term care [7,8].

### 2.1. Participants

The GeroCovid LTCF cohort included 39 sites from 6 Italian regions (n = 2380). For this study analysis, we included nine study sites that reported positive COVID-19 cases from 1 March 2020 to 31 December 2020. For study purposes, we included 586 residents aged $\geq$ 60 years with suspicious signs or symptoms or who were considered at a high risk of a COVID-19 infection.

Onset symptoms included: (i) "typical" (cough, nasal congestion, hoarseness, sore throat, wheezing, sneezing, loss of sense of smell or taste, or high temperature); (ii) "atypical" (diarrhea, vomiting, anorexia, delirium, weakness). High-risk contacts were defined as residents who had direct physical contact with a COVID-19 confirmed case or were in a closed environment with a COVID-19 confirmed case in the absence of suitable personal protective equipment. Furthermore, all new residents admitted to the LTCF or readmitted after a period of hospitalization were considered at risk of infection. Residents with suspicious signs and/or symptoms or at risk of COVID-19 infection were isolated and tested for SARS-CoV-2 positivity using PCR–RNA testing. According to swab results, residents were then categorized as positive or negative for SARS-CoV-2 infection [4].

Mobility assessments over the last month were determined using data from the Frailty Anamnestic Criteria [9]. Low-grade fever was defined as a body temperature ranging from 37 °C to 37.5 °C, while high-grade fever was defined as a body temperature higher than 37.5 °C.

### 2.2. Measures and Data Collection

Data on sociodemographic variables, comorbidities, polypharmacy, mobility, symptoms, SARS-CoV-2 swab testing, and outcome (clinical course, transfer to a different setting, death) were collected.

The Campus Bio-Medico University Ethical Committee approved the overarching protocol of the GeroCovid Observational study on 3 April 2020 (Trial Registration: NCT04379440). All participating investigational sites gained approval from their local Ethical Committee review board. Informed consent was aquired and the data were collected using a national de-identified electronic registry provided by BlueCompanion.

### 2.3. Statistical Analysis

The clinical characteristics of the study participants are reported as means ± standard deviation (SD) or median [25–75th percentile] for quantitative measures and as counts or percentages for categorical variables. The normality of the distributions was evaluated using the Shapiro–Wilk test. Clinical characteristics were summarized and compared among groups (positive vs negative SARS-CoV-2 swab) using the chi-squared or Fisher's exact tests for the categorical variables and the generalized linear model or the Wilcoxon rank-sum test for the quantitative ones. A multivariable logistic regression model adjusted for age, sex, and comorbidity (defined as having three or more comorbidities, according to the median of the sample distribution) evaluated the correlation of having a positive swab with reported signs and symptoms. A stepwise analysis on symptoms was performed with a *p*-value of 0.15 to entry and a *p*-value 0.20 to be retained in the model. Tjur $R^2$ was calculated to evaluate the predictive power of the model [10]. The results are presented as adjusted odds ratios (OR) and 95% confidence intervals (95%CI).

The presence of clusters among COVID-19 symptoms was evaluated using a hierarchical cluster analysis (McQuitty method) as a similarity measure of the proportion of observations when two symptoms were simultaneously present. A dendrogram (a tree-like diagram that illustrates the relationships between symptoms according to the measure of similarity chosen) obtained from cluster analysis was evaluated. The horizontal axis represents the similarity between clusters, while the vertical axis represents the considered symptoms, and each joining of two clusters is represented by the splitting of a horizontal line into two horizontal lines. This analysis started with individual symptoms, and clusters of the most similar symptoms were progressively formed, joining symptoms and clusters until all symptoms were joined into a single large cluster. The association between each cluster and a positive SARS-CoV-2 swab was evaluated using logistic regression models adjusted for age and sex.

Cox proportional hazard models were performed to determine probability risk of short-term mortality, and independent covariates regarding age, sex, number of comorbidities, and COVID-19 positivity were included in models. Additional Cox models with symptom clusters as independent variables adjusted for age, sex, and number of comorbidities were also performed. The results are presented as adjusted hazard ratios (HR) and 95% confidence intervals (95%CI).

All statistical tests were two-tailed, and statistical significance was assumed for *p*-value $< 0.05$. The analyses were performed using SAS, V.9.4 (SAS Institute, Cary, NC, USA).

## 3. Results

The study included 586 residents (mean age 84.8 ± 8.5 years, range 60–100 years, 72.9% women) based on the presence of suspicious signs and/or symptoms of a SARS-CoV-2 infection and those at a high risk of a SARS-CoV-2 infection. SARS-CoV-2 RNA testing using RT-PCR was performed in 583 residents and identified 209 positive SARS-CoV-2 residents. As reported in Table 1, the use of polypharmacy (median number of seven drugs) and having three or more comorbidities were significantly higher in those with a SARS-CoV-2 infection compared with those without infection. Furthermore, mobility worsening in the last month was significantly higher in those with SARS-CoV-2 infection compared with those without (72% vs. 28%) ($p < 0.001$).

**Table 1.** Characteristics of older adults from the GeroCovid LTCFs study: overall population and by SARS-CoV-2 positive or negative swab results.

| | All (n = 586) | SARS-CoV-2 + (n = 209) | SARS-CoV-2 − (n = 374) | *p*-Value |
|---|---|---|---|---|
| Age, year, mean ± SD | 84.8 ± 8.5 | 85.5 ± 8.1 | 84.4 ± 8.6 | 0.19 |
| Sex, female, n (%) | 427 (72.9) | 152 (72.7) | 273 (73.0) | 0.94 |
| Smoking status, n (%) | | | | |
| Current smoker | 11 (3.8) | 1 (1.1) | 9 (4.6) | 0.08 |
| Ex-smoker | 46 (15.8) | 20 (21.3) | 26 (13.3) | |
| Non smoker | 234 (80.4) | 73 (77.7) | 160 (82.0) | |
| Number of drugs, median (Q1, Q3) | 5 (4, 7) | 7 (5, 10) | 5 (3, 7) | <0.001 |
| Total number of chronic diseases, median (Q1, Q3) (available for n = 594) | 3 (2, 5) | 3 (2, 4) | 2 (1, 4) | 0.002 |
| Chronic diseases, n (%) | | | | |
| 0, 1, 2 | 224 (38.2) | 57 (27.3) | 167 (44.7) | <0.001 |
| 3+ | 365 (61.8) | 152 (72.7) | 207 (55.3) | |
| Worsening of mobility in the last month, n (%) (available for n = 271 residents) | 116 (42.8) | 67 (72.0) | 49 (27.5) | <0.001 |

Abbreviations: SD, Standard Deviation; Q1, Quartile 1; Q3, Quartile 3.

An amount of 503 residents had full data regarding any signs and/or symptoms of infection. Of these, approximately 30% of SARS-CoV-2-positive residents did not report any symptoms, while over 70% reported at least one symptom (Table 2). The most common symptom in older residents with a SARS-CoV-2 infection was delirium (41.2%), followed by high-grade fever (39.1%), low-grade fever (36.2%), sudden worsening of health status (35%), weakness (32.1%), low oxygen saturation at rest ($SpO_2 < 90\%$) (29.6%), anorexia (27.0%), dyspnea (26.1%), diarrhea (21.6%), and diuresis contraction (14.2%) (Table 2). According to logistic regression analyses, clinical features associated with RT-PCR positivity were delirium (OR = 9.9; 95%CI: 3.5–27.5; $p < 0.001$), high-grade fever (OR = 7.0; 95%CI: 3.1–16.1; $p < 0.001$), low-grade fever (OR = 4.3; 95%CI: 1.5–12.2; $p = 0.006$), and having three or more comorbidities (OR = 2.0; 95%CI: 1.0–3.7; $p = 0.038$) (Figure 1). The prevalence of delirium as the onset symptom of a SARS-CoV-2 infection was significantly higher in residents with dementia compared with those without dementia (27.1% and 10.5%, respectively; $p = 0.001$).

**Table 2.** Symptoms of older adults from the GeroCovid LTCFs study, according to SARS-CoV-2 infection status.

| | SARS-CoV-2 + (n = 179) | SARS-CoV-2 − (n = 324) | *p*-Value |
|---|---|---|---|
| No symptoms, n (%) | 53 (29.6) | 203 (62.7) | <0.001 |
| At least one symptom, n (%) | 126 (70.4) | 121 (37.3) | <0.001 |
| Fever, n (%) | 70 (39.1) | 21 (6.5) | <0.001 |
| Low-grade fever, n (%) | 64 (36.2) | 8 (2.5) | <0.001 |
| Pharyngodynia, n (%) | 1 (1.3) | 3 (1.0) | 1.000 |
| Cough, n (%) | 21 (12.4) | 16 (5.0) | 0.003 |
| Sneezing, n (%) | 4 (2.3) | 6 (1.9) | 0.72 |
| Dyspnoea, n (%) | 46 (26.1) | 18 (5.7) | <0.001 |
| Low oxygen saturation after walking, n (%) | 2 (2.0) | 6 (2.1) | 1.000 |
| Low oxygen saturation at rest (<90%), n (%) | 37 (29.6) | 15 (4.9) | <0.001 |
| S 02 %, mean±SD | 95 (93, 96) | 97 (96, 98) | <0.001 |
| Weakness/Prostration, n (%) | 52 (32.1) | 41 (12.7) | <0.001 |
| Fall or fainted, n (%) | 1 (0.9) | 7 (2.3) | 0.69 |
| Muscles aching, n (%) | 10 (6.6) | 13 (4.1) | 0.24 |
| Delirium, n (%) | 49 (41.2) | 7 (2.3) | <0.001 |
| Conjunctivitis, n (%) | 3 (1.8) | 5 (1.6) | 1.000 |
| Loss of smell (if new), n (%) | 0 (0.0) | 0 (0.0) | - |
| Loss of taste, n (%) | 3 (2.2) | 2 (0.6) | 0.17 |
| Anorexia, n (%) | 30 (27.0) | 20 (6.6) | <0.001 |
| Nausea/vomiting, n (%) | 12 (7.2) | 4 (1.3) | 0.004 |
| Diarrhea, n (%) | 36 (21.6) | 12 (3.8) | <0.001 |
| Raynaud syndrome, n (%) | 4 (3.5) | 0 (0.0) | 0.005 |
| Cutaneous symptoms, n (%) | 6 (5.1) | 2 (0.7) | 0.007 |
| Sudden worsening of health status, n (%) | 43 (35.0) | 5 (1.6) | <0.001 |
| Aphasia/dysnomia, n (%) | 1 (1.0) | 6 (2.0) | 0.68 |
| Cognitive Impairment, n (%) | 27 (30.0) | 49 (16.3) | 0.004 |
| Diuresis contraction, n (%) | 17 (14.2) | 5 (1.6) | <0.001 |
| Urines of faeces incontinence, n (%) | 5 (4.5) | 47 (15.9) | 0.002 |
| Unable to ask questions, n (%) | 3 (4.4) | 24 (9.2) | 0.21 |
| Unable to fill a self-evaluation questionnaire, n (%) | 7 (10.6) | 35 (13.6) | 0.52 |
| Number of symptoms, median (Q1, Q3) | 2 (0, 6) | 0 (0, 2) | <0.001 |
| Number of symptoms, n (%) | | | |
| 0 | 53 (29.6) | 203 (62.7) | <0.001 |
| 1 | 25 (14.0) | 36 (11.1) | |
| 2+ | 101 (56.4) | 85 (26.2) | |

Abbreviations: Q1, Quartile 1; Q3, Quartile 3.

Cluster analysis identified three symptom clusters (Figure 2): Cluster 1, which included delirium, fever, low-grade fever, diarrhea, anorexia, cough, increased respiratory frequency, dyspnea, low oxygen saturation at rest, and weakness/prostration, was present in 39.6% of the residents; Cluster 2 included recent-onset incontinence, increased blood pressure, and the inability to fill a self-evaluation questionnaire and was present in 20% of the residents; Cluster 3 was defined by new-onset cognitive impairment and included 19.8% of residents. The percentage of residents for each cluster and the association with a positive or negative SARS-CoV-2 swab test are reported in Figure 3. Only Cluster 1 and Cluster 3 symptoms were significantly associated with an increased probability of having a positive PCR swab test (OR = 7.21, 95%CI: 4.8–10.8, $p < 0.001$; OR = 2.05, 95%CI: 1.18–3.56, $p = 0.01$, respectively), while symptoms in Cluster 2 did not correlate with a positive PCR test (OR = 0.75, 95%CI: 0.44–1.29, $p = 0.295$).

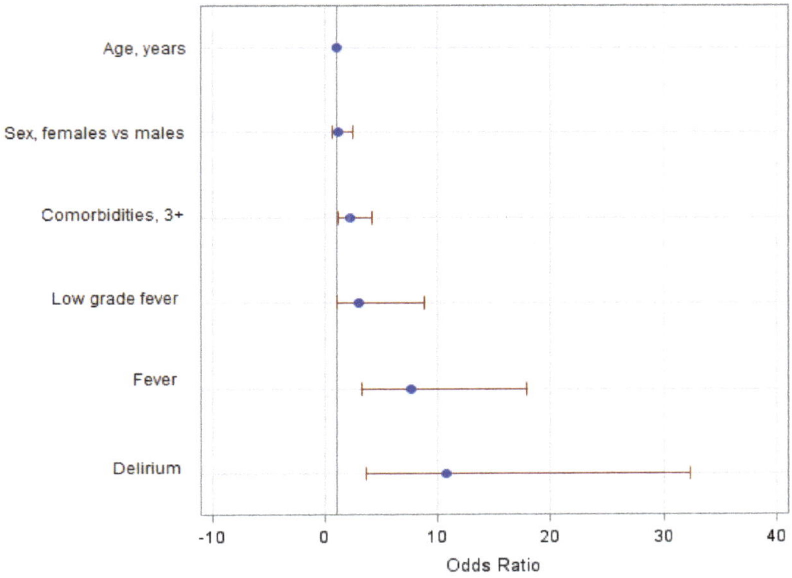


**Figure 1.** The associations between clinical features and SARS-CoV-2 infection (according to PCR swab testing). Logistic regression model using stepwise analysis (sle = 0.15; sls = 0.20), adjusted for age, sex, and comorbidity (defined as having 3+ chronic diseases). Symptoms reported by at least 5% of study participants (including fever, low-grade fever, cough, dyspnea, low oxygen saturation at rest, weakness/prostration, delirium, anorexia, diarrhea, sudden worsening of health status, diuresis contraction, urine or feces incontinence, inability to ask questions, inability to fill a self-evaluation questionnaire) were considered possible independent variables.

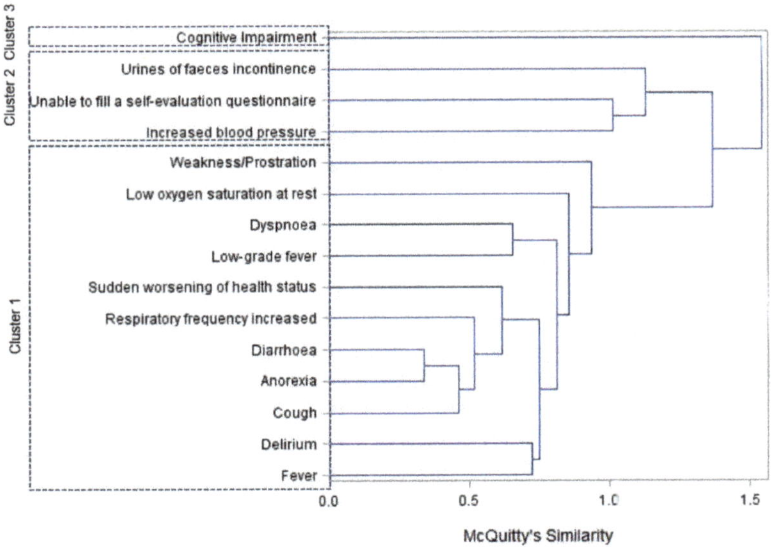


**Figure 2.** The dendrogram of symptom clusters (n = 503 participants independent of swab results; McQuitty method; only symptoms reported for 5% or more of the study participants were included).

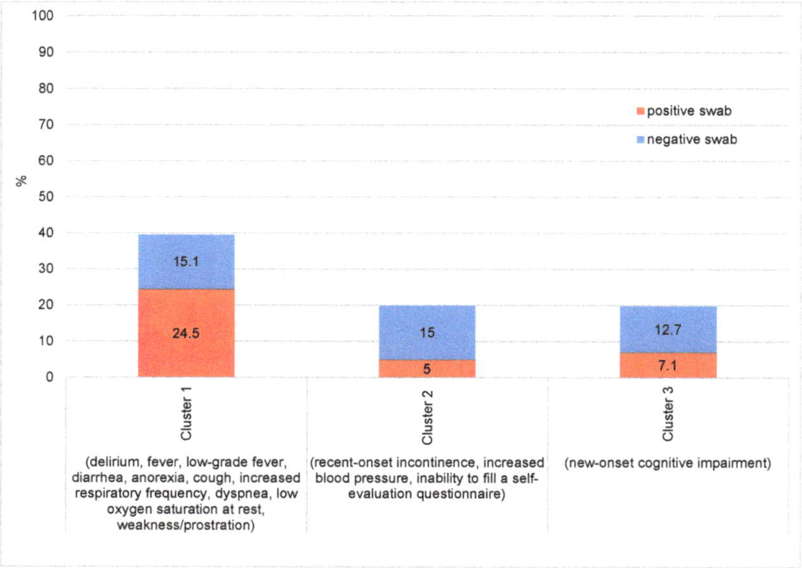


**Figure 3.** Participants (%) in each cluster and SARS-CoV-2 swab test results.

Residents were observed for a median time of 61 days, and those with positive swab test had a median duration of RT-PCR positivity for 20 days. At the end of the observation period, 71.4% of SARS-CoV-2-positive residents who had only one symptom and 47% of those with two or more symptoms showed clinical improvement. No statistical differences were found between SARS-CoV-2 positive and negative residents according to outcomes in all-cause hospitalizations and transfers to different care settings (8% vs 2% respectively; $p$ = 0.115). Mortality probability rates were 19.6% and 9.6% in SARS-CoV-2 positive and negative residents, respectively. Cox regression analysis adjusted for sex and age showed that SARS-CoV-2 positivity (HR = 2.6, 95%CI: 1.8–4.6, $p < 0.001$) and the number of comorbidities (HR = 1.3, 95%CI: 1.1–1.3, $p < 0.001$) were significantly associated with a higher risk of mortality. In additional Cox regression analyses including symptom clusters, we found that Cluster 2 was not related to mortality (HR = 0.82, 95%CI: 0.26–2.56, $p$ = 0.730), while Cluster 3 was significantly associated with an increased mortality rate (HR = 5.41, 95%CI: 1.56–18.8, $p$ = 0.008). All deceased SARS-CoV-2 positive residents had symptoms found in Cluster 1.

## 4. Discussion

Our findings confirm recent reports underlining that the clinical presentation of SARS-CoV-2 infection in older residents differs from those in young and adult individuals [11–13]. Interestingly, we found that older residents often presented atypical and nonspecific symptoms, such as delirium, low-grade fever, and anorexia and were less likely to have dyspnea, ageusia, and anosmia. Indeed, the high prevalence of asymptomatic cases complicates infection identification, control, and the containment of new SARS-CoV-2 infections in LTCFs. Standardized assessments of single or multiple atypical signs and/or symptoms should quickly prompt COVID-19 testing in older LTCF residents. Although high- and low-grade fevers were common findings in our study, fever was not invariably present among residents with a SARS-CoV-2 infection. High-grade fever added specificity compared with low-grade fever for COVID-19 screening in our sample (high-grade fever in 39.1% of residents vs. low-grade fever in 36.2%). According to a previous observation [14], most residents had body temperature elevations when infected with SARS-CoV-2, but rarely over 38.0 °C. Indeed, low-grade fever should be suspicious of an infection due to COVID-19 in older LTCF residents.

Delirium was the most prevalent onset symptom for a SARS-CoV-2 infection. Our finding parallels those of previous studies underlining that environmental and iatrogenic factors such as immobility, social distancing, use of sedative drugs, and quarantine increased the risk of delirium in older people in acute care [15] and in home-dwelling adults with dementia [16]. A literature analysis reported that mechanisms related to hypoxia, inflammation, and hypercoagulability in cerebrovascular events could explain the correlation between SARS-CoV-2 infection and neurological manifestations [17,18]. Along with delirium, anorexia was another prevalent symptom in our cohort and confirmed to be an important indicator of acute illness, including SARS-CoV-2 infection, in nursing home residents [19]. Interestingly, we found that hypoactive delirium in association with low- or high-grade fever, anorexia, and diarrhea was highly predictive of a SARS-CoV-2 infection. Deceased residents with a SARS-CoV-2 infection experienced more symptoms found in Cluster 1 compared with survivors. Moreover, multimorbidity ($\geq$3 conditions) and dementia were significantly associated with SARS-CoV-2 positivity and mortality among residents. We also found that mortality not related to SARS-CoV-2 was significantly higher in residents with a negative RT-PCR test who presented with symptoms suspicious of infection [4]. Similarly, the probability of death was significantly increased in those with new-onset cognitive impairment. This finding suggests a potential role for the use of using standardized screening tools to measure cognitive impairment and delirium in SARS-CoV-2-infected LTCF residents. Future prospective studies are needed to provide important knowledge to this topic.

An additional finding from our study lies in the remarkable number of asymptomatic or paucisymptomatic residents who remained positive for several weeks. At the time of analysis, infected residents underwent prolonged periods of social isolation with negative consequences for psychological and functional status. At the moment, the European Centre for Disease Prevention and Control recommends that isolation can be lifted if one of the following applies: fever no longer present for at least 3 days, symptoms other than fever improved 20 days after the onset of symptoms, or 2 consecutive negative SARS-CoV-2 RT-PCR tests obtained in a 24-h interval from respiratory specimens [20,21]. Although the disease prognosis remains difficult to predict, most residents with a SARS-CoV-2 infection can be treated directly in LTCFs. Expertise in geriatric medicine along with appropriate staff and resources (including PPE and testing capacity) and health care policy support should be implemented in order to manage LTFS populations [22].

LTCFs in Italy have shown progressive reductions in severe SARS-CoV-2 cases, isolations, hospitalizations, and deaths since February 2021, which may be explained by the large implementation of anti-SARS-CoV-2 vaccinations [23]. Despite these encouraging results, outbreaks of COVID-19 among older vaccinated adults continue both in Italy and worldwide. Therefore, knowledge of symptoms and cluster-onset symptoms may assist in early identifying a SARS-CoV-2 infection, especially in older LTCF residents [24].

Due to the observational nature of our study, we cannot identify any cause–effect relationships between SARS-CoV-2 infection and mortality. However, our study provides an important basis for future prospective studies on specific clusters related to higher mortality rates. This research was conducted in LTCF settings, and thus, our findings may not be applicable in all types of care settings. An important strength of our study was the use of an electronic registry dedicated to precise clinical data collection in multiple settings of older persons during the first pandemic wave.

## 5. Conclusions

LTCF residents commonly present an asymptomatic or paucisymptomatic form of SARS-CoV-2 infection. In symptomatic patients, we found that key SARS-CoV-2 infection symptoms included delirium and fever (including low-grade fever), alone or in clusters. Therefore, these symptoms should be considered in early identifying and potentially predicting the prognosis of SARS-CoV-2 infection in LTCF residents. Due to the highly contagious risk of SARS-CoV-2 spread in LTCFs, early recognition of an atypical COVID-19 presentation is pivotal.

**Author Contributions:** Study concept and design: A.M., R.A.I. and S.D.S.; Methodology: A.M., R.A.I., C.T. and S.D.S.; Software: S.D.S. and G.Z.; Investigation and Data Curation: GeroCovid LTCFs Working Group and G.B. (Gilda Borselli); Analysis and interpretation of data: A.M., M.N., A.M.A., C.T. and R.A.I.; Writing-Original Draft Preparation: A.M., R.A.I., M.N., A.M.A. and C.T.; Writing-Review & Editing, Visualization and Supervision: R.A.I., A.M., M.N., P.G., A.M.A. and G.B. (Gilda Borselli), C.C., S.F., E.M., C.T., S.V., A.C. and G.B. (Giuseppe Bellelli), F.M., C.O., S.D.S. and G.Z.; Project Administration: R.A.I. All authors have read and agreed to the published version of the manuscript.

**Funding:** This research received no external funding.

**Institutional Review Board Statement:** The study was conducted in accordance with the Declaration of Helsinki, and approved by the Ethics Committee of Campus Bio-Medico University Ethical Committee (protocol code: 22/20 OSS; date of approval: 3 April 2020).

**Informed Consent Statement:** Informed consent was obtained from all subjects involved in the study.

**Data Availability Statement:** Data are available on the Blue Companion national de-identified clinical data electronic registry.

**Acknowledgments:** The **GeroCovid LTCFs Group** members are as follows (in alphabetical order). Angela Marie Abbatecola, (*RSA INI Città Bianca, Veroli (FR)*), Domenico Andrieri, (*RSA Villa Santo Stefano, S. Stefano di Rogliano (CS)*), Rachele Antognoli, (*RSA Villa Isabella, Pisa*), Paola Bianchi, (*Associazione Nazionale Strutture Territoriali e per la Terza Età, Roma*), Carmine Cafariello, (*RSA Villa Sacra Famiglia, IHG, Roma; I RSA Geriatria, IHG, Guidonia (RM); III RSA Geriatria, IHG, Guidonia (RM); RSA Estensiva, IHG, Guidonia (RM); RSA Intensiva, IHG, Guidonia (RM)*), Valeria Calsolaro, (*RSA Villa Isabella, Pisa*), Francesco Antonio Campagna, (*Centro di Riabilitazione San Domenico, Lamezia Terme (CZ)*), Sebastiano Capurso, (*RSA Bellosguardo, Civitavecchia (RM)*), Silvia Carino, (*RSA San Domenico, Lamezia Terme (CZ); Centro di Riabilitazione San Domenico, Lamezia Terme (CZ); RSA Villa Elisabetta, Cortale (CZ); Casa Protetta Madonna del Rosario, Lamezia Terme (CZ)*), Manuela Castelli, (*ASP Golgi Redaelli, Istituto Geriatrico Camillo Golgi, Abbiategrasso (MI)*), Arcangelo Ceretti, (*ASP Golgi Redaelli, Istituto Geriatrico Camillo Golgi, Abbiategrasso (MI)*), Mauro Colombo, (*ASP Golgi Redaelli, Istituto Geriatrico Camillo Golgi, Abbiategrasso (MI)*), Antonella Crispino, (*RSA Villa Santo Stefano, S. Stefano di Rogliano (CS); RSA Villa Silvia, Altilia Grimaldi (CS)*), Roberta Cucunato, (*RSA Villa Santo Stefano, S. Stefano di Rogliano (CS); RSA Villa Silvia, Altilia Grimaldi (CS)*), Ferdinando D'Amico, (*RSA San Giovanni di Dio, Patti (ME); RSA Sant'Angelo di Brolo (ME)*), Annalaura Dell'Armi, (*III RSA Geriatria, IHG, Guidonia (RM)*), Christian Ferro, (*RSA Sant'Angelo di Brolo (ME)*), Serafina Fiorillo, (*RSA Madonna delle Grazie, Filadelfia (VV); Casa di Riposo Mons. Francesco Luzzi, Acquaro (VV); Casa di Riposo Villa Betania, Mileto (VV); Casa di Riposo Pietro Rosano, Dasà (VV); Casa di Riposo Serena Diocesi, Mileto (VV); Alloggio per Anziani Villa Amedeo, Francavilla Angitola (VV); Casa Albergo Villa Fabiola, Monterosso Calabro (VV); Casa di Riposo Villa Sara, San Nicola da Crissa (VV); Casa di Riposo Don Mottola, Tropea (VV); Casa di Riposo San Francesco, Soriano Calabro (VV); RSA Anziani, Soriano Calabro (VV); Casa di Riposo Suore Missionarie del Catechismo, Pizzo (VV)*), Pier Paolo Gasbarri, (*Associazione Nazionale Strutture Territoriali e per la Terza Età, Roma*), Roberta Granata, (*RSA Villa Sacra Famiglia, IHG, Roma*), Nadia Grillo, (*RSA San Domenico, Lamezia Terme (CZ); Casa di Riposo San Domenico, Lamezia Terme (CZ); RSA Villa Elisabetta, Cortale (CZ)*), Antonio Guaita, (*ASP Golgi Redaelli, Istituto Geriatrico Camillo Golgi, Abbiategrasso (MI)*), Marilena Iarrera, (*RSA Sant'Angelo di Brolo (ME)*), Valerio Alex Ippolito, (*Casa Protetta Villa Azzurra, Roseto Capo Spulico (CS)*), Alba Malara, (*RSA San Domenico, Lamezia Terme (CZ); Casa di Riposo Villa Marinella, Amantea (CS); Casa Protetta Madonna del Rosario, Lamezia Terme (CZ); Casa Protetta Villa Azzurra, Roseto Capo Spulico (CS); Centro di Riabilitazione San Domenico, Lamezia Terme (CZ); RSA Casa Amica, Fossato Serralta (CZ); RSA La Quiete, Castiglione Cosetino (CS); RSA San Domenico, Lamezia Terme (CZ); RSA Villa Elisabetta, Cortale (CZ); RSA Villa Santo Stefano, S. Stefano di Rogliano (CS); RSA Villa Silvia, Altilia Grimaldi (CS)*), Irene Mancuso, (*RSA San Giovanni di Dio, Patti (ME)*), Eleonora Marelli, (*ASP Golgi Redaelli, Istituto Geriatrico Camillo Golgi, Abbiategrasso (MI)*), Paolo Moneti, (*RSA Villa Gisella, Firenze*), Fabio Monzani, (*RSA Villa Isabella, Pisa*), Marianna Noale, (*RSA AltaVita, Istituzioni Riunite di Assistenza, Padova*), Mariasara Osso, (*RSA La Quiete, Castiglione Cosentino (CS)*), Agostino Perri, (*RSA*

*La Quiete, Castiglione Cosentino (CS)*), Maria Perticone, (*Casa di Riposo Villa Marinella, Amantea (CS)*), Francesco Raffaele Addamo, (*RSA San Giovanni di Dio, Patti (ME)*), Giovanni Sgrò, (*RSA Istituto Santa Maria del Soccorso, Serrastretta (CZ); RSA San Vito Hospital, San Vito sullo Jonio (CZ); Casa Protetta Villa Mariolina, Montauro (CZ); Casa Protetta Villa Sant'Elia, Marcellinara (CZ)*), Federica Sirianni, (*Casa di Riposo Villa Marinella, Amantea (CS)*), Deborah Spaccaferro, (*RSA Estensiva, IHG, Guidonia (RM); RSA Intensiva, IHG, Guidonia (RM)*), Fausto Spadea, (*RSA Casa Amica, Fossato Serralta (CZ)*), Rita Ursino, (*I RSA Geriatria, IHG, Guidonia (RM)*).

**Conflicts of Interest:** The authors have no conflict of interest to declare.

## References


1. He, F.; Deng, Y.; Li, W. Coronavirus disease 2019: What we know? *J. Med. Virol.* **2020**, *92*, 719–725. [CrossRef] [PubMed]
2. Morley, J.E.; Vellas, B. COVID-19 and older adults. *J. Nutr. Health Aging* **2020**, *24*, 364–365. [CrossRef] [PubMed]
3. Morley, J.E. 2020: The Year of The COVID-19 Pandemic. *J. Nutr. Health Aging* **2021**, *25*, 1–4. [CrossRef] [PubMed]
4. Malara, A.; Noale, M.; Abbatecola, A.M.; Borselli, G.; Cafariello, C.; Fumagalli, S.; Gareri, P.; Mossello, E.; Trevisan, C.; Volpato, S.; et al. Clinical Features of SARS-CoV-2 Infection in Italian Long-Term Care Facilities: GeroCovid LTCFs Observational Study. *J. Am. Med. Dir. Assoc.* **2022**, *23*, 15–18. [CrossRef]
5. Tang, O.; Bigelow, B.F.; Sheikh, F.; Peters, M.; Zenilman, J.M.; Bennett, R.; Katz, M.J. Outcomes of Nursing Home COVID-19 Patients by Initial Symptoms and Comorbidity: Results of Universal Testing of 1970 Residents. *J. Am. Med. Dir. Assoc.* **2020**, *21*, 1767–1773. [CrossRef]
6. Arons, M.M.; Hatfield, K.M.; Reddy, S.C.; Kimball, A.; James, A.; Jacobs, J.R.; Taylor, J.; Spicer, K.; Bardossy, A.C.; Oakley, L.P.; et al. Presymptomatic SARS-CoV-2 infections and transmission in a skilled nursing facility. *N. Engl. J. Med.* **2020**, *382*, 2081–2090. [CrossRef]
7. Trevisan, C.; Del Signore, S.; Fumagalli, S.; Gareri, P.; Malara, A.; Mossello, E.; Volpato, S.; Monzani, F.; Coin, A.; Bellelli, G.; et al. Assessing the impact of COVID-19 on the health of geriatric patients: The European GeroCovid Observational Study. *Eur. J. Intern Med.* **2021**, *87*, 29–35. [CrossRef]
8. Abbatecola, A.M.; Incalzi, R.A.; Malara, A.; Palmieri, A.; Di Lonardo, A.; Borselli, G.; Russo, M.; Noale, M.; Fumagalli, S.; Gareri, P.; et al. Disentangling the impact of COVID-19 infection on clinical outcomes and preventive strategies in older persons: An Ital. *Perspective. J. Gerontol. Geriatr.* **2021**, *70*, 1–11. [CrossRef]
9. Pedone, C.; Costanzo, L.; Cesari, M.; Bandinelli, S.; Ferrucci, L.; Incalzi, R.A. Are Performance Measures Necessary to Predict Loss of Independence in Elderly People? *J. Gerontol. Ser. A* **2016**, *71*, 84–89. [CrossRef]
10. Tjur, T. Coefficients of determination in logistic regression models—A new proposal: The Coefficient of Discrimination. *Am. Stat.* **2009**, *63*, 366–372. [CrossRef]
11. Bavaro, D.F.; Diella, L.; Fabrizio, C.; Sulpasso, R.; Bottalico, I.; Calamo, A.; Santoro, C.; Brindicci, G.; Bruno, G.; Mastroianni, A.; et al. Peculiar clinical presentation of COVID-19 and predictors of mortality in the elderly: A multicentre retrospective cohort study. *Int. J. Infect Dis.* **2021**, *105*, 709–715. [CrossRef] [PubMed]
12. Carnahan, J.L.; Lieb, K.M.; Albert, L.; Wagle, K.; Kaehr, E.; Unroe, K.T. COVID-19 disease trajectories among nursing home residents. *J. Am. Geriatr. Soc.* **2021**, *69*, 2412–2418. [CrossRef] [PubMed]
13. Ouslander, J.G.; Grabowski, D.C. COVID-19 in Nursing Homes: Calming the Perfect Storm. *J. Am. Geriatr. Soc.* **2020**, *68*, 2153–2162. [CrossRef] [PubMed]
14. Rudolph, J.L.; Halladay, C.W.; Barber, M.; McConeghy, K.W.; Mor, V.; Nanda, A.; Gravenstein, S. Temperature in Nursing Home Residents Systematically Tested for SARS-CoV-2. *J. Am. Med. Dir. Assoc.* **2020**, *21*, 895–899. [CrossRef]
15. Kotfis, K.; Roberson, S.W.; Wilson, J.E.; Dabrowski, W.; Pun, B.T.; Ely, E.W. COVID-19: ICU delirium management during SARS-CoV-2 pandemic. *Crit Care* **2020**, *24*, 176. [CrossRef]
16. Gareri, P.; Fumagalli, S.; Malara, A.; Mossello, E.; Trevisan, C.; Volpato, S.; Coin, A.; Calsolaro, V.; Bellelli, G.; Del Signore, S.; et al. Management of Older Outpatients During The COVID-19 Pandemic: The Gerocovid Ambulatory Study. *Gerontology* **2021**, *28*, 1–6. [CrossRef]
17. Padda, I.; Khehra, N.; Jaferi, U.; Parmar, M.S. The Neurological Complexities and Prognosis of COVID-19. *SN Compr. Clin. Med.* **2020**, *2*, 2025–2036. [CrossRef]
18. Spuntarelli, V.; Luciani, M.; Bentivegna, E.; Marini, V.; Falangone, F.; Conforti, G.; Rachele, E.S.; Martelletti, P. COVID-19: Is it just a lung disease? A case-based review. *SN Compr. Clin. Med.* **2020**, *2*, 1401–1406. [CrossRef]
19. Bianchetti, A.; Rozzini, R.; Guerini, F.; Boffelli, S.; Ranieri, P.; Minelli, G.; Bianchetti, L.; Trabucchi, M. Clinical Presentation of COVID19 in Dementia Patients. *J. Nutr. Health Aging* **2020**, *24*, 560–562. [CrossRef]
20. Cento, V.; Colagrossi, L.; Nava, A.; Lamberti, A.; Senatore, S.; Travi, G.; Rossotti, R.; Vecchi, M.; Casati, O.; Matarazzo, E.; et al. Persistent positivity and fluctuations of SARS-CoV-2 RNA in clinically-recovered COVID-19 patients. *J. Infect.* **2020**, *81*, e90–e92. [CrossRef]
21. European Centre for Disease Prevention and Control. *Guidance for Discharge and Ending Isolation of People with COVID-19, 16 October 2020*; ECDC: Stockholm, Sweden, 2020.

22. Benvenuti, E.; Rivasi, G.; Bulgaresi, M.; Barucci, R.; Lorini, C.; Balzi, D.; Faraone, A.; Fortini, G.; Vaccaro, G.; Del Lungo, I.; et al. Caring for nursing home residents with COVID-19: A "hospital-at-nursing home" intermediate care intervention. *Aging Clin. Exp. Res.* **2020**, *33*, 2917–2924. [CrossRef] [PubMed]
23. Ministero della Salute. Vaccinazione Anti SARS-CoV-2 Piano Strategico. Elementi di Preparazione e Implementazione della Strategia Vaccinale. Available online: https://www.trovanorme.salute.gov.it/norme/renderPdf.spring?seriegu=SG&datagu=24/03/2021&redaz=21A01802&artp=1&art=1&subart=1&subart1=10&vers=1&prog=001 (accessed on 13 June 2022).
24. Faggiano, F.; Rossi, M.A.; Cena, T.; Milano, F.; Barale, A.; Ristagno, Q.; Silano, V. An Outbreak of COVID-19 among mRNA-Vaccinated Nursing Home Residents. *Vaccines* **2021**, *9*, 859. [CrossRef] [PubMed]

*reports*

MDPI

*Article*

# Strategies Addressing the Challenges of the COVID-19 Pandemic in Long-Term, Palliative and Hospice Care: A Qualitative Study on the Perspectives of Patients' Family Members

**Latife Pacolli, Diana Wahidie, Ilknur Özger Erdogdu, Yüce Yilmaz-Aslan and Patrick Brzoska ***

Health Services Research, School of Medicine, Faculty of Health, Witten/Herdecke University, 58455 Witten, Germany; latife.pacolli@uni-wh.de (L.P.); diana.wahidie@uni-wh.de (D.W.); ilknur.oezererdogdu@uni-wh.de (I.Ö.E.); yuece.yilmaz-aslan@uni-wh.de (Y.Y.-A.)

* Correspondence: patrick.brzoska@uni-wh.de

**Abstract:** Patients in long-term, palliative, and hospice care are at increased risk of a severe course of COVID-19. For purposes of infection control, different strategies have been implemented by the respective health care facilities, also comprising visitation and other forms of contact restrictions. The aim of the present study was to examine how these strategies are perceived by family members of patients in these settings. An exploratory, qualitative approach was used to examine perceptions of policies and strategies using partially standardized guided interviews analyzed by means of a thematic approach. Interviews were conducted with 10 family members of long-term, palliative, and hospice care patients. Interviewees were between 30 and 75 years old. Because of the pandemic-related measures, respondents felt that their basic rights were restricted. Results indicate that perceptions of strategies and interventions in long-term, palliative, and hospice care facilities are particularly influenced by the opportunity to visit and the number of visitors allowed. Strict bans on visits, particularly during end-of-life care, are associated with a strong emotional burden for patients and family members alike. Aside from sufficient opportunities for visits, virtual communication technologies need to be utilized to facilitate communication between patients, families, and caregivers.

**Keywords:** palliative; hospice; end-of-life; COVID-19; SARS-CoV-2



**Citation:** Pacolli, L.; Wahidie, D.; Erdogdu, I.Ö.; Yilmaz-Aslan, Y.; Brzoska, P. Strategies Addressing the Challenges of the COVID-19 Pandemic in Long-Term, Palliative and Hospice Care: A Qualitative Study on the Perspectives of Patients' Family Members. *Reports* **2022**, 5, 26. https://doi.org/10.3390/reports5030026

Academic Editors: Toshio Hattori and Yugo Ashino

Received: 30 May 2022
Accepted: 6 July 2022
Published: 8 July 2022



## 1. Introduction

During the COVID-19 pandemic, long-term, palliative, and hospice care facilities have faced numerous challenges [1]. Patients in these health care settings are at an increased risk for a severe course of COVID-19 because of existing co-morbidity and often advanced age [2]. To address the pandemic, different infection control measures were implemented by facilities, including visitation bans and other forms of contact restrictions [3–6].

Visits by family and friends are critical emotional anchors for patients, particularly for those in palliative care. Visitation bans implemented as infection control measures may lead to loneliness and increase the emotional burden for both patients and their loved ones [1,7]. In light of visitation bans, patients in in-patient facilities were encouraged to maintain contact with family members using digital communication services. Patients who are not tech-savvy, however, required assistance, which could often not be provided by staff because of limited personnel resources [1]. In some facilities, this led to patients being isolated and often dying without their relatives being present [8]. Despite exceptions to restrictions occasionally granted, for example for patients at the end of their life, the impact on dying patients was considerable [8]. Additionally, patients' relatives and friends were exposed to additional burden by being confronted with social distancing measures and visitation restrictions in already emotionally tense situations [9]. The grief processes during the COVID-19 pandemic were, thus, compounded by the experience of physical distancing and isolation, as well as feelings of insecurity, anxiety, and frustration affecting their own mental and physical wellbeing [6,10].

With these issues in perspective, the aim of this paper is to examine how family members of patients perceive the strategies and measures that have been used by long-term, palliative, and hospice facilities to address the challenges of the COVID-19 pandemic. The findings provide insight into family members' perspectives and allow to formulate recommendations with respect to how expectations of patients and their families can be better met during the pandemic and can assist health care providers to adapt existing strategies for current and future public health crises.

## 2. Materials and Methods

### *2.1. Study Design*

In the present study, a qualitative research approach was used given that the subjective perspectives were the focus of analysis [11]. Data collection was conducted by means of partially standardized guided interviews [12]. The interview guide was developed jointly by all authors based on existing research in the field. It consisted of four categories and covered, among others, changes due to the COVID-19 pandemic in medical and nursing care, strategies developed for addressing challenges of the COVID-19 pandemic, support measures implemented for patients and relatives, and ethical and social aspects of the strategies developed. Relatives were recruited through the authors with assistance from staff in the health care facilities. In addition, study participants were recruited via open online groups using social media. Eligible participants were 18 years of age or older and relatives of patients who were in long-term care or palliative/hospice care during the COVID-19 pandemic. As a measure of precaution and to prevent any additional infection risks for participants, interviews were carried out via telephone. Interviews were conducted by one of the authors (I.Ö.E.), who has extensive experience in qualitative research. Interviews took place between October 2020 and March 2021 with 10 family members of palliative care patients aged 30–75 years. Interviewees included eight women and two men. Four of the individuals interviewed had a relative in hospice care, three had a relative in palliative care. The other three interviewees had relatives who were first in a palliative care unit and then in a hospice or were first in a hospital and were later transferred to a palliative care unit, a hospice, or home care. Interviewees were related to the palliative/hospice care patients by being daughters ($n$ = 5), wives ($n$ = 3), a husband ($n$ = 1), or a son-in-law ($n$ = 1). Interviews were conducted until a sufficient level of information saturation was reached. The duration of the interviews varied between 40 and 80 minutes. Table 1 provides an overview of the sociodemographic characteristics of the interviewees.

**Table 1.** Sociodemographic data of the study participants.

| Interview ID. | Sex | Age (Years) | Marital Status | Relationship between Study Participant and Patient in Long-Term/Palliative/Hospice Care | Facility/Duration of Stay |
|---|---|---|---|---|---|
| IP01 | female | 75 | married | wife/palliative care husband | Hospice |
| IP02 | female | 53 | married | daughter/deceased mother | Hospital, rehab facility, and most recently home care |
| IP03 | female | 47 | married | daughter/deceased mother | Palliative care unit |
| IP04 | female | 33 | married | daughter/deceased mother | Palliative care unit |
| IP05 | male | 43 | married | son-in-law/ deceased father-in-law | Nursing facility/ palliative care unit |
| IP06 | female | 46 | single | daughter/deceased mother | Hospital, palliative care, hospice facility |
| IP07 | female | 30 | married | daughter/deceased mother | Hospital, hospice facility |
| IP08 | female | 68 | widowed | wife/deceased husband | Hospice |
| IP09 | female | 42 | widowed | wife/deceased husband | Hospice |
| IP10 | male | 66 | widowed | husband / deceased wife | Hospital, palliative care unit |

### *2.2. Data Analysis*

The interviews were transcribed by a research assistant, with verbatim transcription including pauses in the conversation and expressions such as speech disfluency ("ehm", "hmm"), sobs, crying, etc. During transcription, the interviews were anonymized. The data analysis was based on thematic analysis, which enables a mixture of inductive and deductive coding procedures [13]. The deductive category system was created with the help of the main topics of the interview guide and expanded during the analysis with inductive categories based on the data material. The coding was carried out by two authors (I.ÖE. and L.P.) independently from each other; during the analysis, the codes were compiled and discussed among all authors. The analysis was assisted by the software MAXQDA [14].

### 2.3. Ethical Aspects

The study was approved by the ethics committee of Witten/Herdecke University (No. 153/2020; 31 August 2020). The study participants were informed about the study objectives and about the voluntary nature and confidentiality of the study and gave verbal and written informed consent to participate in the study before the interviews were conducted. In addition, consent was obtained for the recording and transcription of the interviews. Study participants did not receive any reimbursement for their participation in the study.

## 3. Results

The analysis allowed to identify central themes with regard to how family members of patients perceive measures and strategies developed by long-term, hospice, and palliative care facilities, and what they expect from health care during the time of the pandemic. Overall, four main themes could be identified. They are presented in the following.

### 3.1. Contact and Visitation Restrictions

A significant factor contributing to family members' perceptions of measures and strategies implemented to address the COVID-19 pandemic were existing contact and visitation restrictions, which increased feelings of stress and added to already existing burdens. Contact and visitation restrictions varied by the type of facility. In hospice and palliative care facilities, restrictions included the number of visitors or the length of time relatives were allowed to stay in the room, while respondents reported to have encountered full visitation bans in long-term nursing facilities. In some facilities, exceptions were allowed so that two or more family members could visit patients simultaneously. Overnight stays were mainly provided by hospices, where relatives had the possibility to use an armchair or bed in the palliative care patient's room. The respondents also encountered the aforementioned regulations in situation involving dying patients. Some relatives were not allowed to enter the room of the dying person together with fellow family members, but had to say their goodbye separately, thus lacking emotional support from each other. According to the respondents, no time limits were set for the farewell, but hygiene regulations had to be observed.

> *"[ ... ] you had to keep to it [ ... ] yes we were asked eh, that we keep to it actually only separately to her in the room to go in, we have of course also done"* IP07

> *"[ ... ] from the time of the pandemic everything was shut down, so it was allowed eh there were no more visits allowed ehm even since he had a first floor room, we were not even allowed to go into the garden of the facility and make contact with him through the window, absolute ban on visits [ ... ]"* IP05

> *"[ ... ] they would have, so if it had only been one night, an armchair, which is not so comfortable for the duration, but they would also have pushed me a whole bed in [ ... ]"* IP06

### 3.2. Impact of the COVID-19 Pandemic and Infection Control Measures

Some respondents described that visitation bans caused the physical condition of their loved ones to deteriorate, contributing to an earlier death. Furthermore, some respondents had the impression that nursing care was neglected during the pandemic, resulting in conflicts with doctors and nursing staff. It became evident from the interviews that infection control measures contributed to emotional strain and stress among family members. In addition, it was stated that due to the restrictions on the number of visitors and on the duration of visits, some family members were unable to visit or say goodbye to their loved ones. Conflicts arose in facilities because of lack of exceptions with respect to protective measures or lack of responsiveness and limited possibilities for communication with health care staff. Some nursing homes also reduced home visits by supervising primary care physicians and scaled back care to basic services further reinforcing relatives' impression about a diminishing quality of health care. However, some respondents also reported being satisfied with the medical and nursing care their loved ones received. They also indicated that care was taken to address the subjective needs of patients as best as possible.

As a result of visitation restrictions, most relatives adopted digital communication tools in order to stay in touch with patients. It was uniformly stated that smartphones, tablets, or laptops were not provided by the facilities but were purchased by relatives themselves. Patients who had problems using such digital communication tools relied on help from nursing staff, who often did not have the time to provide adequate assistance. Relatives had different experiences in communicating with caregivers. Most respondents were positive about communicating with caregivers, stating that they received a lot of support from caregivers, such as being listened to and being offered uplifting words or prayers. In addition, they noted that they could approach the staff at any time and that staff took the time to exchange with relatives. Other participants complained about a lack of proactive communication on the part of the nursing staff.

> *"Yes, the problem was that many people were not able to say goodbye or were not allowed to see them again during that time [ ... ]." IP04*

> *"And that has ultimately certainly contributed to his early death, because ehm when he had visitors, he ate and drank and ehm as I said, it was very very close contact with his daughters and that was then suddenly no longer possible" IP05*

> *"Mhm yes, exactly so by phone was possible, we were also used to that before the pandemic but as I said the handling of the iPad that was, that was already difficult for him because ehm it was also not possible to find a caregiver who could take the time and together with him, to make the iPad ready for use [ ... ]" IP05*

> *"[ ... ] via WhatsApp we have then communicated with each other, we have seen each other and that was wonderful, my husband is even, has even in his old days still learned ehm that just could start video and has seen me then and we could talk twice a day and that was wonderful" IP08*

### 3.3. *Perception of COVID-19 Strategies in Long-Term, Palliative, and Hospice Facilities*

According to some of the interviewees, the COVID-19 pandemic containment strategies were not perceived as a burden. For interviewee IP07, the measures did not play a significant role as long as visitation was possible—irrespective of other protective measures implemented in the facility. In addition, some interviewees stated that they had the feeling that the pandemic "does not exist" in the facility, despite various measures taken by the facility.

Nevertheless, many perceived an overwhelming burden as a result of the pandemic-related protective measures. Providing contact information as a protective strategy to allow contact tracing was perceived as "annoying" because the risk of infection was not considered to be high. Furthermore, waiting outside the hospital in cold temperatures was perceived as an "outrageous" requirement. It became clear from the interviews that particularly visiting bans resulted in a strong emotional burden for relatives and patients. By limiting the number of visitors, relatives felt a lack of emotional support, which resulted in emotional distress.

Respondents uniformly indicated that they felt their basic rights had been restricted due to pandemic-related policies and strategies. Passing away was regarded to be a special situation requiring exceptions to all measures that restrict visits. Respondents who were confronted with a strict ban on visitation perceived it as a strong restriction of their basic rights as well as those of their loved ones.

> *"[ ... ] that ehm yes, the visitor regulations were now limited to one person, maximum 2 on palliative care, I would say yes, it is already very restricted [ ... ] unfortunately my*

*husband had to go out whereby I, where I would have needed him just in the moment, [ ... ] that was where I had to be strong for my sister, although I myself would have needed someone [ ... ]" IP04*

*"[ ... ] So he was mentally very unwell and as I said his daughters were very very sad and depressed as well, that was a huge burden that was actually dominating everyday life [ ... ]" IP05*

*"[ ... ] Freedom to make decisions and to move freely and to do what you want, that is of course restricted [ ... ] what we already felt as very restrictive was just that we were not allowed to visit them, I would have wished that differently [ ... ]" IP07*

*"[ ... ] she was segregated in a single room and that was a condition that I don't wish to happen to anyone, that has shaped me so much [ ... ] my wife and I were married for 42 years and eh that has affected me, still hits me hard today, that is a condition that is simply inhumane [ ... ]" IP10*

### 3.4. Need and Expectations for Better Support

To improve care in long-term, palliative, and hospice facilities, interviewees considered higher staffing levels to enable nurses to also take the time during care to provide support to relatives. It was often mentioned that dying is an exceptional situation in which visitors should be allowed access without restriction and also that the number of visitors should not be pre-determined by the facility. Relatives stated that they felt left alone. They said they required more support and preparation, for example by being told what to expect and what dying will look like. In addition, it was stated that psycho-oncological care and other palliative services for patients and their relatives should be maintained, especially in times of pandemics, as the emotional state of relatives and patients can change greatly as a result of the measures implemented.

Furthermore, continuous staff education and the development of appropriate pandemic plans were mentioned as recommendations for care in long-term, palliative, and hospice facilities. In addition to maintaining visits as well as ensuring support from staff, it was recommended that no palliative care units be closed, as support by medical and nursing staff during the dying phase is necessary, especially during the pandemic.

*"Maybe a little more staff and a little more ... Encouragement and a little more comfort and a nice word [at times] ... a smile" IP01*

*"[ ... ] I would have liked it just that everyone who wants, no matter how many people there are, as long as the patient wants it and does not explicitly say, [ ... ] to allow to receive visitors, just when the person is simply dying, yes he feels alone otherwise. There are so many people who would like to see my mom [ ... ] a better concept in this respect simply ehm I mean clearly there are hygiene concepts everywhere, but this does not have to be done by only one person per day, so I don't understand why it has to be throttled down so much [ ... ]". IP04*

*"So I think, seriously ill and dying, in the palliative situations I think patients must have unrestricted access to relatives [ ... ] I think it needs a lot of knowledge and education, constant education, I also don't think that this was the last pandemic we had to deal with and ehm that is actually reason enough to fundamentally think about how we want to deal with our seriously ill people and that ehm, I hope that we learn the lessons from this current pandemic that we are smarter next time and ehm do justice to it and and ehm make sure that people can be adequately cared for in every respect" IP05*

## 4. Discussion

This study used a qualitative research approach to examine how strategies implemented in long-term, palliative, and hospice care facilities during the COVID-19 pandemic are perceived by family members of patients who receive palliative care. The findings show that perceptions of strategies are particularly influenced by the extent to which visitation restrictions are in place. They highlight that strict bans on visits are associated with a strong emotional burden for patients and family members. These findings are in line with the results of a study from the US, in which social workers in hospice facilities were interviewed about the pandemic situation [15]. The study found that isolation is an additional challenge and emotional burden for both hospice patients and their families, especially when a ban on visitation is maintained even during the patients' dying phase [15]. In another study from the US, in which the relatives of palliative patients were interviewed, it was shown that visitation restrictions or bans, poor communication with staff, and inadequate quality of care resulted in despair among relatives and feelings of anxiety about the patient dying alone [16]. In a study from the United Kingdom, more than half of the relatives surveyed stated that they were not allowed to visit their loved ones during the dying phase. The study also revealed that relatives who were allowed to visit were more likely to feel supported than those without possibilities for visits [17]. In the present study, it was shown that by limiting the number of visitors, relatives lack emotional support during their loved ones' dying process, corroborating findings from previous research in Germany [18].

High-quality communication with nursing staff during the pandemic is characterized by two components: (1) easy access to staff to address concerns and questions about the patient's care and (2) involvement of family members in decision-making processes about nursing care [16]. Various studies have highlighted the increased relevance of adequate communication during pandemic periods when visits are no longer possible or limited as a result of infection control measures. Staff that is difficult to reach or inaccessible, as well as lack of information about the health status of patients and the impression that family members are kept out of decision-making processes, led to fear and uncertainty among relatives, as well as the perception of inadequate end-of-life care [16,19]. These findings are consistent with the results of the present study, given that in cases where interviewees perceived poor communication, they also criticized the quality of nursing care and support. Pre-pandemic studies show that both family members and patients consider communication to be essential in palliative care [20–24].

Visitation bans and restricted in-person communication require alternative communication tools to meet needs of patients and their relatives. Video or at least telephone calls make it possible for relatives to see or talk to patients when visits are not possible. Furthermore, video or phone calls allow relatives to receive assurance that their loved ones are well [25]. Limited access to virtual communication technologies or communication tools that are difficult to use without assistance can lead to family members' perception of inferior care and result in frustration about lack of support and poor exchange [16].

Respondents' needs and expectations with respect to better support during a pandemic included more comfort and encouragement from caregivers and the removal of visitation restrictions and bans. The death of a family member is seen as a special situation in which family members and friends consider it essential to say goodbye to the patient not only in person but together with fellow relatives. Saying goodbye together provides resources of mutual emotional support, which in many cases was not available during the pandemic. The reported needs of the relatives are in line with results from other studies and are also reflected in recommendations in national and international guidelines [3,6,17,26,27].

Some limitations of the present study need to be considered. Only two of the ten interviewees were men and most of the participants were over 40 years old, potentially not sufficiently covering the perspective of male relatives and younger individuals, respectively. Insights gained by the present study therefore need to be complemented by investigations that can provide a contrasting perspective between men and women. Additionally, the sample was not diverse in terms of culture, ethnicity, and migration status. Considering that individuals from collectivistic cultures may be more affected by contact restrictions than individuals from individualistic cultures, and thus, preexisting health disparities could be further exacerbated, future studies need to examine how well strategies are able to take into account diversity in the society.

## 5. Conclusions

Open communication is an important factor in long-term, palliative, and hospice care. Since face-to-face interaction between patients, families, and health care staff may be limited as a result of infection control measures, alternative communication methods need to be used [19]. Different guidelines exist aiming to assist health care facilities with implementation [3,28,29]. Visits by relatives play an important role, particularly in end-of-life care, for both patients as well relatives themselves and should, therefore, be facilitated during pandemics and balanced with measures of infection control [30]. In addition, the potential for virtual communication must be utilized. Representatives of patients and relatives must be involved in the development of appropriate support strategies in order to ensure that measures implemented consider patients' and relatives' needs as best as possible.

**Author Contributions:** Conceptualization, Y.Y.-A. and P.B.; funding acquisition, Y.Y.-A. and P.B.; project administration Y.Y.-A. and P.B.; methodology, L.P., I.Ö.E., D.W., Y.Y.-A. and P.B.; investigation, L.P., I.Ö.E., Y.Y.-A. and P.B.; writing—original draft preparation, L.P.; writing—review and editing, D.W., Y.Y.-A. and P.B.; Data curation I.Ö.E.; Formal analysis L.P. and I.Ö.E. All authors have read and agreed to the published version of the manuscript.

**Funding:** The project upon which this publication is based was funded by the Federal Minister of Education and Research, Germany (grant number 01 KI20126).

**Institutional Review Board Statement:** The study was conducted in accordance with the Declaration of Helsinki and approved by the Ethics Committee) of Witten/Herdecke University (No. 153/2020, 31 August 2020).

**Informed Consent Statement:** Informed consent was obtained from all subjects involved in the study.

**Data Availability Statement:** The data are available from the corresponding author upon reasonable request.

**Conflicts of Interest:** The authors declare no conflict of interest.

## References

1. Ong, K.J.; Lim, M.Y.Y.; Chng, J.X.R.; Wong, Y.P.; Koh, L.H. Collateral Damage: How the COVID-19 Pandemic Has Affected the Dying Process of Palliative Care Patients in Hospitals-Our Experience and Recommendations. *Ann Acad. Med. Singap.* **2020**, *49*, 616–620. [PubMed]
2. Jordan, R.E.; Adab, P.; Cheng, K.K. COVID-19: Risk factors for severe disease and death. *BMJ* **2020**, *368*, m1198. [CrossRef] [PubMed]
3. Wahidie, D.; Altinok, K.; Yılmaz-Aslan, Y.; Brzoska, P. Strategien, Richtlinien und Empfehlungen zur Bewältigung der COVID-19-Pandemie in Einrichtungen der Palliativ- und Hospizversorgung. *Ergebnisse eines Scoping-Reviews. Z. Gerontol. Geriatr.* **2022**, *55*, 151–156. [CrossRef]
4. Hsu, Y.-C.; Liu, Y.-A.; Lin, M.-H.; Lee, H.-W.; Chen, T.-J.; Chou, L.-F.; Hwang, S.-J. Visiting Policies of Hospice Wards during the COVID-19 Pandemic: An Environmental Scan in Taiwan. *Int. J. Environ. Res. Public Health* **2020**, *17*, 2857. [CrossRef]
5. Bolt, S.R.; van der Steen, J.T.; Mujezinović, I.; Janssen, D.J.A.; Schols, J.M.G.A.; Zwakhalen, S.M.G.; Khemai, C.; Knapen, E.P.A.G.M.; Dijkstra, L.; Meijers, J.M.M. Practical nursing recommendations for palliative care for people with dementia living in long-term care facilities during the COVID-19 pandemic: A rapid scoping review. *Int. J. Nurs. Stud.* **2021**, *113*, 103781. [CrossRef]
6. Münch, U.; Müller, H.; Deffner, T.; von Schmude, A.; Kern, M.; Kiepke-Ziemes, S.; Radbruch, L. Empfehlungen zur Unterstützung von belasteten, schwerstkranken, sterbenden und trauernden Menschen in der Corona-Pandemie aus palliativmedizinischer Perspektive: Empfehlungen der Deutschen Gesellschaft für Palliativmedizin (DGP), der Deutschen Interdisziplinären Vereinigung für Intensiv- und Notfallmedizin (DIVI), des Bundesverbands Trauerbegleitung (BVT), der Arbeitsgemeinschaft für Psychoonkologie in der Deutschen Krebsgesellschaft, der Deutschen Vereinigung für Soziale Arbeit im Gesundheitswesen (DVSG) und der Deutschen Gesellschaft für Systemische Therapie, Beratung und Familientherapie (DGSF). *Schmerz* **2020**, *34*, 303–313. [CrossRef]
7. Gosch, M.; Altrichter, D.; Pflügner, M.; Frohnhofen, H.; Steinmann, J.; Schmude-Basic, I.; Adamek, A.; Johnscher, I.; Kandler, U.; Wunner, C.; et al. Langzeitpflegeeinrichtungen in der COVID-19-Pandemie: Überlegungen auf dem Weg zurück in die Normalität. *Z. Gerontol. Geriatr.* **2021**, *54*, 377–383. [CrossRef]
8. Downar, J.; Kekewich, M. Improving family access to dying patients during the COVID-19 pandemic. *Lancet Respir. Med.* **2021**, *9*, 335–337. [CrossRef]
9. Mehnert, A. Clinical psychology in palliative care. In *Oxford Textbook of Palliative Medicine*; Oxford University Press: Oxford, UK, 2015; pp. 221–227.

10. Wallace, C.L.; Wladkowski, S.P.; Gibson, A.; White, P. Grief During the COVID-19 Pandemic: Considerations for Palliative Care Providers. *J. Pain Symptom Manag.* **2020**, *60*, e70–e76. [CrossRef]
11. Helfferich, C. *Die Qualität Qualitativer Daten*; VS Verlag für Sozialwissenschaften: Wiesbaden, Germany, 2011; ISBN 978-3-531-17382-5.
12. Misoch, S. *Qualitative Interviews*; De Gruyter: Berlin, Germany, 2019; ISBN 9783110545982.
13. Vaismoradi, M.; Turunen, H.; Bondas, T. Content analysis and thematic analysis: Implications for conducting a qualitative descriptive study. *Nurs. Health Sci.* **2013**, *15*, 398–405. [CrossRef] [PubMed]
14. VERBI Software. MAXQDA 12 Reference Manual, Berlin. Available online: https://www.maxqda.com/download/manuals/MAX12_manual_eng.pdf (accessed on 30 May 2022).
15. Gergerich, E.; Mallonee, J.; Gherardi, S.; Kale-Cheever, M.; Duga, F. Strengths and Struggles for Families Involved in Hospice Care During the COVID-19 Pandemic. *J. Soc. Work End Life Palliat. Care* **2021**, *17*, 198–217. [CrossRef] [PubMed]
16. Feder, S.; Smith, D.; Griffin, H.; Shreve, S.T.; Kinder, D.; Kutney-Lee, A.; Ersek, M. "Why Couldn't I Go in To See Him?" Bereaved Families' Perceptions of End-of-Life Communication During COVID-19. *J. Am. Geriatr. Soc.* **2021**, *69*, 587–592. [CrossRef] [PubMed]
17. Mayland, C.R.; Hughes, R.; Lane, S.; McGlinchey, T.; Donnellan, W.; Bennett, K.; Hanna, J.; Rapa, E.; Dalton, L.; Mason, S.R. Are public health measures and individualised care compatible in the face of a pandemic? A national observational study of bereaved relatives' experiences during the COVID-19 pandemic. *Palliat. Med.* **2021**, *35*, 1480–1491. [CrossRef]
18. Schloesser, K.; Simon, S.T.; Pauli, B.; Voltz, R.; Jung, N.; Leisse, C.; van der Heide, A.; Korfage, I.J.; Pralong, A.; Bausewein, C.; et al. "Saying goodbye all alone with no close support was difficult"- Dying during the COVID-19 pandemic: An online survey among bereaved relatives about end-of-life care for patients with or without SARS-CoV2 infection. *BMC Health Serv. Res.* **2021**, *21*, 998. [CrossRef] [PubMed]
19. Ersek, M.; Smith, D.; Griffin, H.; Carpenter, J.G.; Feder, S.L.; Shreve, S.T.; Nelson, F.X.; Kinder, D.; Thorpe, J.M.; Kutney-Lee, A. End-Of-Life Care in the Time of COVID-19: Communication Matters More Than Ever. *J. Pain Symptom Manag.* **2021**, *62*, 213–222.e2. [CrossRef] [PubMed]
20. Steinhauser, K.E.; Christakis, N.A.; Clipp, E.C.; McNeilly, M.; McIntyre, L.; Tulsky, J.A. Factors considered important at the end of life by patients, family, physicians, and other care providers. *JAMA* **2000**, *284*, 2476–2482. [CrossRef]
21. Teno, J.M.; Clarridge, B.R.; Casey, V.; Welch, L.C.; Wetle, T.; Shield, R.; Mor, V. Family perspectives on end-of-life care at the last place of care. *JAMA* **2004**, *291*, 88–93. [CrossRef] [PubMed]
22. Thorpe, J.M.; Smith, D.; Kuzla, N.; Scott, L.; Ersek, M. Does Mode of Survey Administration Matter? Using Measurement Invariance to Validate the Mail and Telephone Versions of the Bereaved Family Survey. *J. Pain Symptom Manag.* **2016**, *51*, 546–556. [CrossRef]
23. Anhang Price, R.; Stucky, B.; Parast, L.; Elliott, M.N.; Haas, A.; Bradley, M.; Teno, J.M. Development of Valid and Reliable Measures of Patient and Family Experiences of Hospice Care for Public Reporting. *J. Palliat. Med.* **2018**, *21*, 924–932. [CrossRef]
24. Virdun, C.; Luckett, T.; Davidson, P.M.; Phillips, J. Dying in the hospital setting: A systematic review of quantitative studies identifying the elements of end-of-life care that patients and their families rank as being most important. *Palliat. Med.* **2015**, *29*, 774–796. [CrossRef]
25. Hanna, J.R.; Rapa, E.; Dalton, L.J.; Hughes, R.; Quarmby, L.M.; McGlinchey, T.; Donnellan, W.J.; Bennett, K.M.; Mayland, C.R.; Mason, S.R. Health and social care professionals' experiences of providing end of life care during the COVID-19 pandemic: A qualitative study. *Palliat. Med.* **2021**, *35*, 1249–1257. [CrossRef] [PubMed]
26. Gesell, D.; Lehmann, E.; Gauder, S.; Wallner, M.; Simon, S.; Bausewein, C. National and international non-therapeutic recommendations for adult palliative and end-of-life care in times of pandemics: A scoping review. *Palliat. Support. Care* **2021**, *31*, 1–13. [CrossRef]
27. Schwartz, J.; Reuters, M.C.; Schallenburger, M.; Meier, S.; Roch, C.; Ziegaus, A.; Werner, L.; Fischer, M.; van Oorschot, B.; Neukirchen, M. Allgemeine Palliativversorgung in Pandemiezeiten. *Onkologe* **2021**, *27*, 686–690. [CrossRef] [PubMed]
28. Chua, I.S.; Jackson, V.; Kamdar, M. Webside Manner during the COVID-19 Pandemic: Maintaining Human Connection during Virtual Visits. *J. Palliat. Med.* **2020**, *23*, 1507–1509. [CrossRef]
29. de Lima Thomas, J.; Leiter, R.E.; Abrahm, J.L.; Shameklis, J.C.; Kiser, S.B.; Gelfand, S.L.; Sciacca, K.R.; Reville, B.; Siegert, C.A.; Zhang, H.; et al. Development of a Palliative Care Toolkit for the COVID-19 Pandemic. *J. Pain Symptom Manag.* **2020**, *60*, e22–e25. [CrossRef]
30. Selman, L.E.; Chao, D.; Sowden, R.; Marshall, S.; Chamberlain, C.; Koffman, J. Bereavement Support on the Frontline of COVID-19: Recommendations for Hospital Clinicians. *J. Pain Symptom Manag.* **2020**, *60*, e81–e86. [CrossRef]

*reports*

MDPI

*Article*

# Social Determinants Contribute to Disparities in Test Positivity, Morbidity and Mortality: Data from a Multi-Ethnic Cohort of 1094 GU Cancer Patients Undergoing Assessment for COVID-19

**Rebecca A. Moorhead [1], Jonathan S. O'Brien [1,2], Brian D. Kelly [1,2,3,4], Devki Shukla [5], Damien M. Bolton [4], Natasha Kyprianou [5], Peter Wiklund [5], Anna Lantz [6], Nihal Mohamed [5], Heather H. Goltz [7], Dara J. Lundon [5,*] and Ashutosh Tewari [5]**

1 Peter MacCallum Cancer Centre, Division of Cancer Surgery, Melbourne, VIC 3000, Australia; rebecca.a.moorhead@gmail.com (R.A.M.); jonathan.s.obrien@gmail.com (J.S.O.); drbriankelly@gmail.com (B.D.K.)
2 Sir Peter MacCallum Department of Oncology, University of Melbourne, Melbourne, VIC 3000, Australia
3 Department of Urology, Eastern Health, Melbourne, VIC 3000, Australia
4 Department of Urology, Austin Health, Melbourne, VIC 3000, Australia; damienmbolton@gmail.com
5 Department of Urology, Icahn School of Medicine, Mount Sinai Hospitals, New York, NY 10029, USA; devki.shukla@mountsinai.com (D.S.); natasha.kyprianou@mountsinai.com (N.K.); peter.wiklund@mountsinai.org (P.W.); n.mohamed@mountsinia.org (N.M.); ashutosh.tewari@mountsinai.org (A.T.)
6 Department of Medical Epidemiology and Biostatistics, Karolinska Institutet, 17177 Stockholm, Sweden; a.lantz@gmail.com
7 College of Public Service, University of Houston-Downtown, Houston, TX 77204, USA; h.goltz@gmail.com
* Correspondence: dara.lundon@mountsinai.org



**Citation:** Moorhead, R.A.; O'Brien, J.S.; Kelly, B.D.; Shukla, D.; Bolton, D.M.; Kyprianou, N.; Wiklund, P.; Lantz, A.; Mohamed, N.; Goltz, H.H.; et al. Social Determinants Contribute to Disparities in Test Positivity, Morbidity and Mortality: Data from a Multi-Ethnic Cohort of 1094 GU Cancer Patients Undergoing Assessment for COVID-19. *Reports* **2022**, 5, 29. https://doi.org/10.3390/reports5030029

Academic Editors: Toshio Hattori and Yugo Ashino

Received: 23 May 2022
Accepted: 6 July 2022
Published: 20 July 2022



**Abstract:** Background: The COVID-19 pandemic exploits existing inequalities in the social determinants of health (SDOH) that influence disease burden and access to healthcare. The role of health behaviours and socioeconomic status in genitourinary (GU) malignancy has also been highlighted. Our aim was to evaluate predictors of patient-level and neighbourhood-level factors contributing to disparities in COVID-19 outcomes in GU cancer patients. Methods: Demographic information and co-morbidities for patients screened for COVID-19 across the Mount Sinai Health System (MSHS) up to 10 June 2020 were included. Descriptive analyses and ensemble feature selection were performed to describe the relationships between these predictors and the outcomes of positive SARS-CoV-2 RT-PCR test, COVID-19-related hospitalisation, intubation and death. Results: Out of 47,379 tested individuals, 1094 had a history of GU cancer diagnosis; of these, 192 tested positive for SARS-CoV-2. Ensemble feature selection identified social determinants including zip code, race/ethnicity, age, smoking status and English as the preferred first language—being the majority of significant predictors for each of this study's four COVID-19-related outcomes: a positive test, hospitalisation, intubation and death. Patient and neighbourhood level SDOH including zip code/ NYC borough, age, race/ethnicity, smoking status, and English as preferred language are amongst the most significant predictors of these clinically relevant outcomes for COVID-19 patients. Conclusion: Our results highlight the importance of these SDOH and the need to integrate SDOH in patient electronic medical records (EMR) with the goal to identify at-risk groups. This study's results have implications for COVID-19 research priorities, public health goals, and policy implementations.

**Keywords:** COVID-19; SARS-CoV-2; urologic oncology; genitourinary cancer; social determinants of health

## 1. Introduction

The current COVID-19 pandemic, caused by the severe acute respiratory syndrome coronavirus 2 (SARS-CoV-2), represents the third occurrence of widespread disease caused by a coronavirus in 20 years [1]. First identified in Wuhan, China, in December 2019, the rapid spread of SARS-CoV-2 has produced over 7 million cases and over 350,000 deaths worldwide as of June 2020 [2]. Emerging global data indicates older age, male sex, and several underlying conditions/diseases are predisposing factors to higher severity COVID-19 disease [3,4]. Furthermore, immunocompromised patients with cancer appear to be more susceptible to infection, have a higher risk of severe events, and ultimately poorer outcomes [5]. Pathogenesis of SARS-CoV-2 infection is mediated, in part, by angiotensin-converting enzyme 2 (ACE-2) and transmembrane protease serine 2 (TMPRSS2). SARS-CoV-2 host cell entry is facilitated by viral spike proteins, primed by TMPRSS2-mediated cleavage, which bind to ACE-2 and gain access [6]. TMPRSS2 is highly expressed in prostate epithelial cells; a minor percentage of the prostate club and hillock cells express both ACE-@ and TMPRSS2 [7]. Additionally, prostate adenocarcinoma cells may have the highest TMPRSS2 expression of all cancers, highlighting the need to further examine the relationship between genitourinary (GU) cancer and COVID-19 [8].

First described over 100 years ago by sociologists such as W.E.B. DuBois, social determinants of health (SDOH) are conditions in which people are born, raised, and currently live in, and the greater socioecological systems creating the economic policies, political systems, and social norms that shape the conditions of daily life. SDOH are primarily responsible for the severe health inequities seen today [9,10]. Factors such as race and socioeconomic status have been repeatedly linked to differences in overall health and survival of communities in all medical literature, including in the field of urology [9,11]. Mortality rates for GU malignancies also vary in rural and urban dwellings [12–14]. Disparities related to prostate cancer, bladder cancer, and kidney cancer—three of the most commonly diagnosed malignancies in the United States—are heavily linked to patient and community (i.e., neighbourhood) levels SDOH. As examples, low SES communities have high prostate cancer mortality rates (e.g., Appalachian, Kentucky residents) and the mortality rate of African American men with prostate cancer is 2.4 times higher than White men; men with less than high school education have a 20% increased risk of bladder cancer compared to those with postgraduate education; and kidney cancer mortality directly correlates to lower-ranked healthcare systems and lower healthcare expenditures [15–18].

To explore the potential impact of patient and neighbourhood level SDOH on COVID-19 outcomes, we propose to adapt Nicholas and colleagues' Socioeconomic Deprivation and Chronic Kidney Disease model to examine potential clinical (e.g., comorbidities), behavioural (e.g., smoking, obesity), and neighbourhood predictors (zip code), of COVID-19 outcomes. This conceptual framework emphasises the importance of socioeconomic factors as a mediator of key disease prevention and treatment pathways and highlights its vast impact on urologic disease outcomes (Figure 1). The figure shows that many of the determinants of disparities, such as comorbidities including diabetes and hypertension, may have their foundation in socioeconomic deprivation and its consequences. These include, but are not limited to, discrimination and segregation, substandard living conditions, limited access to quality healthcare among the uninsured or underinsured, limited health literacy, and chronic stress resulting in measurable and quantifiable pathologic factors that contribute to and enhance the development of urologic disease and eventually premature mortality [9,11,15]. Increasing evidence from the COVID-19 reports and emerging data points to potential overlaps in drivers of health disparities in both urologic cancer and COVID-19, suggested that factors fuelling cancer disparities also rendered this patient population more vulnerable to worse COVID-19 outcomes (i.e., morbidity and mortality).

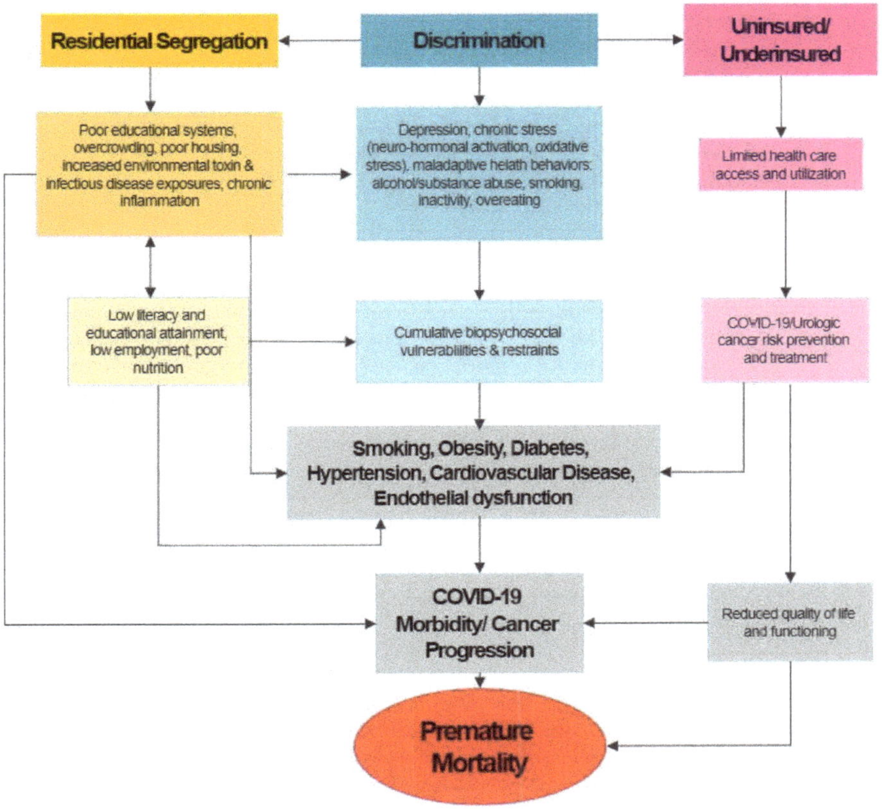


**Figure 1.** Theoretical framework for the potential of socioeconomic, behavioral, psychosocial and medical co-morbidities as drivers of GU cancers and COVID-19 disparities in the United States (adapted from Nicholas et al.) [11].

This current analysis of a multi-ethnic cohort of GU cancer patients aims to delineate the patient- and neighbourhood-level factors contributing to disparities in COVID-19 test positivity, morbidity and mortality.

## 2. Materials and Methods

### *2.1. Patient Data*

Symptomatic patients presenting to the Mount Sinai Healthcare System (MSHS), a network of 10 institutes and facilities across New York City, were tested and included in this dataset ($n$ = 47,379). SARS-CoV-2 testing was performed by reverse transcriptase PCR assay following a nasopharyngeal swab. The MSHS Ethics Committee approved a waiver of documentation of informed consent.

De-identified patient data was obtained from the MSHS Data Warehouse (https://msdw.mountsinai.org/). Demographic and social determinants available for analysis included age, sex, and first language preference being English, as well as race/ethnicity and smoking status. City borough of residence, hereafter referred to as "zip -code", was derived from the first three digits of a patient's zip code and included in models.

The MSHS Ethics Committee approved a waiver of documentation of informed consent; de-identified patient data was obtained from the MSHS Data Warehouse (https://msdw.mountsinai.org/).

### 2.2. Statistical Analysis

Continuous data were presented as medians (interquartile range [IQR]) and categorical data were presented as numbers (percentage). The $\chi 2$ test was used to compare differences in clinical outcomes between COVID test-Positive and COVID test-Negative groups. No single feature selection methodology seems capable of ensuring optimal results in predictive performance and stability in medical datasets, therefore, ensemble feature selection (EFS) was utilised to overcome these limitations. EFS reduces data dimensionality, removing irrelevant, redundant, or confounding features, leaving only those most relevant to the outcome [16,17].

Briefly; six feature selection methods for binary classifications were utilised; namely median, Pearson, Spearman-correlation, logistic regression, and two variable importance measures embedded in the random forest algorithm. The median method compares positive samples with negative samples by a Mann–Whitney U Test; the smaller the p-value, the higher the importance. Spearman-correlation was used to select features that are highly correlated with the dependent variable, but showed low correlation with other features and avoids multi-collinearity. Logistic regression involves a pre-processing step (Z-transformation) to ensure comparability between the different ranges of feature values and the $\beta$-coefficients of the resulting regression equation represent the importance measure. The random forest are themselves ensembles of multiple decision trees, which gain their randomness from the randomly chosen starting feature for each tree [19]. The random forest approach provides an importance measure based on the Gini-index (Gini_RF), which measures the node impurity in the trees and the error rate-based method (ER_RF) measure the difference before and after permuting the class variable. Each feature selection method was normalised to a common scale—an interval from 0 to 1/n—where n is the number of conducted feature selection methods (Figure 2).

A simple social determinants risk scale was computed by assigning equal weight to each of the five identified features per respective COVID-19 outcome: testing positive, hospitalisation, intubation and death. Calculated scores for each patient were determined and charted against the proportion of patients who experienced each outcome (Figure 3). All analyses were performed using R software [20].

## 3. Results

Of 47,379 tested patients, 10,444 (22%) tested positive for SARS-CoV-2. There were 1094 GU cancer patients in this cohort with 192 (17.6%) who tested positive. This cohort includes 659 prostate cancer patients with 134 (20.3%) who tested positive; bladder cancer patients ($n$ = 283) with 37 (13.1%) confirmed positive; kidney cancer patients ($n$ = 194) with 10.3%, 16% ($n$ = 31) tested positive, and testis ($n$ = 29) cancer patients of whom 10.3% ($n$ = 3) tested positive for SARS-CoV-2. Of all 192 GU cancer patients who tested positive for SARS-CoV-2, 128 were hospitalised, 19 were intubated, and 39 died of the disease (Table 1).

Of the 1094 GU cancer patients that presented to MSHS for testing, 997 (91.1%) were male. Regarding their race/ethnicity, 459 (42%) were White, 273 (25.5%) were of African ancestry, 204 (18.6%) were Hispanic/Latinx, 41 (37.5%) were Asian, and 117 (10.7%) were Other/Unknown. There was a significant difference in the rate of positive tests between these groups ($p < 0.001$), with the highest proportion of positive tests occurring in Hispanic/Latinx patients with GU cancer (31.3%). There were no significant statistical differences in the rates of hospitalisation, intubation, or death between these groups.

**Table 1.** Urologic cancer patient social and clinical demographics. * indicates $p < 0.05$; † indicates $p < 0.001$. Total percentages for prostate, bladder, kidney and testis cancer do not sum to 100% as patients may have had a diagnosis of more than one malignancy.

| Parameter | COVID-19 Test | | Hospitalisation | | Intubation | | Mortality | |
|---|---|---|---|---|---|---|---|---|
| | Negative ($n$ = 902) | Positive ($n$ = 192) | No ($n$ = 64) | Yes ($n$ = 128) | No ($n$ = 173) | Yes ($n$ = 19) | Alive ($n$ = 153) | Deceased ($n$ = 39) |
| **Age (years)** | | * | | * | | | | * |
| Mean (SD) | 69.3 (10.9) | 71.9 (11.0) | 68.8 (12.9) | 73.5 (9.53) | 71.6 (11.4) | 74.5 (6.18) | 71.0 (11.2) | 75.5 (9.40) |
| Median (Min, Max) | 70.0 (26.0, 90.0) | 72.5 (32.0, 90.0) | 69.0 (32.0, 90.0) | 74.0 (39.0, 90.0) | 71.0 (32.0, 90.0) | 74.0 (67.0, 90.0) | 71.0 (32.0, 90.0) | 76.0 (55.0, 90.0) |
| **Sex** | | | | | | | | |
| Female | 84 (86.6%) | 13 (13.4%) | 3 (23.1%) | 10 (76.9%) | 13 (100.0%) | 0 (0%) | 10 (76.9%) | 3 (23.1%) |
| Male | 818 (82.0%) | 179 (18.0%) | 61 (34.1%) | 118 (65.9%) | 160 (89.4%) | 19 (10.6%) | 143 (79.9%) | 36 (20.1%) |
| **Race/Ethnicity** | | † | | | | | | |
| African ancestry | 221 (81.0%) | 52 (19.0%) | 13 (25.0%) | 39 (75.0%) | 51 (98.1%) | 1 (1.9%) | 42 (80.8%) | 10 (19.2%) |
| Asian | 35 (85.4%) | 6 (14.6%) | 2 (33.3%) | 4 (66.7%) | 6 (100.0%) | 0 (0.0%) | 4 (66.7%) | 2 (33.3%) |
| Hispanic/Latinx | 144 (70.6%) | 60 (29.4%) | 23 (38.3%) | 37 (61.7%) | 53 (88.3%) | 7 (11.7%) | 52 (86.7%) | 8 (13.3%) |
| White | 409 (89.1%) | 50 (10.9%) | 17 (34.0%) | 33 (66.0%) | 42 (84.0%) | 8 (16.0%) | 37 (74.0%) | 13 (26.0%) |
| Other/Unknown | 93 (79.5%) | 24 (20.5%) | 9 (37.5%) | 15 (62.5%) | 21 (87.5%) | 3 (12.5%) | 18 (75.0%) | 6 (25.0%) |
| **Zip code** | | * | | | | * | | |
| Bronx | 53 (81.5%) | 12 (41.7%) | 5 (58.3%) | 7 (5.5%) | 12 (100.0%) | 0 (0.0%) | 9 (75.0%) | 3 (25.0%) |
| Brooklyn | 137 (80.1%) | 34 (23.5%) | 8 (23.5%) | 26 (20.3%) | 26 (76.5%) | 8 (23.5%) | 29 (85.3%) | 5 (14.7%) |
| Manhattan | 405 (78.9%) | 108 (21.1%) | 34 (23.5%) | 74 (68.5%) | 101 (93.5%) | 7 (6.5%) | 90 (83.3%) | 18 (16.7%) |
| Nassau | 24 (96.0%) | 1 (4.0%) | 0 (0.0%) | 1 (100.0%) | 1 (100.0%) | 0 (0.0%) | 1 (100.0%) | 0 (0.0%) |
| Queens | 180 (86.5%) | 28 (13.5%) | 13 (46.4%) | 15 (53.6%) | 26 (92.9%) | 2 (7.1%) | 16 (57.1%) | 12 (42.9%) |
| Staten Island | 23 (88.5%) | 3 (11.5%) | 1 (33.3%) | 2 (66.7%) | 3 (100.0%) | 0 (0.0%) | 2 (66.7%) | 1 (33.3%) |
| Suffolk | 21 (95.5%) | 1 (4.5%) | 1 (100%) | 0 (0%) | 1 (100.0%) | 0 (0.0%) | 1 (100.0%) | 0 (0.0%) |
| Outside NYS | 19 (82.6%) | 4 (17.4%) | 2 (50.0%) | 2 (50.0%) | 2 (50.0%) | 2 (50.0%) | 4 (100.0%) | 0 (0.0%) |
| **English as Preferred 1st Language** | | | | | | | | |
| | 777 (83.3%) | 156 (16.7%) | 55 (85.9%) | 101 (78.9%) | 143 (91.7%) | 13 (8.3%) | 127 (81.4%) | 29 (18.6%) |
| **Current/Former Smoker** | | | | | | | | |
| | 559 (85.2%) | 97 (14.8%) | 31 (34.0%) | 66 (68.0%) | 86 (88.7%) | 11 (11.3%) | 74 (76.3%) | 23 (23.7%) |
| **Asthma** | 41 (74.5%) | 14 (25.5%) | 6 (42.9%) | 8 (57.1%) | 14 (100.0%) | 0 (0.0%) | 12 (85.6%) | 2 (14.3%) |
| **COPD** | 59 (76.6%) | 18 (23.4%) | 7 (38.9%) | 11 (61.1%) | 17 (94.4%) | 1 (5.6%) | 15 (83.3%) | 3 (16.7%) |
| **Hypertension** | 443 (80.3%) | 109 (19.7%) | 31 (28.4%) | 78 (71.6%) | 101 (92.7%) | 8 (7.3%) | 86 (78.9%) | 23 (21.1%) |
| **Obesity** | 61 (73.5%) | 22 (26.5%) * | 7 (31.8%) | 15 (68.2%) | 22 (100.0%) | 0 (0.0%) | 19 (86.4%) | 3 (13.6%) |
| **Diabetes** | 166 (74.4%) | 57 (25.6%) † | 17 (29.8%) | 40 (70.2%) | 52 (91.2%) | 5 (8.8%) | 43 (75.4%) | 14 (24.6%) |
| **C.K.D** | 157 (78.1%) | 44 (21.9%) | 16 (36.4%) | 28 (63.6%) | 42 (95.5%) | 2 (4.5%) | 36 (81.8%) | 8 (18.2%) |
| **Prostate Cancer** | 525 (79.7%) | 134 (20.3%) * | 39 (29.1%) | 95 (70.9%) | 120 (89.6%) | 14 (10.4%) | 101 (75.4%) | 33 (24.6%) * |
| **Bladder Cancer** | 246 (86.9%) | 37 (13.1%) | 16 (43.2%) | 21 (64.5%) | 34 (91.9%) | 3 (8.1%) | 32 (86.5%) | 5 (13.5%) |
| **Kidney Cancer** | 163 (84.0%) | 31 (16.0%) | 11 (35.5%) | 20 (64.5%) | 29 (93.5%) | 2 (6.5%) | 27 (87.1%) | 4 (12.9%) |
| **Testis Cancer** | 26 (89.7%) | 3 (10.3%) | 2 (66.7%) | 1 (33.3%) | 3 (100.0%) | 0 (0.0%) | 3 (100.0%) | 0 (0.0%) |

Older age was associated with a significantly higher risk of testing positive ($p = 0.002$), being hospitalised ($p=0.01$) and death due to COVID-19 in this cohort ($p = 0.01$) but not intubation ($p = 0.09$) (Table 1).

The majority of patients (933; 85%) in this cohort spoke English as their preferred first language. While there were no statistical differences between those who did and did not speak English as their first language for each of the outcomes on univariate analysis, English was the preferred first language of 81% of patients who tested positive and 74.4% who expired due to COVID-19 in this cohort.

The borough of residence was significantly associated with testing positive for COVID-19 and intubation ($p = 0.009$), but not hospitalisation or death. Manhattan had the highest rate of positive tests (108/513; 21.1%) and Queens had the highest mortality rate (12/28; 42.9%). There was a significant difference in ever smokers vs. never smokers receiving COVID-19 diagnosis ($p = 0.004$). Additionally, while the rates of hospitalisation (68% vs. 65.3%), intubation (11.3% vs. 8.4%) and death (23.7% vs. 16.8%) were higher amongst ever smokers, these were not significant.

Figure 2 outlines the results of EFS analysis, where age, race/ethnicity, diabetes, current/former smoker and prostate cancer diagnosis were the top five features selected as the most parsimonious, and biologically reasonable model to describe the relationship between those testing positive, and the features from social, demographic and medical co-morbidities. In a similar manner, the identified features in this cohort predicting the risk of hospitalisation were: older age, prostate and bladder cancer diagnosis, hypertension, and zip code. For risk of intubation, the identified factors were zip code, age, obesity, English as the preferred 1st language, and hypertension. For risk of death, the identified factors were: age, zip code, race/ethnicity, prostate cancer, and smoking status.

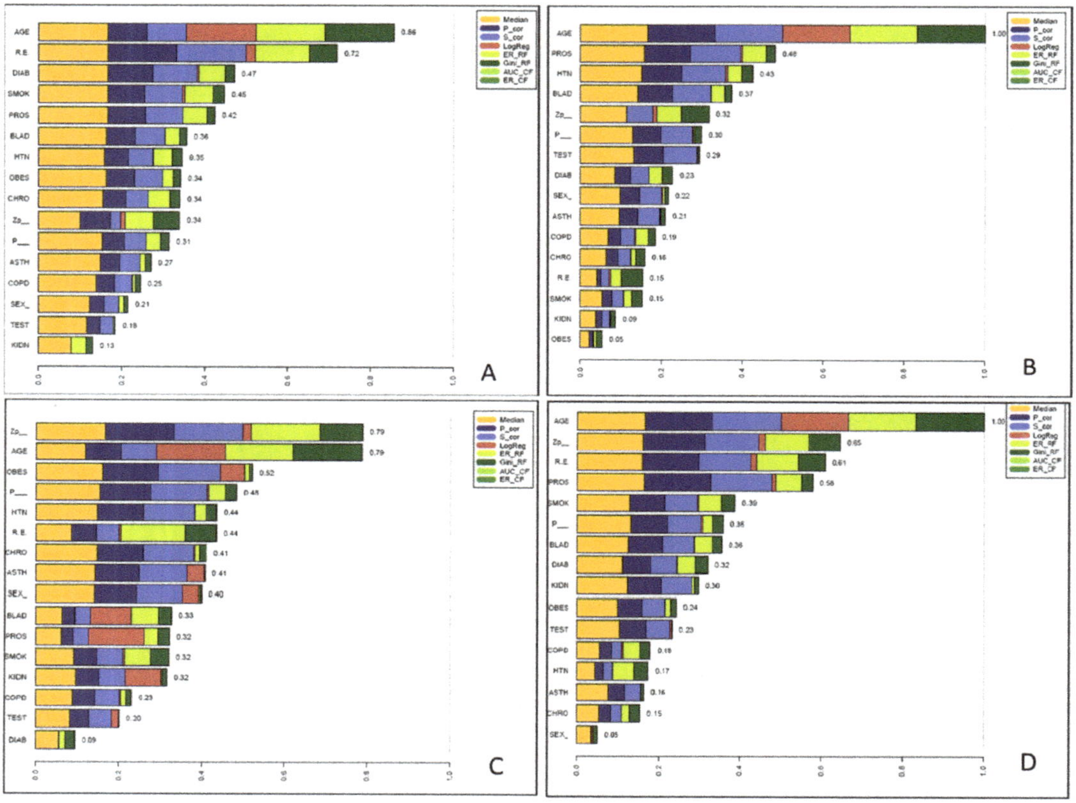


**Figure 2.** Ensemble feature analysis (EFS) of social, demographic and medical co-morbidities of GU cancer patients for the risk of (**A**) Positive COVID-19 test, (**B**) hospitalisation, (**C**) intubation and (**D**) death from COVID-19. EFS combined six feature selection methods—namely median, Pearson (P_cor), Spearman-correlation (S_cor), logistic regression (LogReg) and two two variable importance measures embedded in the random forest algorithm; the Gini index (Gini_RF) and error rate based detection (ER_RF). Each selection method was normalised to a common scale; a score of 1 indicates this parameter is the most prominent parameter selected by every method. R.E = race/ethnicity; DIAB = diabetes mellitus; SMOK= current/former smoker; PROS = prostate cancer diagnosis; BLAD = bladder cancer diagnosis; HTN = hypertension; OBES = obese; CHRO = chronic HIV infection; Zp_= zip code; P_ = English as the preferred 1st language; ASTH = asthma; COPD = chronic obstructive pulmonary disease; KIDN = chronic kidney disease.

Figure 3 demonstrates progressive increases in the risk for each outcome across the scale from 0 through to ≥4 for the risk of a positive test, risk of intubation, and risk of death. Factors comprising each scale are also displayed in Table 2. For GU cancer patients who scored ≥4 points or more on these scales, more than 30% tested positive for COVID-19, 10% were hospitalised, more than 80% were intubated, and over 50% died. (Figure 3).

**Table 2.** The most parsimonious parameters as identified EFS analysis for each of this study's outcomes: risk of testing positive for SARS-CoV-2 infection and COVID-19-related hospitalisation, intubation and death in a cohort of patients with genitourinary cancers.

| Outcome | Positive COVID-19/SARS-C0V-2 Test | Hospitalisation | Intubation | Death |
|---|---|---|---|---|
| **Parameter** | Age<br>Race/Ethnicity<br>Diabetes<br>Ever Smoker<br>Prostate Cancer | Age<br>Zip code<br>Hypertension<br>Prostate Cancer<br>Bladder Cancer | Age<br>Zip code<br>Hypertension<br>English as Preferred 1st Language<br>Obesity | Age<br>Zip code<br>Race/Ethnicity<br>Ever Smoker<br>Prostate Cancer |

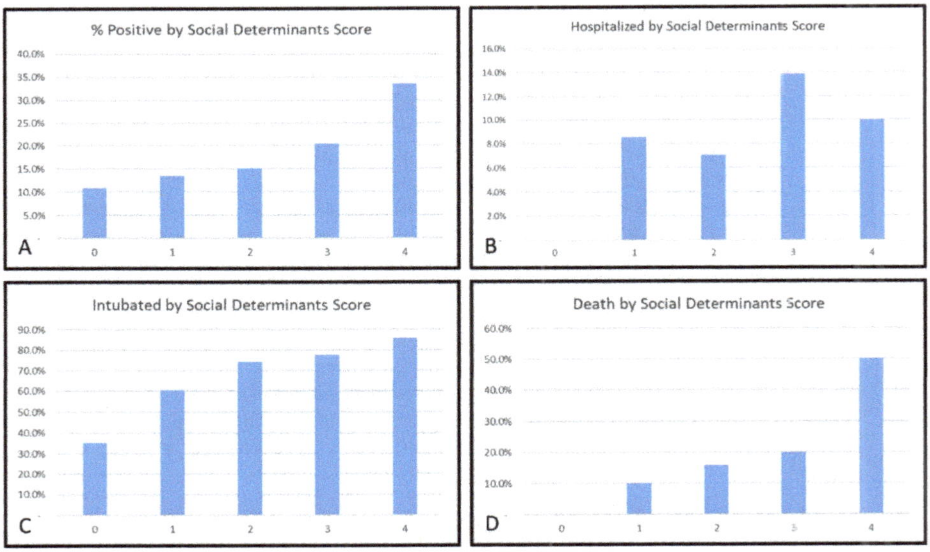


**Figure 3.** Relationship between social and medical determinants and COVID-19 outcomes: (**A**) positive COVID-19 test, (**B**) hospitalisation, (**C**) intubation and (**D**) mortality for patients with urologic cancers. A unique social determinant scale of (**A**) age, race/ethnicity, diabetes, current/former smoker, prostate cancer; (**B**) age, prostate cancer, hypertension, bladder cancer, zip code, (**C**) zip code, age, obesity, English as preferred 1st language, hypertension and (**D**) age, zip code, race/ethnicity, prostate cancer, current/former smoker was created—in which each determinant was awarded 1 point. Of those urologic cancer patients who scored 4 points on these scales, >30% tested positive for COVID-19; 10% were hospitalised, >80% were intubated and >50% died.

## 4. Discussion

This is one of the first studies to report on the impact of SDOH on COVID-19 outcomes for patients with urologic cancers. Our study findings provide evidence for the effects of patient and neighbourhood levels of SDOH on COVID-19 test positivity, morbidity, and mortality. The diverse cohort and geographic variation within New York City allowed for novel identification of underlying SDOH patient and neighbourhood-specific factors influencing COVID-19 outcomes.

Our results show that patient and neighbourhood-SDOH-specific factors (e.g., age, race, zip Code) play decisive roles in GU cancer morbidity and mortality from COVID-19. As this data reveals, zip code and race/ethnicity, established proxies for socioeconomic class, are strongly associated with urologic cancer patient outcomes following COVID-19 diagnosis. These findings highlight the importance of SDOH and the need to comprehensively address individual patient's risk factors among GU-cancer patients.

### 4.1. *Urological Cancer Outcomes and Social Determinants*

The relationship between urologic cancer outcomes and socioeconomic class has been well described in the literature. In regards to bladder cancer, more patients present with advanced-stage disease in countries with the highest poverty levels; white-collar workers with bladder cancer have a longer length of survival than blue-collar workers; and even when adjusted for smoking status, people with less than high school education have a 20% higher risk of bladder cancer compared to those with postgraduate education [21–23]. Similar data have been published regarding prostate and kidney cancer, ultimately demonstrating that lower income is a predictor of more advanced-stage cancer and worse postoperative outcomes [24–26].

Not only is socioeconomic class itself largely impactful on urologic cancer outcomes, it is also uniquely linked to behavioural factors that also correlate to more severe outcomes. Behavioural factors such as diet, physical activity, and smoking all contribute to the development of co-morbidities such as hypertension and obesity, which are associated with worse outcomes in this analysis. In this cohort, smoking was also associated with testing positive and death after COVID-19 diagnosis. As one of the largest risk factors for bladder and kidney cancer diagnosis, smoking is two times more prevalent in those who are below the poverty level versus those above it [27]. Additionally, poor diet and nutritional deficiency at the time of cystectomy or nephrectomy predicts perioperative mortality and 90-day mortality [28]. These health behaviours develop from far more than just individual decision-making; they are influenced by many systemic, socioeconomic and cultural factors critical for urologists to recognise.

Large disparities also exist regarding physical and built environments in relation to urologic cancers. As shown in this analysis as well, location and zip code significantly impact health outcomes for urologic cancer patients. The role of occupational environment on urologic cancer diagnosis has been extensively studied. Blue-collar workers such as car mechanics, construction workers, painters, and factory workers have much higher exposure to bladder and renal carcinogens [29]. Furthermore, environmental pollutants such as low levels of arsenic in drinking water have been associated with increased bladder, prostate, and kidney cancer risk [30,31].

A communities' built environments are also one of the major factors contributing to differing access to healthcare. Non-insured patients and those with Medicaid have 60% greater odds of presenting with more locally-advanced cancer and 50–70% greater mortality, compared to privately insured patients. This may be explained in part by Schrag and colleagues' analysis of Medicare/Medicaid data that found that only 40% of non-privately insured patients received adequate follow-up after bladder cancer diagnosis [32]. Even if patients are insured, factors such as distrust in the medical community, inadequate transportation, and provider density contribute to treatment delays. Additionally, higher hospital volume, specifically in New York State, is tied to better outcomes, including decreased operative mortality and decreased length of stay, after major cancer surgeries such as prostatectomy and cystectomy [33]. As reflected in this study, where a person with urologic cancer lives, it significantly impacts their mortality through multiple avenues. Especially when considering the well-documented differences in geographic access and availability of care in the COVID-19 era, this analysis further supports that where one lives directly impacts one's health.

### 4.2. Social Disparities in COVID-19

Understanding COVID-19-related racial/ethnic disparities can be challenging, as they are often rooted in historic, socio-structural inequalities. Minorities are often subjected to living in segregated, suboptimal neighbourhoods with poor housing and environmental conditions, as well as limited economic mobility and access to healthcare—a complex interplay of factors that may contribute to increased susceptibility and vulnerability to COVID-19. Racial/ethnic disparities in COVID-19 may also stem from labour inequalities, lack of workplace protections, and large household size, which decrease the ability to adhere to social distancing. Additionally, racial/ethnic minorities are more likely to have respiratory and cardio-metabolic comorbidities due to suboptimal built environments that reduce opportunities for engaging in health promoting activities and may be in close proximity to petrochemical and manufacturing plants or superfund sites.

This study also demonstrated that non-modifiable determinants such as age and race/ethnicity were among the top predictors of worse outcomes following COVID-19 diagnosis. This finding, specifically for urologic cancer patients, echoes numerous recent reports of racial disparities in COVID-19 outcomes in the general population. In the United States, African Americans and Hispanic people have experienced significantly higher COVID-19 mortality than White people [34]. Along with race, increasing age was another non-modifiable factor found to significantly impact COVID-19 outcomes for urologic cancer patients. While these older adults are more likely to be diagnosed with a urologic malignancy, there are other social determinants closely associated with ageing, which negatively impacts health outcomes for older adults [18]. Differences in employment, caretaker roles, language barriers, and transportation access are just a few of the many SDOH that can be attributed to worse health outcomes among older patients. The evident influence that these non-modifiable individual factors have on health outcomes highlights the need for the medical field to address these disparities and actively work towards reducing them.

Our results confirm shared demographic and clinical characteristics between COVID-19 risk and documented urologic cancer health disparities in the U.S. (e.g., race, older age, comorbidities). In order to reduce the effect of COVID-19 on existing urologic cancer disparities and to improve the health of vulnerable patients, healthcare systems must invest in optimising clinical cancer care and reducing the risk of infection and worse outcomes of COVID-19. A recent COVID-19 paper argued that parameters for the prediction of the need for admission to ICUs are urgently needed for patients with nephritis to enable timely management and appropriate resource allocation [35]. Routine data collection of differential clinical (morbidity, mortality) and SDOH (socioeconomic factors, healthcare access, physical environment, individual and collective health behaviours) within electronic medical records and health equity surveillance systems are necessary to optimise understanding of the cancer–COVID-19 double burden [36–40]. The surveillance system would benefit from local knowledge and active involvement of clinical supportive care staff (e.g., oncology and medical social workers) to facilitate understanding of broader contextual factors that can drive mortality and morbidity associated with outbreaks, including COVID-19 [35–37,41].

### 4.3. Strengths and Limitations

Our study presents important findings. With the largest sample size to date, of over 47,000 patients from the epicentre of the pandemic in the U.S., our study is reflective of a broad patient demographic and outcomes in New York City. However, our study does have limitations. The specific cancer clinical information (e.g., time since diagnosis and treatment received) is not available in the dataset, therefore, the severity of the cancer's stage cannot be determined. Nor do we have data on the long-term outcomes for these patients to assess for post-intensive care syndrome [42]. Another limitation is that our study does not account for cases and deaths outside of the MSHS system, such as patients who were homebound or in nursing homes and other care facilities.

## 5. Conclusions

This large population-based cohort of patients tested for COVID-19 was taken from the epicentre of the pandemic in the U.S. Our results show that SDOH, including zip code/ NYC borough, age, race/ethnicity, smoking status, and English as the preferred language are significant predictors of COVID-19 outcomes in patients with GU cancers. Our results highlight the importance of taking SDOH into consideration when addressing each individual patient's risk factors in patients with GU cancers.

We found that various medical and social determinants, when used together in a point scoring system, can risk stratify those GU cancer patients susceptible to COVID-19 diagnosis, hospitalisation, intubation, and death. Urologists, oncologists and others involved in the care of GU cancer patients should consider and account for the importance of social determinants when managing patients.

**Author Contributions:** R.A.M.: manuscript writing and editing; J.S.O.: manuscript writing and editing; B.D.K.: project development, data management, data analysis, manuscript writing; D.S.: manuscript writing; D.M.B.: project development, manuscript writing and editing; N.K.: project development, manuscript writing and editing; P.W.: project development, manuscript writing and editing; A.L.: project development, manuscript writing and editing; N.M.: project development, manuscript writing and editing; H.H.G.: project development, manuscript writing and editing; D.J.L.: project development, data management, data analysis, manuscript writing; A.T.: project development, manuscript writing and editing. All authors have read and agreed to the published version of the manuscript.

**Funding:** Nihal E. Mohamed is supported by scholar grants from the Department of Defense (W81XWH-17-1-0590 Log#PC160194), and the National Institute of Nursing Research (1R21 NR016518-01A1).

**Institutional Review Board Statement:** The study was conducted according to the guidelines of the Declaration of Helsinki and approved by the MSHS Ethics Committee.

**Informed Consent Statement:** The MSHS Ethics Committee approved a waiver of documentation of informed consent as de-identified patient data was used.

**Data Availability Statement:** Data managed by msdw.mountsinai.org.

**Acknowledgments:** This work was supported in part through the computational and data resources and staff expertise provided by Scientific Computing at the Icahn School of Medicine at Mount Sinai.

**Conflicts of Interest:** A.K. Tewari: CONFLICTS OF INTEREST. COMPANY RELATIONSHIP TYPE FINANCIAL. Uretheral Catheterless Radical Prostatectomy: Patent No. DNA-Based Bicistronic Vectors with Inducible and Constitutive Promoters—ID#: 160608: Patent No. High-Intensity Focus Ultrasound and CPG-BrachyurysiRNA for Treatment of Prostate Cancer—ID# 160403: Patent No. Patent for a Catheterless Device and Approach Patent No. *Promaxo Leadership Position Yes. *Promaxo Equity Ownership YES. Global Prostate Cancer Research Foundation Leadership Position No. Kalyani Prostate Cancer Institute Leadership Position No. Prostate Cancer Foundation: Leadership Position No. Roivant Consultant No. Blank Family Foundation Grant Yes. Intuitive Surgical Scientific Study or Trial Yes. Department of Defense (DOD) Scientific Study or Trial Yes. AxoGen, Inc. Scientific Study or Trial Yes. Oncovir, Inc—Poly ICLC Scientific Study or Trial Yes. National Institute of Health (NIH/DHHS) Scientific Study or Trial Yes. National Cancer Institute Scientific Study or Trial Yes. National Institute on Drug Abuse Scientific Study or Trial Yes. Kite Pharma Scientific Study or Trial Yes. Lumicell, Inc. Scientific Study or Trial Yes. Dendreon Scientific Study or Trial Yes.

## References

1. Zhou, P.; Yang, X.-L.; Wang, X.-G.; Hu, B.; Zhang, L.; Zhang, W.; Si, H.-R.; Zhu, Y.; Li, B.; Huang, X.-L.; et al. A pneumonia outbreak associated with a new coronavirus of probable bat origin. *Nature* **2020**, *579*, 270–273. [CrossRef] [PubMed]
2. Dong, E.; Du, H.; Gardner, L. An interactive web-based dashboard to track COVID-19 in real time. *Lancet Infect. Dis.* **2020**, *20*, 533–534. [CrossRef]
3. Kannan, S.; Ali, P.S.S.; Sheeza, A.; Hemalatha, K. COVID-19 (Novel Coronavirus 2019)—Recent trends. *Eur. Rev. Med. Pharmacol. Sci.* **2020**, *24*, 2006–2011. [PubMed]
4. Yuki, K.; Fujiogi, M.; Koutsogiannaki, S. COVID-19 pathophysiology: A review. *Clin. Immunol.* **2020**, *215*, 108427. [CrossRef]

5. Liang, W.; Guan, W.; Chen, R.; Wang, W.; Li, J.; Xu, K.; Li, C.; Ai, Q.; Lu, W.; Liang, H.; et al. Cancer patients in SARS-CoV-2 infection: A nationwide analysis in China. *Lancet Oncol.* **2020**, *21*, 335–337. [CrossRef]
6. Hoffmann, M.; Kleine-Weber, H.; Schroeder, S.; Krüger, N.; Herrler, T.; Erichsen, S.; Schiergens, T.S.; Herrler, G.; Wu, N.-H.; Nitche, A.; et al. SARS-CoV-2 Cell Entry Depends on ACE2 and TMPRSS2 and Is Blocked by a Clinically Proven Protease Inhibitor. *Cell* **2020**, *181*, 271–280.e8. [CrossRef]
7. Song, H.; Seddighzadeh, B.; Cooperberg, M.R.; Huang, F.W. Expression of ACE2, the SARS-CoV-2 Receptor, and TMPRSS2 in Prostate Epithelial Cells. *Eur. Urol.* **2020**, *78*, 296–298. [CrossRef]
8. Katopodis, P.; Anikin, V.; Randeva, H.S.; Spandidos, D.A.; Chatha, K.; Kyrou, I.; Karteris, E. Pancancer analysis of transmembrane protease serine 2 and cathepsin L that mediate cellular SARSCoV2 infection leading to COVID-19. *Int. J. Oncol.* **2020**, *57*, 533–539. [CrossRef]
9. Norris, K.; Nissenson, A.R. Race, gender, and socioeconomic disparities in CKD in the United States. *J. Am. Soc. Nephrol.* **2008**, *19*, 1261–1270. [CrossRef]
10. Lundon, D.J.; Mohamed, N.; Lantz, A.; Goltz, H.H.; Kelly, B.D.; Tewari, A.K. Social Determinants Predict Outcomes in Data From a Multi-Ethnic Cohort of 20,899 Patients Investigated for COVID-19. *Front. Public Health* **2020**, *8*, 571364. [CrossRef]
11. Nicholas, S.B.; Kalantar-Zadeh, K.; Norris, K.C. Socioeconomic disparities in chronic kidney disease. *Adv. Chronic Kidney Dis.* **2015**, *22*, 6–15. [CrossRef] [PubMed]
12. Colla Ruvolo, C.; Stolzenbach, L.F.; Nocera, L.; Deuker, M.; Wenzel, M.; Tian, Z.; La Rocca, R.; Creta, M.; Capece, M.; Saad, F.; et al. Higher Cancer Mortality in Rural Upper Urinary Tract Urothelial Carcinoma Patients. *Urol. Int.* **2021**, *105*, 624–630. [CrossRef] [PubMed]
13. Deuker, M.; Stolzenbach, L.F.; Ruvolo, C.C.; Nocera, L.; Tian, Z.; Roos, F.C.; Becker, A.; Kluth, L.A.; Tilki, D.; Shariat, S.F.; et al. Bladder cancer stage and mortality: Urban vs. rural residency. *Cancer Causes Control* **2021**, *32*, 139–145. [CrossRef]
14. Stolzenbach, L.F.; Deuker, M.; Collà-Ruvolo, C.; Nocera, L.; Tian, Z.; Maurer, T.; Tilki, D.; Briganti, A.; Saad, F.; Mirone, V.; et al. Differences between rural and urban prostate cancer patients. *World J. Urol.* **2021**, *39*, 2507–2514. [CrossRef]
15. Calderon, J.L.; Zadshir, A.; Norris, K. A survey of kidney disease and risk-factor information on the World Wide Web. *MedGenMed* **2004**, *6*, 3. [PubMed]
16. Neumann, U.; Genze, N.; Heider, D. EFS: An ensemble feature selection tool implemented as R-package and web-application. *BioData Min.* **2017**, *10*, 21. [CrossRef]
17. Polikar, R. Ensemble based systems in decision making. *IEEE Circ. Syst. Mag.* **2006**, *6*, 21–45. [CrossRef]
18. Buac, N.P.; Khusid, J.A.; Sturgis, M.R.; Gupta, M.; Lundon, D.J.; Chow, A.K.; Becerra, A.Z. Disparities in patient and system factors explain racial/ethnic disparities in delayed time to treatment in muscle invasive bladder cancer. *Urol. Oncol.* **2022**, *40*, 343.e15–343.e20. [CrossRef]
19. Breiman, L. Random Forests. *Mach. Learn.* **2001**, *45*, 5–32. [CrossRef]
20. R Core Team. *A Language and Environment for Statistical Computing*; R Foundation for Statistical Computing: Vienna, Austria, 2015.
21. Mouw, T.; Koster, A.; Wright, M.; Blank, M.M.; Moore, S.C.; Hollenbeck, A.; Schatzkin, A. Education and risk of cancer in a large cohort of men and women in the United States. *PLoS ONE* **2008**, *3*, e3639. [CrossRef]
22. Greenlee, R.T.; Howe, H.L. County-level poverty and distant stage cancer in the United States. *Cancer Causes Control* **2009**, *20*, 989–1000. [CrossRef] [PubMed]
23. Vagero, D.; Persson, G. Cancer survival and social class in Sweden. *J. Epidemiol. Commun. Health* **1987**, *41*, 204–209. [CrossRef] [PubMed]
24. Weprin, S.A.; Parker, D.C.; Jones, J.D.; Kaplan, J.R.; Giusto, L.L.; Mydlo, J.H.; Yu, S.-J.S.; Lee, D.I.; Eun, D.D.; Reese, A.C. Association of Low Socioeconomic Status With Adverse Prostate Cancer Pathology Among African American Men Who Underwent Radical Prostatectomy. *Clin. Genitourin. Cancer* **2019**, *17*, e1054–e1059. [CrossRef]
25. Maurice, M.J.; Zhu, H.; Kiechle, J.E.; Kim, S.P.; Abouassaly, R. Nonclinical Factors Predict Selection of Initial Observation for Renal Cell Carcinoma. *Urology* **2015**, *86*, 892–899. [CrossRef]
26. Izadmehr, S.; Lundon, D.J.; Mohamed, N.; Katims, A.; Patel, V.; Eilender, B.; Mehrazin, R.; Badani, K.K.; Sfakianos, J.P.; Tsao, C.-K.; et al. The Evolving Clinical Management of Genitourinary Cancers Amid the COVID-19 Pandemic. *Front. Oncol.* **2021**, *11*, 734963. [CrossRef] [PubMed]
27. Ward, E.; Jemal, A.; Cokkinides, V.; Singh, G.K.; Cardinez, C.; Ghafoor, A.; Thun, M. Cancer disparities by race/ethnicity and socioeconomic status. *CA Cancer J. Clin.* **2004**, *54*, 78–93. [CrossRef]
28. Ko, K.; Park, Y.H.; Lee, J.W.; Ku, J.H.; Kwak, C.; Kim, H.H. Influence of nutritional deficiency on prognosis of renal cell carcinoma (RCC). *BJU Int.* **2013**, *112*, 775–780. [CrossRef]
29. Michalek, I.M.; Martinsen, J.I.; Weiderpass, E.; Kjaerheim, K.; Lynge, E.; Sparen, P.; Tryggvadottir, L.; Pukkala, E. Occupation and risk of cancer of the renal pelvis in Nordic countries. *BJU Int.* **2019**, *123*, 233–238. [CrossRef]
30. Tsuji, J.S.; Alexander, D.D.; Perez, V.; Mink, P.J. Arsenic exposure and bladder cancer: Quantitative assessment of studies in human populations to detect risks at low doses. *Toxicology* **2014**, *317*, 17–30. [CrossRef]
31. Bulka, C.M.; Jones, R.M.; Turyk, M.E.; Stayner, L.T.; Argos, M. Arsenic in drinking water and prostate cancer in Illinois counties: An ecologic study. *Environ. Res.* **2016**, *148*, 450–456. [CrossRef]
32. Schrag, D.; Hsieh, L.J.; Rabbani, F.; Bach, P.B.; Herr, H.; Begg, C.B. Adherence to surveillance among patients with superficial bladder cancer. *J. Natl. Cancer Inst.* **2003**, *95*, 588–597. [CrossRef] [PubMed]

33. Omidele, O.O.; Finkelstein, M.; Omorogbe, A.; Palese, M. Radical Prostatectomy Sociodemographic Disparities Based on Hospital and Physician Volume. *Clin. Genitourin. Cancer* **2019**, *17*, e1011–e1019. [CrossRef] [PubMed]
34. Yancy, C.W. COVID-19 and African Americans. *JAMA* **2020**, *323*, 1891–1892. [CrossRef]
35. Deng, Y.; Liu, W.; Liu, K.; Fang, Y.-Y.; Shang, J.; Zhou, L.; Wang, K.; Leng, F.; Wei, S.; Chen, L.; et al. Clinical characteristics of fatal and recovered cases of coronavirus disease 2019 in Wuhan, China: A retrospective study. *Chin. Med. J.* **2020**, *133*, 1261–1267. [CrossRef] [PubMed]
36. Sohn, H. Racial and Ethnic Disparities in Health Insurance Coverage: Dynamics of Gaining and Losing Coverage over the Life-Course. *Popul. Res. Policy Rev.* **2017**, *36*, 181–201. [CrossRef] [PubMed]
37. Yang, J.; Zheng, Y.; Gou, X.; Pu, K.; Chen, Z.; Guo, Q.; Ji, R.; Wang, H.; Wang, Y.; Zhou, Y. Prevalence of comorbidities and its effects in patients infected with SARS-CoV-2: A systematic review and meta-analysis. *Int. J. Infect. Dis.* **2020**, *94*, 91–95. [CrossRef]
38. Lundon, D.J.; Kelly, B.D.; Nair, S.; Bolton, D.M.; Kyprianou, N.; Wiklund, P.; Tewari, A. Early mortality risk stratification after SARS-CoV-2 infection. *Med. Intensiva* **2020**, *45*, e40–e42. [CrossRef]
39. Lundon, D.J.; Kelly, B.D.; Nair, S.; Bolton, D.M.; Patel, G.; Reich, D.; Tewari, A. A COVID-19 Test Triage Tool, Predicting Negative Results and Reducing the Testing Burden on Healthcare Systems During a Pandemic. *Front. Med.* **2021**, *8*, 563465. [CrossRef]
40. Lundon, D.J.; Kelly, B.D.; Shukla, D.; Bolton, D.M.; Wiklund, P.; Tewari, A. A Decision Aide for the Risk Stratification of GU Cancer Patients at Risk of SARS-CoV-2 Infection, COVID-19 Related Hospitalization, Intubation, and Mortality. *J. Clin. Med.* **2020**, *9*, 2799. [CrossRef]
41. Gross, O.; Moerer, O.; Weber, M.; Huber, T.B.; Scheithauer, S. COVID-19-associated nephritis: Early warning for disease severity and complications? *Lancet* **2020**, *395*, e87–e88. [CrossRef]
42. Nakanishi, N.; Liu, K.; Kawakami, D.; Kawai, Y.; Morisawa, T.; Nishida, T.; Sumita, H.; Unoki, T.; Hifumi, T.; Iida, Y.; et al. Post-Intensive Care Syndrome and Its New Challenges in Coronavirus Disease 2019 (COVID-19) Pandemic: A Review of Recent Advances and Perspectives. *J. Clin. Med.* **2021**, *10*, 3870. [CrossRef] [PubMed]

reports

MDPI

Article

# Diagnostic Accuracy of Routine Laboratory Tests for COVID-19

Joshua Davis [1,*] and Gina Gilderman [2]

[1] Department of Emergency Medicine, University of Kansas School of Medicine and Vituity, 929 N. St. Francis Ave, Wichita, KS 67214, USA
[2] Burrell College of Osteopathic Medicine, Las Cruces, NM 88001, USA; gina.gilderman@burrell.edu
* Correspondence: jjvwd@udel.edu

**Abstract:** Objectives: COVID-19 has ravaged healthcare systems across the globe. Availability of and timely results for PCR testing have made diagnosis in the Emergency Department challenging. Therefore, we sought to determine if routine serum laboratory tests could be diagnostic of COVID-19. Methods: All patients tested for COVID-19 at an academic hospital in Pennsylvania between 1 March 2020–28 April 2020, were retrospectively analyzed. Results of COVID-19 PCR testing and laboratory tests were recorded. Mean difference was used to determine which tests demonstrated a significant difference, with $p < 0.01$ used, due to multiple observations. The tests that met these criteria had ROC curves and sensitivity and specificity determined. Results: Of the patients identified, 553 had had any laboratory test. All tests that showed a statistically significant mean difference were lower in COVID-19 positive patients. These included white blood cell count, platelets, absolute neutrophil count, absolute lymphocyte count, absolute eosinophil count, alkaline phosphatase, albumin, troponin T, lactic acid, D-DIMER, and procalcitonin. D-Dimer was excluded for only having four tests completed in COVID-19 positive patients. The remaining tests had a specificity of 88–96%, with a sensitivity of 5–50%. Discussion: No single serum laboratory test demonstrated sensitivity for COVID-19. Some tests might be moderately specific, but this was of limited clinical use. Future research should focus on a combination of tests to diagnose COVID-19, and healthcare systems should work to obtain rapid and accurate PCR tests to diagnose COVID-19.

**Keywords:** COVID-19; coronavirus; laboratory; serum markers; diagnostic accuracy; SARS-CoV-2



**Citation:** Davis, J.; Gilderman, G. Diagnostic Accuracy of Routine Laboratory Tests for COVID-19. *Reports* **2022**, 5, 25. https://doi.org/10.3390/reports5030025

Academic Editors: Toshio Hattori and Yugo Ashino

Received: 24 May 2022
Accepted: 18 June 2022
Published: 22 June 2022



## 1. Introduction

The novel coronavirus disease 2019 (COVID-19) has ravaged and overwhelmed many healthcare systems during its initial pandemic, with over 500 million cases leading to over 6 million deaths worldwide [1]. It is caused by Severe Acute Respiratory Distress Syndrome Coronavirus 2 (SARS-CoV-2). This novel viral pathogen is associated with high rates of both infectivity [2,3]. and mortality, which has led to the need to allocate scarce healthcare resources in many settings [4].

Testing for COVID-19 is typically done via nasopharyngeal, or oral, PCR, or, more recently, antigen testing. PCR tests do not have rapid turnaround times at many facilities [5], and antigen tests are known to have limited sensitivity [6]. Even PCR tests are known to be imperfect, with sensitivities near 73–85% [7,8]. The lack of universally available rapid and accurate tests leads to a diagnostic dilemma for many clinicians, especially those in acute care, like emergency medicine, urgent care, and primary care. Incorrect guidance regarding quarantining and isolation can lead to ongoing spread of this deadly virus. Recommendations for quarantining that are over-excessive can lead to lack of compliance and social and financial burdens for patients.

Serum laboratory tests are routinely available in most acute care settings with a rapid turnaround time. If there is a single or combination of laboratory tests that could strongly suggest whether a patient had COVID-19, it could allow more accurate quarantine and isolation recommendations. Therefore, we sought to determine the diagnostic accuracy of serum laboratory tests for COVID-19.

## 2. Methods

We conducted a retrospective review of all patients who had viral testing from 1 March 2020, to 28 April 2020, at a tertiary academic medical center in central Pennsylvania. This study was approved by the Institutional Review Board of Penn State Milton S. Hershey Medical Center.

Charts were identified using the specific order for COVID-19 testing. All patients who met this criterion and had any serum laboratory test result were included.

Availability and policies regarding COVID-19 testing at our hospital have changed often during the study period. Four different tests have been available: ARUP® Laboratories (Salt Lake City, UT, USA), Quest Diagnostics® (Secaucus, NJ, USA), Pennsylvania Department of Health (Harrisburg, PA, USA), and in-house testing at our clinical laboratory (Hershey, PA, USA). PCR testing for in house COVID-19, approved under FDA Emergency Use Authorization, was targeted against two different regions of the SARS-CoV-2 genome, ORF1ab and S gene. An RNA internal control is used to detect RT-PCR failure and/or inhibition.

Data abstracted included age and sex of patients, results of COVID-19 testing, date of testing, and results of laboratory tests. Mean difference was used to determine which tests demonstrated a significant difference, with an alpha of 0.01 selected as significant, due to multiple observations. The tests that met this criterion had receiver-operator characteristic (ROC) curves and sensitivity and specificity determined. Diagnostic accuracy was determined using standard definitions. Data was managed and statistically analyzed in Microsoft® Excel (Seattle, WA, USA).

## 3. Results

Of the 1024 patients identified who had COVID-19 testing during the study period, 553 (54%) had any laboratory testing performed. Of these, 488 (88%) were negative for COVID-19 and 65 (12%) were positive. The mean age was 54 years (SD = 22 years) and the average weight was 84 kg (SD = 28 kg). Males were 45% of the sample (248/553). Of the patients where race was provided, 77% were white (422/549), 10% Other race (58/549), 9% Black (51/549), and 3% Asian (18/549). Ten percent (59/552) were Hispanic. Among patients who tested positive for COVID-19, 45% were white (29/64), 31% Other race (20/64), 14% (9/64) Asian, and 9% (6/64) Black. Among COVID-19 positive patients, 25% were Hispanic (16/64) and 48% were male (32/66). All tests that showed a mean difference were lower in COVID-19 positive patients (Table 1). These included white blood cell count, platelets, absolute neutrophil count, absolute lymphocyte count, absolute eosinophil count, alkaline phosphatase, albumin, troponin T, lactic acid, D-DIMER, and procalcitonin. D-Dimer was excluded post hoc for only having four tests completed in COVID-19 positive patients. The remaining tests had a specificity of 88–96% with a sensitivity of 5–50% (Table 2).

**Table 1.** Mean Difference of Laboratory Tests for COVID-19.

| Laboratory Value | COVID (+) *n* | COVID (+) Mean | SD of (+) Group | COVID (−) *n* | COVID (−) Mean | SD of (−) Group | SD Both Groups | *p* Value |
|---|---|---|---|---|---|---|---|---|
| **White Blood Cell Count** | 65 | 6.09 | 2.54 | 487 | 10.46 | 5.92 | 3.09 | **<0.001** |
| **Hemoglobin** | 65 | 12.87 | 1.93 | 487 | 12.36 | 2.30 | 0.36 | 0.054 |
| **Platelet** | 64 | 178.47 | 68.73 | 480 | 247.26 | 106.84 | 48.64 | **<0.001** |
| **Abs Neutrophil Count** | 64 | 4.1 | 5.30 | 469 | 7.7 | 2.29 | 2.55 | **<0.001** |
| **Abs Lymphocyte Count** | 64 | 0.94 | 0.61 | 468 | 1.72 | 1.52 | 0.55 | **<0.001** |
| **Abs Eosinophil Count** | 64 | 0.03 | 0.06 | 468 | 0.14 | 0.19 | 0.08 | **<0.001** |
| **AST** | 64 | 45.59 | 46.13 | 436 | 47.49 | 115.52 | 1.34 | 0.812 |

**Table 1.** *Cont.*

| Laboratory Value | COVID (+) *n* | COVID (+) Mean | SD of (+) Group | COVID (−) *n* | COVID (−) Mean | SD of (−) Group | SD Both Groups | *p* Value |
|---|---|---|---|---|---|---|---|---|
| ALT | 64 | 33.05 | 30.69 | 443 | 43.7 | 138.15 | 7.53 | 0.162 |
| Alkaline Phosphatase | 64 | 70.94 | 30.20 | 443 | 113.8 | 93.44 | 30.31 | **<0.001** |
| Total Bilirubin | 64 | 0.49 | 0.67 | 441 | 1.39 | 7.91 | 0.64 | 0.02 |
| Albumin | 63 | 3.66 | 0.48 | 438 | 4.02 | 0.60 | 0.25 | **<0.001** |
| Lactate Dehydrogenase | 38 | 330.05 | 219.38 | 263 | 307.81 | 218 07 | 15.73 | 0.562 |
| Troponin T | 36 | 0.01 | 0.03 | 240 | 0.06 | 0.30 | 0.04 | **0.013** |
| Lactate | 43 | 1.38 | 0.64 | 299 | 1.81 | 1.08 | 0.30 | **<0.001** |
| D-DIMER | 4 | 0.43 | 0.14 | 81 | 1.57 | 2.98 | 0.81 | **0.001** |
| INR | 4 | 1.4 | 0.67 | 93 | 1.54 | 0.76 | 0.10 | 0.708 |
| Thromboplastin Time | 1 | 36 | 36.00 | 27 | 31.78 | 6.72 | 2.98 | - |
| C Reactive Protein | 37 | 5.32 | 5.57 | 306 | 5.55 | 8.12 | 0.16 | 0.824 |
| Erythrocyte Sedimentation Rate | 37 | 39.51 | 22.25 | 278 | 42.66 | 31.11 | 2.23 | 0.446 |
| Procalcitonin | 52 | 0.14 | 0.19 | 356 | 1.64 | 7.1[illegible] | 1.06 | **<0.001** |
| Ferritin | 37 | 915.49 | 1125.75 | 301 | 542.01 | 1188.54 | 264.09 | 0.065 |

COVID-19: novel coronavirus disease 2019; AST: aspartate aminotransferase; ALT: alanine transferase; INR: International Normalized Ratio

**Table 2.** Diagnostic Accuracy of Select Laboratory Tests for COVID-19.

| | Direction | Sensitivity | Specificity | Area Under Curve | Cutoff |
|---|---|---|---|---|---|
| White Blood Cell | Decr. | 26.7% | 95.8% | 82.7% | 7000 cells/hpf |
| Platelet | Decr. | 14.6% | 95.0% | 73.2% | 250,000 cells/hpf |
| Abs Neutrophil Count | Decr. | 18.1% | 95.6% | 77.2% | 6000 cellls/hpf |
| Abs Lymphocyte Count | Decr. | 13.9% | 96.0% | 76.8% | 2000 cells/hpf |
| Abs Eosinophil Count | Decr. | 23.1% | 96.1% | 94.0% | 25 cells/hpf |
| Alkaline Phosphatase | Decr. | 50.0% | 93.4% | 81.4% | 80 Units/L |
| Albumin | Decr. | 11.9% | 88.6% | 74.2% | 4.0 g/dL |
| Troponin T | Decr. | 10.9% | 95.3% | 96.0% | 0.015 ng/mL |
| Lactate | Decr. | 13.1% | 96.6% | 59.2% | 2.5 mmol/L |
| Procalcitonin | Decr. | 13.6% | 93.5% | 61.2% | 0.16 ug/mL |

COVID-19: novel coronavirus disease 2019.

## 4. Discussion

Our study reviewed the diagnostic accuracy of laboratory testing for COVID-19. Many specific findings were identified, but none of these findings were sensitive. Statistically significant findings associated with COVID-19 included leukopenia, thrombocytopenia, lymphopenia, neutropenia, eosinopenia, low alkaline phosphatase, low albumin, low troponin T, low lactic acid, and low procalcitonin. These findings were specific, but not sensitive.

Leukopenia, thrombocytopenia, and lymphopenia have previously been reported in many viral illnesses and are known to be commonly seen in COVID-19 [9] and have been shown to be negative prognostic markers [10,11]. Several mechanisms for lymphopenia and thrombocytopenia have been proposed. For lymphopenia, the following mechanisms have been proposed: hyperimmune response to IL-6 may lead to lymphocyte death, SARS-CoV-2 may directly infect T cells via ACE-2 receptors or ACE-2 independent pathways, SARS-CoV-2 may directly infect the bone marrow, or COVID-19 infection may lead to exhaustion of T cells or restrict their expansion [12]. For thrombocytopenia, the theory of bone marrow infection by SARS-CoV2 remains, but there are also theories of bone marrow suppression for hemophagocytic lymphohistiocytosis, like reaction, autoimmune platelet destruction, or platelet consumption due to microthrombi and lung damage in a mechanism similar to that seen in disseminated intravascular coagulation [13]. Our study showed that eosinopenia is associated with COVID-19 diagnosis, which has been reported previously, but is less widely known [14,15].

Our study is the first study to suggest that low alkaline phosphatase is associated with the diagnosis of COVID-19. A prior meta-analysis has shown that elevated liver functions are not associated with diagnosis of COVID-19 at presentation [16]. Interestingly, prior studies have shown elevated liver enzymes, namely alanine aminotransferase and aspartate transaminase, to be poor prognostic markers in COVID-19 [10,11]. Acute viral hepatitis from COVID-19 has also been reported, similar to other viruses [17]. The mechanism of this viral-associated hepatitis in COVID-19 is unknown, but widely accepted theories include direct viral injury, micro-thombosis, causing ischemic hepatitis, cholestasis from systemic inflammation, and non-hepatic causes of elevation in liver enzymes (i.e., muscle damage). Hypoalbuminemia has previously been reported as a poor prognostic, but not a diagnostic, marker [18]. This has been suggested to reflect endothelial damage or pulmonary capillary leakage playing a significant role in the pathogenesis of severe COVID-19 [19].

The fact that low lactate, troponin, and procalcitonin are associated with COVID-19 is likely more reflective of ruling out alternative pathologies for COVID-19 symptoms. Many patients with COVID-19 have fever, tachycardia, and tachypnea. Thus, a normal procalcitonin and lactate may be indicative of COVID-19 in a pandemic as it makes bacterial sepsis unlikely when COVID-19 has high prevalence in the population. Similarly, chest pain is also a common complaint in patients with COVID-19. During times of high prevalence, a normal troponin may be specific to COVID-19 because it makes cardiac causes of chest pain unlikely. While classic understanding of sensitivity and specificity is that they do not vary with prevalence of disease, more recent analyses have brought this concept into question [20,21].

Unfortunately, our study did not have enough positive D-DIMER tests to evaluate this as a diagnostic marker for COVID-19. Elevated D-DIMER has been associated with COVID-19 diagnosis and prognosis, with markedly elevated levels reported, even in the absence of known confirmed thrombosis [10,22].

Given the low sensitivity of each laboratory test in isolation, they really have no clinical value in ruling out COVID-19. In resource limited settings, some of these findings may suggest COVID-19 as a diagnosis, especially in times of high prevalence of the disease. Future research should focus on identifying a combination of laboratory markers to aid in the diagnosis of COVID-19 for settings in which access to rapid direct testing is unavailable. However, it is important to note that our study was not carried out in this setting, where the prevalence of other disease processes may affect the accuracy of laboratory tests for this diagnosis (e.g., malaria and thrombocytopenia). Given the lower prevalence of disease and increased availability of PCR and antigen tests for COVID-19, there will hopefully not be a need to use surrogate laboratory markers to assist in diagnosis.

## 5. Limitations

Our study was a single site retrospective review. It has the inherent limitations of both, including the possibility of limited generalizability. We included every patient who had COVID-19 testing, thus we included patients with at least moderate pretest probability of disease. Our study occurred in the Northeast United States at an academic medical center, so populations in other settings may be different. As mentioned above, the value of some tests may vary with lower disease prevalence. Since our COVID-19 testing changed and we used PCR testing as the reference standard, the differences in the test characteristics of the different PCR tests may also affect the diagnostic accuracy of laboratory tests in our analysis.

## 6. Conclusions

Based on our data, no single serum laboratory test demonstrates sensitivity for COVID-19. Some tests may be moderately specific, but are of limited clinical use, given lower prevalence and increased availability of direct antigen and PCR testing for COVID-19. Future research should focus on a combination of tests to aid in the diagnosis of COVID-19, particularly for low resource settings without access to direct rapid COVID-19 testing. Healthcare systems should work to obtain rapid and accurate PCR tests to diagnose COVID-19, as relying on laboratory findings alone is inaccurate.

**Author Contributions:** Conceptualization, J.D.; Data curation, J.D. and G.G.; Formal analysis, J.D. and G.G.; Investigation, J.D.; Project administration, J.D.; Supervision, J.D.; Writing—original draft, J.D.; Writing—review and editing, G.G. All authors have read and agreed to the published version of the manuscript.

**Funding:** This research received no external funding.

**Institutional Review Board Statement:** This study was granted exemption by the Institutional Review Board at Penn State Milton S. Hershey Medical Center.

**Informed Consent Statement:** Not applicable.

**Data Availability Statement:** Data is available from the authors upon reasonable request.

**Conflicts of Interest:** The authors have no conflict of interest relevant to this article to disclose.

## References

1. Johns Hopkins University. Coronavirus Resource Center. Available online: https://coronavirus.jhu.edu/data/mortality (accessed on 20 May 2022).
2. Zhang, S.; Diao, M.; Yu, W.; Pei, L.; Lin, Z.; Chen, D. Estimation of the reproductive number of novel coronavirus COVID-19) and the probable outbreak size on the Diamond Princess cruise ship: A data-driven analysis. *Int. J. Infect. Dis.* **2020**, *93*, 201–204. [CrossRef] [PubMed]
3. Sayampanathan, A.A.; Heng, C.S.; Pin, P.H.; Pang, J.; Leong, T.Y.; Lee, V.J. Infectivity of asymptomatic versus symptomatic COVID-19. *Lancet* **2021**, *397*, 93–94. [CrossRef]
4. Kirkpatrick, J.N.; Hull, S.C.; Fedson, S.; Mullen, B.; Goodlin, S.J. Scarce-resource allocation and patient triage during the COVID-19 pandemic: JACC review topic of the week. *J. Am. Coll. Cardiol.* **2020**, *76*, 85–92. [CrossRef] [PubMed]
5. Ward, S.; Lindsley, A.; Courter, J.; Assa'ad, A. Clinical testing for COVID-19. *J. Allergy Clin. Immunol.* **2020**, *146*, 23–34. [CrossRef] [PubMed]
6. Dinnes, J.; Deeks, J.J.; Berhane, S.; Taylor, M.; Adriano, A.; Davenport, C.; Dittrich, S.; Emperador, D.; Takwoingi, Y.; Cunningham, J.; et al. Rapid, point-of-care antigen and molecular-based tests for diagnosis of SARS-CoV-2 infection. *Cochrane Database Syst. Rev.* **2021**, *3*, CD013705. [CrossRef]
7. Gopaul, R.; Davis, J.; Gangai, L.; Goetz, L. Practical Diagnostic Accuracy of Nasopharyngeal Swab Testing for Novel Coronavirus Disease 2019 (COVID-19). *West. J. Emerg. Med.* **2020**, *21*, 1–4. [CrossRef]
8. Böger, B.; Fachi, M.M.; Vilhena, R.O.; Cobre, A.F.; Tonin, F.S.; Pontarolo, R. Systematic review with meta-analysis of the accuracy of diagnostic tests for COVID-19. *Am. J. Infect. Control* **2021**, *49*, 21–29. [CrossRef]
9. Araya, S.; Wordofa, M.; Mamo, M.A.; Tsegay, Y.G.; Hordofa, A.; Negesso, A.E.; Fasil, T.; Berhanu, B.; Begashaw, H.; Atlaw, A.; et al. The magnitude of hematological abnormalities among COVID-19 patients in Addis Ababa, Ethiopia. *J. Multidiscip. Healthc.* **2021**, *14*, 545–554. [CrossRef]
10. Davis, J.; Umeh, U.; Saba, R. Treatment of SARS-CoV-2 (COVID-19): A safety perspective. *World J. Pharmacol.* **2021**, *10*, 1–32. [CrossRef]
11. United States Centers for Disease Control and Prevention. Interim Clinical Guidance for Management of Patients with Confirmed Coronavirus Disease (COVID-19). 2020. Available online: https://stacks.cdc.gov/view/cdc/88624 (accessed on 19 May 2022).
12. Tavakolpour, S.; Rakhshandehroo, T.; Wei, E.X.; Rashidian, M. Lymphopenia during the COVID-19 infection: What it shows and what can be learned. *Immunol. Lett.* **2020**, *225*, 31–32. [CrossRef] [PubMed]
13. Xu, P.; Zhou, Q.; Xu, J. Mechanism of thrombocytopenia in COVID-19 patients. *Ann. Hematol.* **2020**, *99*, 1205–1208. [CrossRef] [PubMed]
14. Tanni, F.; Akker, E.; Zaman, M.M.; Figueroa, N.; Tharian, B.; Hupart, K.H. Eosinopenia and COVID-19. *J. Am. Osteopath. Assoc*, 2020, *Epub ahead of print*. [CrossRef]
15. Djangang, N.N.; Peluso, L.; Talamonti, M.; Izzi, A.; Gevenois, P.A.; Garufi, A.; Goffard, J.-C.; Henrard, S.; Severgnini, P.; Vincent, J.-L.; et al. Eosinopenia in COVID-19 patients: A retrospective analysis. *Microorganisms* **2020**, *8*, 1929. [CrossRef] [PubMed]

16. Bzeizi, K.; Abdulla, M.; Mohammed, N.; Alqamish, J.; Jamshidi, N.; Broering, D. Effect of COVID-19 on liver abnormalities: A systematic review and meta-analysis. *Sci. Rep.* **2021**, *11*, 10599. [CrossRef] [PubMed]
17. Wander, P.; Epstein, M.; Bernstein, D. COVID-19 Presenting as Acute Hepatitis. *Am. J. Gastroenterol.* **2020**, *115*, 941–942. [CrossRef] [PubMed]
18. Huang, J.; Cheng, A.; Kumar, R.; Fang, Y.; Chen, G.; Zhu, Y.; Lin, S. Hypoalbuminemia predicts the outcome of COVID-19 independent of age and co-morbidity. *J. Med. Virol.* **2020**, *92*, 2152–2158. [CrossRef] [PubMed]
19. Wu, M.A.; Fossali, T.; Pandolfi, L.; Carsana, L.; Ottolina, D.; Frangipane, V.; Rech, R.; Tosoni, A.; Lopez, G.; Agarossi, A.; et al. Hypoalbuminemia in COVID-19: Assessing the hypothesis for underlying pulmonary capillary leakage. *J. Intern. Med.* **2021**, *289*, 861–872. [CrossRef] [PubMed]
20. Leeflang, M.M.; Rutjes, A.W.; Reitsma, J.B.; Hooft, L.; Bossuyt, P.M. Variation of a test's sensitivity and specificity with disease prevalence. *CMAJ* **2013**, *185*, E537–E544. [CrossRef] [PubMed]
21. Li, J.; Fine, J.P. Assessing the dependence of sensitivity and specificity on prevalence in meta-analysis. *Biostatistics* **2011**, *12*, 710–722. [CrossRef] [PubMed]
22. Conte, G.; Cei, M.; Evangelista, I.; Colombo, A.; Vitale, J.; Mazzone, A.; Mumoli, N. The Meaning of D-Dimer value in COVID-19. *Clin. Appl. Thromb. Hemost.* **2021**, *27*, 10760296211017668. [CrossRef] [PubMed]

*reports*

MDPI

*Article*

# Deep Learning Methods to Reveal Important X-ray Features in COVID-19 Detection: Investigation of Explainability and Feature Reproducibility

**Ioannis D. Apostolopoulos [1,*], Dimitris J. Apostolopoulos [2] and Nikolaos D. Papathanasiou [2]**

[1] Department of Medical Physics, School of Medicine, University of Patras, 265-00 Patras, Greece
[2] Laboratory of Nuclear Medicine, University Hospital of Patras, 265-00 Patras, Greece; dimap@med.upatras.gr (D.J.A.); nikopapath@upatras.gr (N.D.P.)
* Correspondence: ece7216@upnet.gr

**Abstract:** X-ray technology has been recently employed for the detection of the lethal human coronavirus disease 2019 (COVID-19) as a timely, cheap, and helpful ancillary method for diagnosis. The scientific community evaluated deep learning methods to aid in the automatic detection of the disease, utilizing publicly available small samples of X-ray images. In the majority of cases, the results demonstrate the effectiveness of deep learning and suggest valid detection of the disease from X-ray scans. However, little has been investigated regarding the actual findings of deep learning through the image process. In the present study, a large-scale dataset of pulmonary diseases, including COVID-19, was utilized for experiments, aiming to shed light on this issue. For the detection task, MobileNet (v2) was employed, which has been proven very effective in our previous works. Through analytical experiments utilizing feature visualization techniques and altering the input dataset classes, it was suggested that MobileNet (v2) discovers important image findings and not only features. It was demonstrated that MobileNet (v2) is an effective, accurate, and low-computational-cost solution for distinguishing COVID-19 from 12 various other pulmonary abnormalities and normal subjects. This study offers an analysis of image features extracted from MobileNet (v2), aiming to investigate the validity of those features and their medical importance. The pipeline can detect abnormal X-rays with an accuracy of 95.45 ± 1.54% and can distinguish COVID-19 with an accuracy of 89.88 ± 3.66%. The visualized results of the Grad-CAM algorithm provide evidence that the methodology identifies meaningful areas on the images. Finally, the detected image features were reproducible in 98% of the times after repeating the experiment for three times.

**Keywords:** deep learning; COVID-19; explainable artificial intelligence



**Citation:** Apostolopoulos, I.D.; Apostolopoulos, D.J.; Papathanasiou, N.D. Deep Learning Methods to Reveal Important X-ray Features in COVID-19 Detection: Investigation of Explainability and Feature Reproducibility. *Reports* **2022**, *5*, 20. https://doi.org/10.3390/reports5020020

Academic Editors: Toshio Hattori and Yugo Ashino

Received: 21 April 2022
Accepted: 27 May 2022
Published: 31 May 2022



## 1. Introduction

Deep learning has already demonstrated superiority to conventional methods in a variety of medical imaging tasks, including the classification of important diseases using different imaging modalities, such as Computed Tomography (CT), Positron Emission Tomography (PET), and X-ray [1]. The recent human coronavirus disease (COVID-19) poses new challenges for deep learning experts, such as the automatic segmentation and classification of CT or X-ray images that can lead to a timely, accurate, and cost-effective diagnosis. Limitations related to data scarcity have been a major obstacle in designing deep and robust frameworks [2]. Since March 2020, the available X-ray image datasets included no more than 500 images of COVID-19 disease.

Typical imaging findings of COVID-19 lung infection include bilateral, patchy, lower-lobe-predominant, and peripheral ground-glass opacities and/or consolidation. These are mainly identified on CT imaging rather than X-ray, which has lower sensitivity for COVID-19 diagnosis at the level of ≈67–100% [3]. Nevertheless, the scientific community has responded to the aforementioned challenge and has provided first answers as to whether this disease can indeed be detected solely from X-ray images. Several works suggest the utilization of deep learning models, such as Convolutional Neural Networks (CNNs) for diagnosis [4–10]. In most cases, either handcrafted CNNs, or established CNNs in other domains, yield precise and promising results, at least in cases where the COVID-19 disease is adequately visualized in the particular imaging modality. All those networks have been evaluated utilizing approximately the same image sources.

Deep learning has already demonstrated its effectiveness in distinguishing COVID-19 using the particular image datasets. However, the assumption that through deep learning it is possible to diagnose COVID-19 solely on the basis of X-ray images is not valid yet. This is because the available datasets are heavily incomplete due to the following reasons:

a. The samples are too few for deep model training
b. The image information is not accompanied by clinical outcomes.
c. There are few multicenter studies to support the conclusions.
d. The samples commonly illustrate COVID-19 disease of patients showing disease symptoms. Asymptomatic cases are under-represented.

The above issues motivated the scientific community towards applying data augmentation techniques to expand the training sets, add diversity to the data distributions, and enable their models to become robust to transformations.. Nevertheless, the data scarcity issue is not circumvented completely. The question arising at this point is the following: "Besides their undeniably strong predictive power, are the developed deep learning models capable of providing explanations regarding their decisions, informing the actual user of their image findings so as to be trustworthy and accountable?".

Motivated by our previous studies on the automatic identification of COVID-19 from X-rays [5,9] and aiming to shed light on the explainability of deep learning, we performed a deeper analysis on the decision mechanisms of mobile network, a state-of-the-art CNN, that exhibited promising results in our recent study [5]. In previous work of our group [9], the effectiveness of training from scratch strategy against transfer learning is demonstrated, showing that training from scratch may discover potential image biomarkers extracted from X-ray images. This conclusion is based on the comparison of transfer learning with training from scratch. The reader should note that with transfer learning, the classification is mainly based on pre-learned feature extraction knowledge of a particular CNN. This knowledge is obtained by performing an independent training on large-scale datasets of a completely different domain task. Although transfer learning also yields good results, training from scratch improves the classification accuracy. This led the authors to the conclusion that novel and vital image features were extracted from the latter strategy.

In the present work, the feature extraction capabilities of MobileNet (v2) were further analyzed by performing extensive experiments and visualizing the output feature maps. The Grad-CAM algorithm [11] was utilized to reveal the regions where MobileNet (v2) seeks for important features. In this way, a better understanding of the decision mechanism of the network is achieved.

The contributions of this paper can be summarized as follows:

- The successful state-of-the-art network (MobileNet v2) was extensively evaluated in performing multi-class and two-class classification of X-ray images with the aim of identifying images related to the coronavirus disease. Further, the consistency of the reported metrics was assessed by running a 25-times 10-fold cross-validation
- The explainability algorithm (Grad-CAM) was employed to inspect the consistency of the suggested areas of interest across a three-run experiment.
- We present a staged approach for the detection of COVID-19 from X-ray images that exhibited an accuracy of 89.88 $\pm$ 3.66%.

## 2. COVID-19 Detection Based on X-ray Imaging: Recent Studies

The research community has put an enormous effort in developing deep learning pipelines for COVID-19 detection from either computed tomography (CT) scans or X-ray scans. In addition, a large amount of attention has been paid to leveraging explainability methods to visualize the suggested areas of interest as proposed by the models. Hence, model assessment can be based not only on quantitative metrics (such as the accuracy, the sensitivity, and the specificity scores), but also on qualitative evaluation. In this section, we briefly describe major findings and trends found in the latest literature.

Hou and Gao [12] proposed a deep CNN-based platform for COVID-19 detection that could identify COVID-19 cases with an accuracy of 96%. Their model has been trained using a dataset of 1400 chest X-ray images, which includes 400 normal images, 400 images of pneumonia infection from bacteria, 400 images of pneumonia infection by other viruses, and 200 images of pneumonia infection by COVID-19. The authors used the Grad-CAM algorithm to visualize the suggested areas of interest.

Ahsan et al. [13] proposed the utilization of the state-of-the-art networks named Virtual Geometry Group (VGG) and MobileNet (v2) to distinguish between COVID-19 and non-COVID-19 X-rays from an imbalanced dataset of 2191 X-rays. The networks achieved remarkable accuracy, stretching between 91% and 96% and an AUC score of approximately 0.82. The authors used the local interpretable model-agnostic explanations (LIME) [14] method for the visualization of important image areas.

Brunese et al. [4] analyzed 6523 X-ray scans and developed a pipeline for an incremental detection of COVID-19. Their framework identifies pulmonary-disease-related X-rays and then further distinguishes between COVID-19 cases and non-COVID-19 cases. Their model reached an accuracy of 97%. The authors adopted the Grad-CAM algorithm to visualize the feature maps and verified that their model did not focus on irrelevant locations of the image.

In [9], which is a previous study by the authors of this study, a first attempt to evaluate the extracted features of deep learning methods for COVID-19 detection from X-rays revealed evidence that training MobileNets from scratch can extract problem-specific features that could be if medical importance. In addition, an accuracy of 99% in distinguishing between COVID-19 and non-COVID-19 cases from an imbalanced dataset of 3905 scans.

Wang et al. [15] proposed COVID-Net, a tailored CNN trained on a dataset of 13,975 X-ray scans. They achieved an accuracy of 93.3% in distinguishing between normal, common pneumonia, and COVID-19-related pneumonia images. The authors employed the GSInquire method [16] to plot the associated critical factors on the image. COVID-Net primarily leveraged areas in the lungs in the X-ray images as the main critical factors in determining whether an X-ray image is of a patient with COVID-19.

Thorough interpretation and examination of the explainability methods is missing from the majority of the related studies, although particular explainability methods have been employed.

## 3. Materials and Methods

### 3.1. Deep Learning with Mobile Networks

The main advantage of CNNs lies in extracting new features from the input data distributions (i.e., images), thereby bypassing the manual feature extraction process, which is traditionally performed in image analysis task with machine learning methods [17].

Each convolution layer in a CNN is processing the output of the previous layer by applying new filters and extracting new features. Due to the fact that the convolutional layers are hierarchically ordered, features directly from the original image are only extracted by the first convolutional layer, whereas the other layers process the outputs of each other [18]. In this way, a slow introduction to large amounts of filters is achieved, whilst underlying features may be revealed during the later layers. The general rule of thumb relates the effectiveness of the network with the number of convolutional layers. This is why deep networks are generally superior, provided that adequate amounts of image data are present. In cases where the dataset's size is not large enough to feed a deep network, three solutions are commonly proposed:

(a) The selection of a simpler CNN, which contains less trainable parameters and fits in the particular data well.

(b) Transfer learning [19], utilizing deep and complex CNNs, but freezing their layers, thereby decreasing the trainable parameters and allowing for knowledge transfer, following their training on large image datasets.
(c) Data augmentation methods to increase the training set size, such as geometric transformation (rotation, sheer) and pixel-level transformations (equalizations, grey-level alterations) [20].

In this study, MobileNet (v2) [21] was selected for the classification task, which is a state-of-the-art CNN and has been recently employed and evaluated by the authors [9]. In that particular study, MobileNet (v2) was found to be superior for false negative reduction in COVID-19 detection, in comparison with a variety of famous CNNs, including Inception (v3) [22] and Xception [23].

The superiority of MobileNet (v2) in reducing the false negatives for the detection of COVID-19, compared to other famous CNNs, is demonstrated in [5,9]. Moreover, this CNN introduces a smaller number of parameters compared to other CNNs, which makes it appropriate for swift training and portable applications. The inventors of this network made use of depth-wise separable convolution [22] to drastically reduce the number of learnable parameters in CNNs, thereby reducing the computational cost.

MobileNet (v2) is employed and trained from scratch, letting it fit in the training set completely and without making any adjustments to its structure. Every parameter is made trainable. In essence, the obtained weights from its training on ImageNet challenge dataset [24] are erased. This methodology is selected to allow for problem-specific feature extraction. At the top of the network, wherein the final feature maps are produced, a global average pooling [25] layer is applied to reduce overfitting. This layer connects the final feature map directly to the dense layer at the top of the CNN, which consists of 2500 nodes. Another dense layer of two outputs is inserted for the binary classification of the inputs. Batch normalization and dropout layers aid in the reduction of overfitting and are part of the densely connected layers at the top of the network.

### 3.2. *Image Dataset*

#### 3.2.1. COVID-19, Common Bacterial and Viral Pneumonia X-ray Scans

X-ray images corresponding to confirmed cases infected by the virus SARS-CoV-2 were selected. Through extensive research, a collection of 1281 well-visualized, confirmed pathological X-ray images was created. The final collection included X-rays from a publicly available repository [26]. Contributing institutions of this repository include the Indian Institute of Science, the PES University, the M. S. Ramaiah Institute of Technology, and Concordia University. The publishers of this data did not include important clinical information, which could be useful for a more robust analysis.

#### 3.2.2. Pulmonary Diseases Detected from X-ray Scans

The National Institutes of Health (NIH) X-ray repository was accessed and analyzed. It comprises 112.120 frontal-view X-ray images of 30.805 unique patients with the text-mined 14 disease image labels [27].

Those images were extracted from the clinical PACS database at the National Institutes of Health Clinical Center in USA. The contents of this archive contained 14 common thoracic pathologies, namely, atelectasis, consolidation, infiltration, pneumothorax, edema, emphysema, fibrosis, effusion, pneumonia, pleural thickening, cardiomegaly, nodule, mass, and hernia. This dataset is significantly more representative of the real patient population distributions and realistic clinical diagnosis challenges than any previous chest X-ray datasets. The medical reports were analyzed by an automatic text-mining model that assigned the corresponding labels according to its text-mining procedure. This method has been initially adopted by the creators of the dataset and is not part of this work.

The final dataset characteristics are summarized in Table 1. In Figure 1, selected samples from major classes are presented.

**Table 1.** Characteristics of the dataset.

| Dataset Name | Classes | Description | Total Number of Images |
|---|---|---|---|
| Multiclass | 14 | Huge dataset including normal, COVID-19, and 12 categories of abnormal X-ray scans. | 11,984 |
| Abnormality detection | 2 | Huge dataset consisting of normal and abnormal X-ray scans. In the abnormal class, X-rays corresponding to COVID-19 were also included. | 13,320 |
| Abnormality discrimination | 13 | Dataset containing 13 classes corresponding to 13 abnormalities, including COVID-19. | 8714 |
| COVID-19 detection | 2 | Dataset containing COVID-19 X-ray scans and a second class of both normal and abnormal X-ray scans (selected samples). | 2935 |

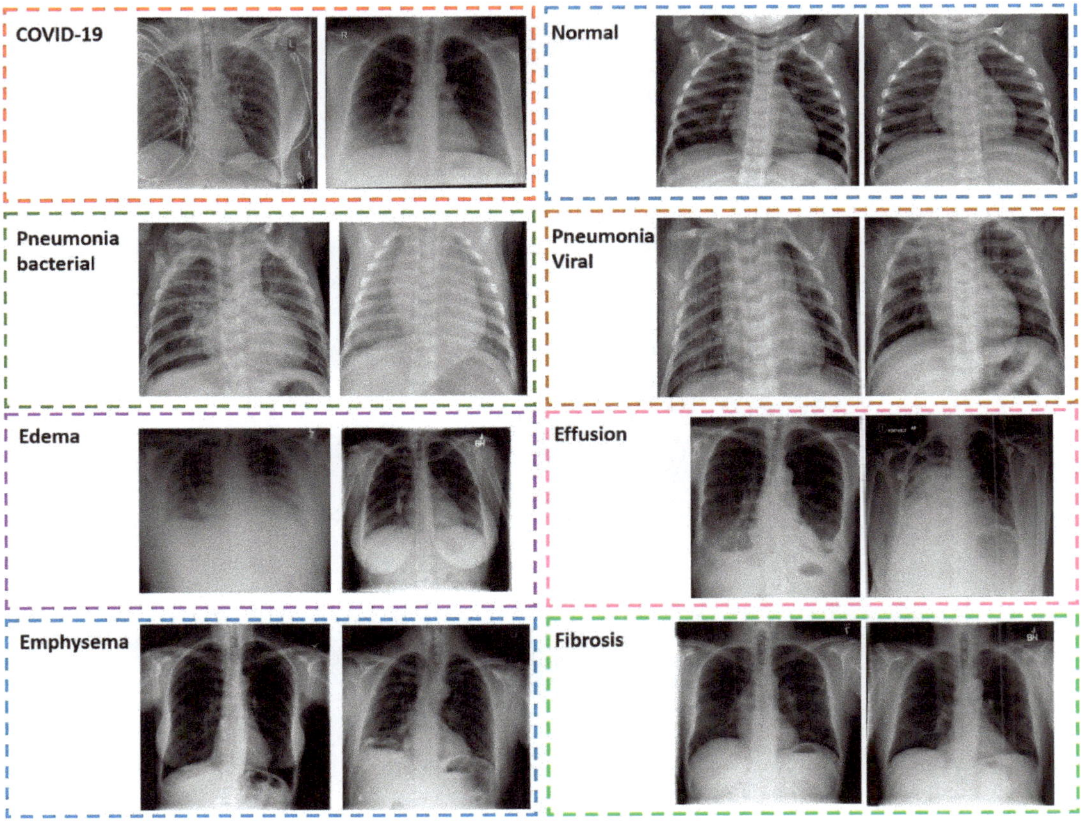


**Figure 1.** Samples of some classes belonging to abnormalities.

For the normal class in the abnormality detection dataset, we added some more images to make the classes approximately even in terms of number of images included. All image sizes were adjusted to 400 × 400 pixels (height, width). The resolution of the images varied from 72 to 150 pixels/inch, and the bit depth if the image was 8 bits.

### 3.3. Data Augmentation Techniques

Data augmentation is an important method in deep learning applications and research, mainly utilized for two reasons. The first reason is the data scarcity, which impedes deep learning models adoption to the domain of interest. Few images are usually not enough for a deep learning framework to train on [28], especially in cases where the classification should be based on deep features and not obvious and low-level characteristics (e.g., colors). With data augmentation, the initial training set can be broadly expanded by applying a variety of transformations on the original images. In this way, the model learns to ignore irrelevant characteristics and improves its spatial capabilities [29]. For example, applying random rotations directs the model towards seeking for patterns in moving positions.

In the present research, the following augmentations to the training sets to expand the available data and to increase the generalization capabilities of the experimental deep learning network were applied:

a. Random rotations;
b. Horizontal flips;
c. Height and width shifts.

The reader should note that data augmentation was performed on-line. During each 10-fold repetition, the augmented images were supplied to the classification model, whilst the test sets remained untouched. In this way, each training image was augmented to produce contextual images by performing the abovementioned augmentations.

Random rotations were restricted to −20 to 20 degrees, and height and width shifts were restricted to ±20 pixels. The ±20 degree of rotation was empirically selected to avoid excessive rotations, whilst letting the model develop robustness to spatial discrepancies between the image findings, for example, the position of the lungs.

### 3.4. Experiments

The initial dataset included 14 classes. On the basis of this dataset, subsets were created according to Figure 2 and Table 2. The intention of the experimental phases and the methods utilized are summarized in Table 2.

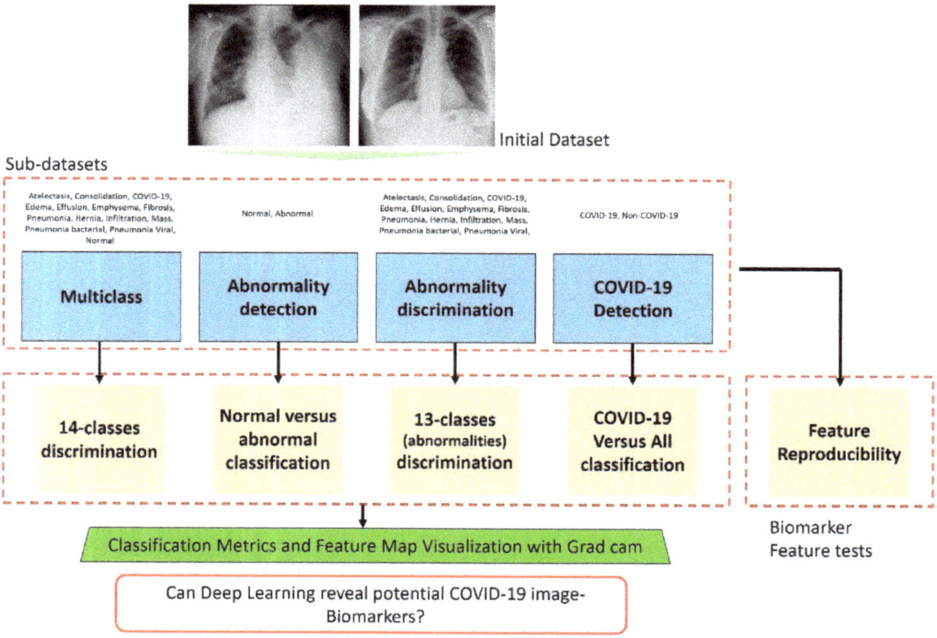


**Figure 2.** Overview of the experiments of this study.

**Table 2.** Overview of the experiments.

| Experiment Name | Aim | Classes Utilized |
|---|---|---|
| Multiclass | Evaluate the effectiveness of MobileNet (v2) in multiclass discrimination | 13 respiratory infections and the class normal. |
| Abnormality detection | Evaluate the effectiveness of MobileNet (v2) in abnormality detection | All respiratory infection classes, including COVID-19, were joined together into a big class. Normal X-ray scans constituted the second class. |
| Abnormality discrimination | Evaluate the effectiveness of MobileNet (v2) in distinguishing between various diseases, including COVID-19 | 13 classes of X-rays corresponding to 13 respiratory infections |
| COVID-19 detection | Evaluate the effectiveness of MobileNet (v2) in distinguishing between COVID-19 and non-COVID-19 X-ray scans | Selected samples from the 12 respiratory diseases constituted the first class, whereas the second class referred to COVID-19. |
| Reproducibility | Evaluate the reproducibility of features when MobileNet is trained distinguishing between COVID-19 and non-COVID-19 X-ray scans | Selected samples from the 12 respiratory diseases constituted the first class, whereas the second class referred to COVID-19. |

For all the experiments, the parameters of the model were retained. The batch size was 16 and the number of epochs varied from 30 to 40 according to the validation loss. All experiments were performed in a Python programming language environment making use of the Tensorflow library. An Intel Core i5-9400F CPU at 2.90 GHz computer equipped with 64 Gb RAM and a GeForce RTX 2060 Super was the main infrastructure for the experiments. In Figure 2, an overview of the study is presented.

## 4. Results

### 4.1. Results of Multiclass Classification

For the multiclass classification, MobileNet (v2) achieved sub-optimal performance, as presented in Table 3. The model achieved good classification for the bacterial pneumonia, normal, mass, COVID-19, and consolidation classes (confusion matrix is available in the Supplementary Material). Especially for COVID-19, 1095 true positives were recorded (out of 1281), corresponding to 85.48% accuracy. Moreover, only 12 false negatives were reported. This observation indicates that, despite the overall sub-optimal performance, the model correctly captured COVID-19 image characteristics that distinguish these images from the rest. Moreover, the normal class was adequately predicted, with 2439 true normal predictions and 36 predictions that were mistakenly identified as normal.

**Table 3.** Classification results. The mean accuracy for the complete 10-fold and standard deviation for the performance between the 10-fold are also reported.

| Dataset | Accuracy (%) | AUC Score (%) |
|---|---|---|
| Multiclass | $73.11 \pm 2.21$ | $94.07 \pm 1.45$ |
| Abnormality detection | $95.45 \pm 1.54$ | $98.92 \pm 0.83$ |
| Abnormality discrimination | $62.26 \pm 4.21$ | $90.93 \pm 1.57$ |
| COVID-19 detection | $89.88 \pm 3.66$ | $96.26 \pm 2.14$ |

Figure 3 illustrates the results of the multiclass classification and selected samples from the outputs of the Grad-CAM algorithm. The red areas of the image suggest the region where the model has captured significant features. Blue areas are considered neutral regions, where no features, or insignificant features, are found. The reader can observe that COVID-19 features were mainly discovered in the center of the respiratory system and that those regions indeed contained COVID-19 findings. Moreover, Figure 3 illustrates misclassified instances. For COVID-19, it was observed that the misclassified image did not contain any information in the center of the respiratory system, perhaps leading the model to falsely recognize specific patterns. In fact, it was observed that the model looked for patterns in the upper right of the image, which was a completely irrelevant region. This issue highlights the flaws of the model and its decision mechanism.

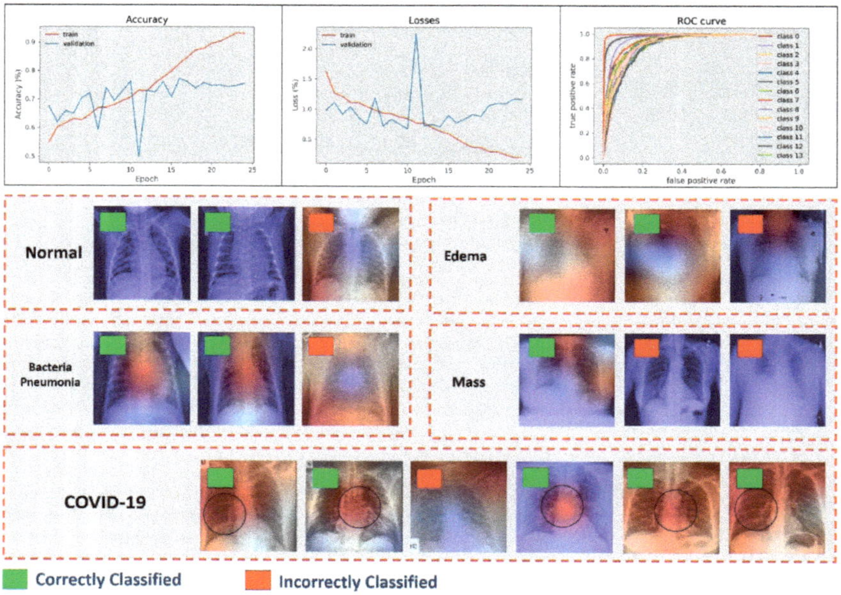


**Figure 3.** Visualized results for the multiclass classification. Train-validation accuracy and loss over the training epochs and AUC scores for the classes are presented in the top graph. Selected output images of the Grad-CAM implementation are visualized. Each dashed-line box presents a true class, while the green and red boxes distinguish between correctly classified samples and mistakes, respectively.

Taking into consideration both the good classification accuracy in distinguishing the COVID-19 class from the other classes and the Grad-CAM visualizations, it can be assumed that in the majority of COVID-19 X-rays, potential biomarkers are discovered. However, this assumption requires further investigation.

### *4.2. Results of Abnormality Detection (Two-Class)*

Abnormality detection tests produce excellent results. As observed in Table 3, 95.45% accuracy was achieved. The total number of false negatives was 211, as the confusion matrix of Figure 4 suggests. It is clearly concluded that the model achieved great capability in distinguishing normal from abnormal X-ray scans. In Figure 4, it is observed that the Grad-CAM results confirmed the assumption that the model seeks for patterns in the correct regions of the respiratory system.

Due to the fact that all types of infections were grouped together in one class (abnormal), the model learned global features explaining the presence of any disease and did not learn the visual differences that each disease may display in the image. However, there are still images were the Grad-CAM exposed some limitations and flaws of the model. In essence, there were images where the model was unable to locate the region of interest correctly, despite the correct classification.

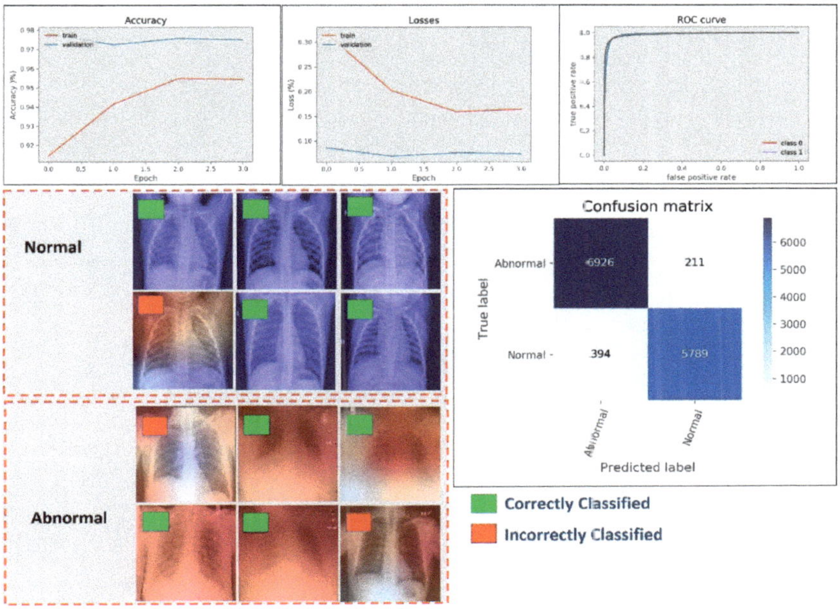


**Figure 4.** Visualized results for the abnormality detection. Train-validation accuracy and loss over the training epochs and AUC scores for the classes are presented in the top graph. Selected output images of the Grad-CAM implementation are visualized. Each dashed-line box presents a true class, while the green and red boxes distinguish between correctly classified samples and mistakes, respectively.

### *4.3. Results of Abnormality Discrimination*

The abnormality discrimination experiment produced poor performance due to the presence of many respiratory diseases, many of which produce overlapping X-ray results. Specifically, 62.26% accuracy was achieved. In the Supplementary Material, the confusion matrix is provided. It is observed that MobileNet (v2) achieved good classification results for COVID-19 (1110 true positives, 171 false negatives, 168 false positives), mass (2427 true positives, 78 false negatives, 14 false positives), and bacterial pneumonia (1108 true positives, 25 false negatives, 14 false positives). For the rest of the diseases, the discrimination task performed sub-optimally. As is observed in Figure 5, the validation accuracy did not improve, despite the improvement in the training accuracy. The same phenomenon applied to the validation loss. Those results highlighted the inability of the model to capture and learn discriminant features. Data augmentation has not been beneficial enough to improve its discrimination ability for the majority of the diseases. However, due to the fact that the aim of this study was focused on COVID-19, the reason behind the sub-optimal performance for multi-class classification was not further investigated in terms of the type of the extracted features. Moreover, the imbalance of the dataset hindered thorough and extensive evaluation. Several classes were underrepresented. As a result, a deep analysis on the extracted features of those classes would yield negligible outcomes.

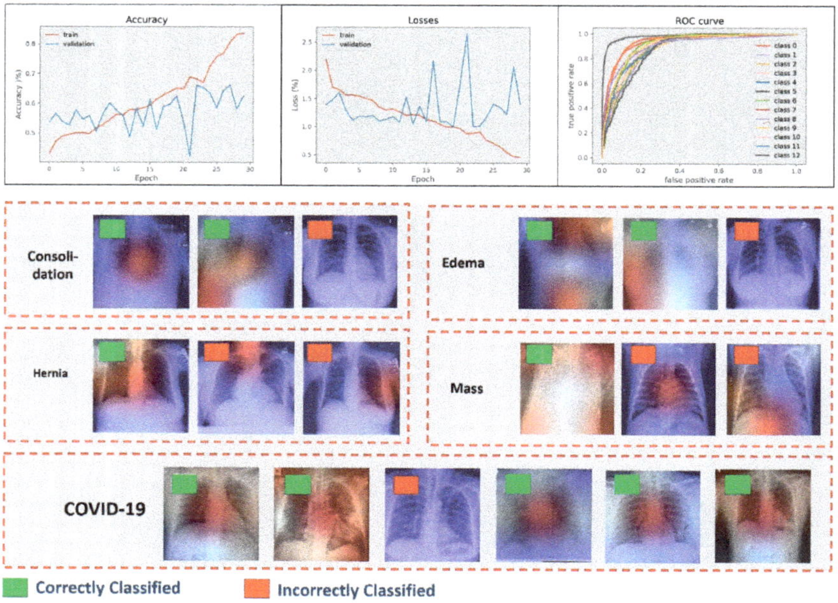


**Figure 5.** Visualized results for the abnormality discrimination. Train-validation accuracy and loss over the training epochs and AUC scores for the classes are presented in the top graph. Selected output images of the Grad-CAM implementation are visualized. Each dashed-line box presents a true class, while the green and red boxes distinguish between correctly classified samples and mistakes, respectively.

### *4.4. Results of COVID-19 Detection*

For the COVID-19 detection experiment, top performance was observed, with the classification accuracy reaching 89.88%. Specifically, as the confusion matrix of Figure 6 suggests, 1154 COVID-19 X-ray images were correctly identified out of 1281. The total number of false negatives was 127, whilst the total number of false positives was 170. The Grad-CAM output suggested that the model looked for COVID-19 related features, focusing on the upper respiratory system. For the non-COVID-19 class, the model based its predictions on the collection of different features found in various regions of the image.

A significant observation is that in every experiment, COVID-19 images were correctly classified, either as part of a multiclass dataset or as the major class in a two-class dataset. There is significant evidence that this stability derives from unique image features discovered by the model in those processes. The results of the upcoming reproducibility test favor this assumption.

### *4.5. Results of Feature Reproducibility in COVID-19 Detection*

The two-class classification routine has been repeated for 25 times, and the reported accuracy is assessed for statistical significance. A one-sample t-test was performed, assuming that there is no difference in the mean accuracy score between the 25 runs (i.e., setting the second variable equal to the first obtained accuracy). Table 4 presents the accuracy of each run. As can be observed from Table 5, the $p$-value was greater than 0.05. Hence, there is no evidence that the mean accuracy obtained from the 25 runs deviated from the expected values. To summarize, the t-test results suggest that the model is stable in reproducing the particular results in terms of accuracy.

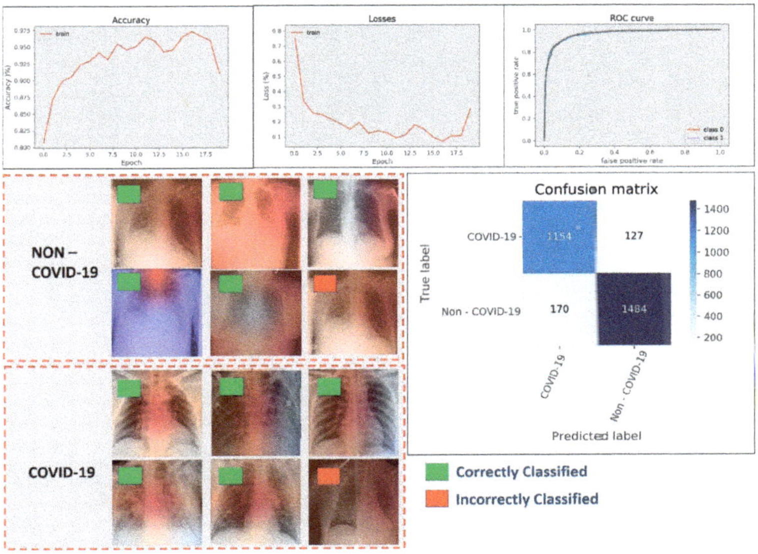


**Figure 6.** Visualized results for COVID-19 detection. Train-validation accuracy and loss over the training epochs and AUC scores for the classes are presented in the top graph. Selected output images of the Grad-CAM implementation are visualized. Each dashed-line box presents a true class, while the green and red boxes distinguish between correctly classified samples and mistakes, respectively.

**Table 4.** Classification results of 25-run 10-fold cross-validation when training and testing MobileNet (v2) using the COVID-19 detection dataset (two classes).

| Run | Mean Accuracy (%) |
|---|---|
| 1 | 89.88 |
| 2 | 91.23 |
| 3 | 88.54 |
| 4 | 92.14 |
| 5 | 89.24 |
| 6 | 89.36 |
| 7 | 88.53 |
| 8 | 88.86 |
| 9 | 90.76 |
| 10 | 88.86 |
| 11 | 91.23 |
| 12 | 90.37 |
| 13 | 92.43 |
| 14 | 89.02 |
| 15 | 89.67 |
| 16 | 88.54 |
| 17 | 90.79 |
| 18 | 89.36 |
| 19 | 87.13 |
| 20 | 91.23 |
| 21 | 86.98 |
| 22 | 88.86 |
| 24 | 92.41 |
| 24 | 90.66 |
| 25 | 91.23 |
| Overall | 89.89 |
| Std | ±1.49 |

**Table 5.** Statistical significance results of 25-run 10-fold cross-validation when training and testing MobileNet (v2) using the COVID-19 detection dataset (two classes).

| Factor | Result for Accuracy |
|---|---|
| Mean | 89.89 |
| Variance | 2.24 |
| Observations | 25 |
| T-statistic | 0.0413 |
| *p*-value | 0.4836 |

It was observed that there was no significant variation of the accuracy over the 25 runs. As a result, the comparison between the Grad-CAM visualization outputs of the 25 runs was performed using the outputs of three runs. We performed a case-to-case examination of the similarity of the produced Grad-CAM images to inspect whether the suggested areas of interest remained consistent across the three independent trainings. The evaluation was conducted by two of the authors (J.A. and N.P.) by visually inspecting the suggested areas in terms of their relative position inside the image. The methodology of this experiment is better understood in Figure 7. Figure 8 illustrates the Grad-CAM outputs obtained by three independent trainings of MobileNet (v2). All parameters, hyper-parameters, and image sets were retained during the three separate trainings.

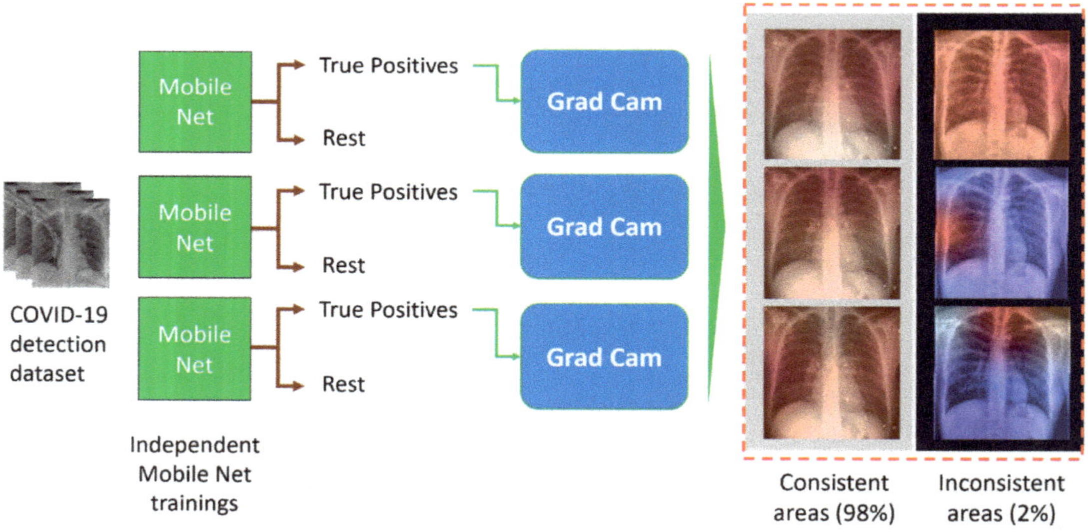


**Figure 7.** Reproducibility of test methodology.

In approximately 98% of the visualized Grad-CAM maps, the features were reproduced and the suggested areas remained the same. It was noted that there was a disagreement between the three independent training–testing results for 2% of the images. The reader should note that Figure 8 illustrates only true positive (true COVID-19) images, aiming to investigate whether the features were reproduced for the specific examples and not for the incorrectly classified instances.

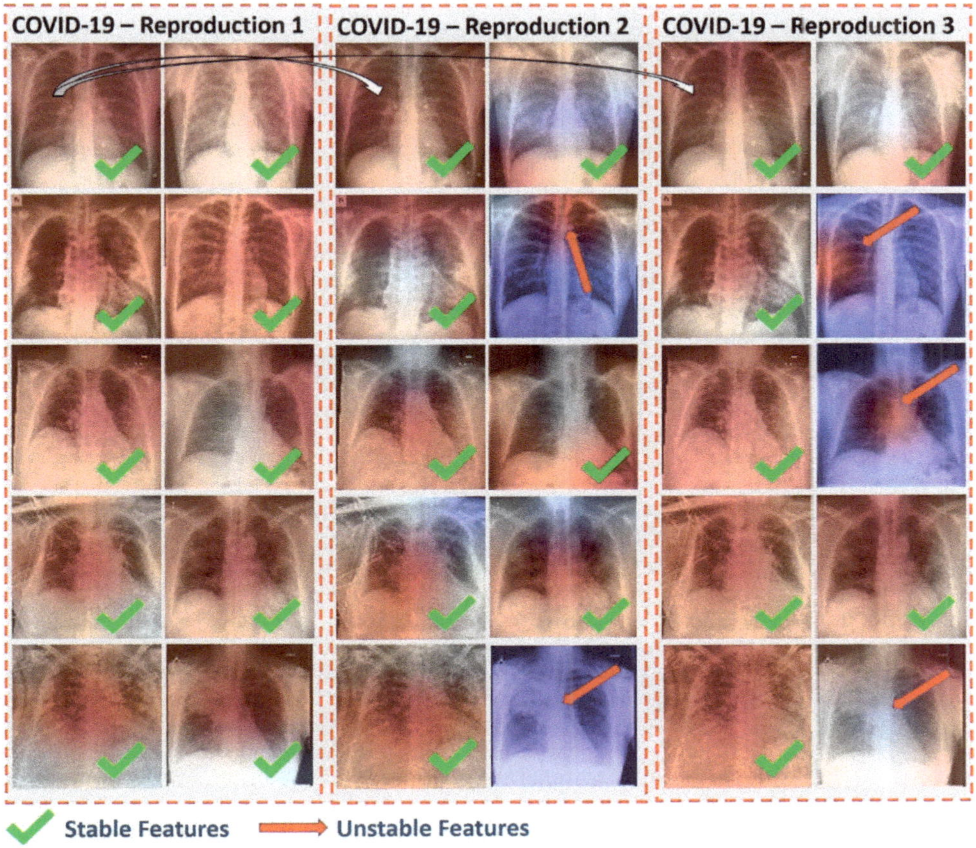


**Figure 8.** Results of the reproducibility tests. Each dashed-line box presents Grad-CAM results for 10 images of COVID-19 infection. The visualized maps correspond to the same images for each group. The green tick mark suggests feature reproducibility and the red arrow suggests failure to reproduce specific features, leading to misclassification.

It was observed that a few discovered features are not always reproducible (2%). Figure 8 provides regions of specific images where the discovered features in the first training were not re-discovered during the second or third training. The classification accuracy remained top-level (approximately 90%) for each repetition. This is a conflicting situation. The reasons behind this phenomenon can vary:

(a) Some of the COVID-19 images may contain annotations that are recognized by the model as features. Although the data were tested, the non-official nature of the dataset source led us to not be completely sure about the origin of the images and the pre-processing that may have taken place.
(b) The learning capacity of MobileNet (v2) is not enough to capture all significant features, leading to the exclusion of some of them.
(c) Data augmentation fails to improve the model's capability in capturing global and important features completely, thereby allowing for irrelevant feature discovery.

## 5. Discussion

Deep Learning enabled the extraction of a massive amount of low- and high-level features from medical images. Those features may represent important biomarkers, closely related to the corresponding diseases. However, deep learning methods lack the ability to specifically assess these features. The extracted features are not well-defined and usually refer to combinations of findings inside the image. This issue derives from the millions of complex mathematical procedures incorporated into deep models. Tracking the extracted features is not an easy task. The above issue raises concern about the trustfulness of such models for medical image classification tasks. For the recent COVID-19 disease, deep learning has been proven to be helpful in early detection, utilizing only X-ray scans. Little has been yet investigated as to why all deep learning models yield top results in a variety of scientific papers.

This study was focused on revealing evidence supporting the assumption that COVID-19 imprints specific pattern-stamps on the X-rays, which testify to its existence. The results provide strong evidence that MobileNet (v2) can capture those underlying signatures and reveal them. However, in many occasions, the MobileNet (v2) model was unable to locate the proper regions of interest, even if the classification was correct. In essence, the decision outcome was not verified on a correct basis. It is fair to assume that the model was deceived, and the associated features were irrelevant. This behavior raises many questions and mandates future research. Nevertheless, the majority of samples demonstrated a correct model reasoning and require further attention.

The experiments were based on the recently introduced Grad-CAM algorithm, which kept track of the learned weights in a way similar to backpropagation of a trained model. The experimental tests have been repeated three times to investigate the reproducibility of those regions, which contained the suggested features. It was found that in 98% of the samples, the suggested areas remained consistent. Moreover, the model insists on suggesting specific regions of the image that helped in distinguishing COVID-19 from both normal X-rays and X-rays corresponding to other respiratory and lung diseases. With the aid of those experiments, it is fair to assume that, out of the millions of extracted image features, there are potential features of medical importance.

Besides the demonstrated effectiveness of MobileNet (v2), this network is also suitable for mobile applications due to its inherently low computational requirements [21]. In the present work, it took approximately 70 min for a complete 40-epoch training of MobileNet (v2) using a dataset of 11,984 images (of size $400 \times 400$) and whilst performing online data augmentation. The reader shall recall that the experiments were performed using an ordinary computer. The trained model can process a new image input and provide both classification and Grad-CAM generation in less than one second. The latter boosts the significance of our work because limited computational costs and low model complexity are highly desirable in modern medical technology solutions, which can operate in real time.

This study has a number of limitations. Firstly, due to COVID-19 data scarcity, every publicly available image dataset related to COVID-19 is incomplete it terms of clinical data, verification, specific annotations, demographic details, and more. Those issues hinder the development of models that will approach the problem holistically. For example, Tartaglione et al. [30] highlight that either missing or imbalanced demographic information can result in biased models. Moreover, real-life evaluation is mandatory to verify the validity of the results, due to the above issue. Secondly, the experts' opinion regarding each sample of the image involved in this study was also missing from the image datasets. Hence, it is not possible to compare the model's decisions with that of the medical experts. This is an important limitation of the study, and we intend to suggest solutions in future research. Thirdly, this study used only the Grad-CAM algorithm for visualizing the suggested areas of interest. Although Grad-CAM is extensively used in related works, its performance can sometimes be sub-optimal [31]. Future studies can consider employing more explainability tools, such as saliency maps visualization [31] and the LIME [14] and the Shapley Additive explanations (SHAP) methods [32]. Moreover, the reader shall recall that the model underperformed in abnormality discrimination, failing to provide acceptable classification metrics for a number of pulmonary defects and diseases. Although this study is focused on COVID-19 detection rather than abnormality discrimination, the inability of the model to discriminate other pulmonary diseases is a limitation that cannot be overlooked.

During the experiments, it has also been revealed that a more accurate diagnosis of COVID-19 involves a two-stage approach (Figure 9). During the first stage, the input X-ray is analyzed for pathological findings, with 95.45% certainty. If the image is abnormal, the second stage takes place. The X-ray is further analyzed for COVID-19 detection, with 89.89% certainty. If the corresponding X-ray is not identified as COVID-19 class, an optional third stage may take place, where the image is analyzed for other abnormalities. The latter stage was not further explored in the particular research study.

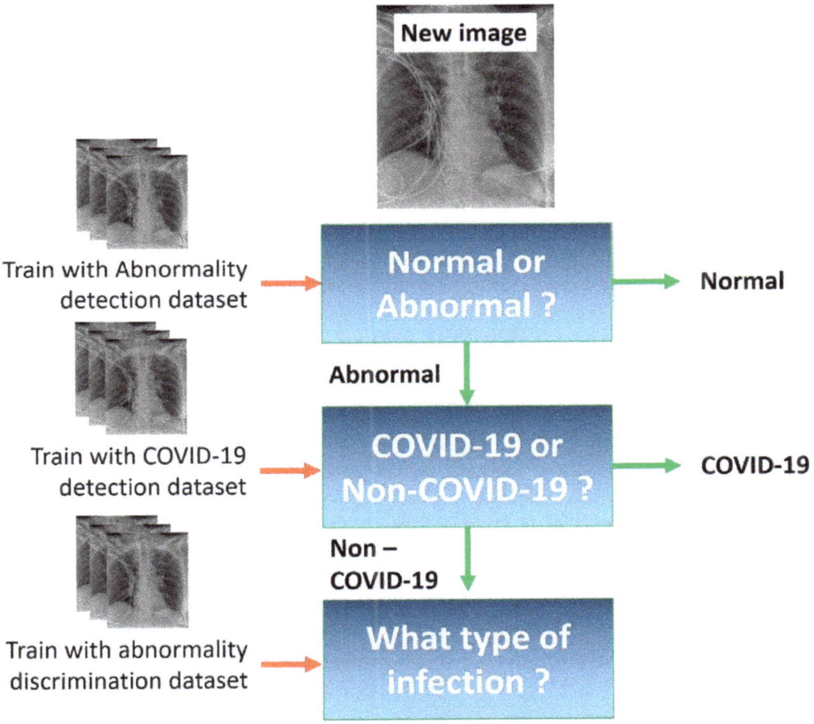


**Figure 9.** Suggestion for more accurate classification based on the results of the study.

The scope of the study is not to present a framework that exhibits classification metrics superior to the related works but to investigate the extracted image features as to their validity and importance. Nevertheless, the classification accuracy of the presented framework competes with the recent literature (Table 6). The reader shall recall that this work utilizes a large collection of X-ray images that belong to many classes. This poses additional challenges to the classification model.

**Table 6.** Comparison with related studies.

| Study | Method | Test Data Size | Classes | Accuracy |
|---|---|---|---|---|
| Hou and Gao [12] | Deep CNN | 400 | 4 (normal, bacterial pneumonia, viral pneumonia, COVID-19) | 96% (COVID-19 vs. ALL) |
| Ahsan et al. [13] | VGG, MobilNet (v2) | 518 | 2 (COVID-19, non-COVID-19) | 95% |
| Brunese et al. [4] | VGG-16 | 1100 | 2 (COVID-19, other disease) | 97% |
| Apostolopoulos et al. [5] | MobileNet (v2) | 1428 | 3 (normal, pneumonia, COVID-19) | 93% |
| Apostolopoulos et al. [5] | MobileNet (v2) | 1428 | 2 (COVID-19, non-COVID-19) | 93% |
| Apostolopoulos et al. [9] | MobileNet (v2) | 3905 | 2 (COVID-19, non-COVID-19) | 99% |
| Apostolopoulos et al. [9] | MobileNet (v2) | 3905 | 7 (COVID-19, normal, 6 abnormal classes) | 87% |
| Wang et al. [15] | tailored CNN (COVID-Net) | 300 | 3 (normal, pneumonia, COVID-19) | 93% |
| This study | MobileNet (v2) | 13,320 | 2 (COVID-19, other abnormal X-ray) | 90% |
| This study | MobileNet (v2) | 11,984 | 7 (normal, COVID-19, 5 abnormal classes) | 73% |

## 6. Conclusions

For the present study, a collection of 11,984 images corresponding to 12 different respiratory–lung abnormalities, including COVID-19 and normal X-ray scans, was utilized. Five independent experiments were performed. In the first experiment, the 14-class dataset is used to evaluate MobileNet (v2) in distinguishing between the complete dataset classes. MobileNet (v2) was found to be superior to other relative state-of-the-art CNNs in previous studies conducted by the authoring team [4,8]. In the second experiment, two-class (normal vs. abnormal) classification was performed. In the third experiment, a 13-class dataset was utilized to distinguish between abnormal classes. In the fourth experiment, two-class (COVID-19 vs. non-COVID-19) classification was performed. Finally, the last experiment was repeated three times in order to investigate the reproducibility of the extracted features and to assess the explainability of the model. Grad-CAM visualizations and accuracy metrics yielded strong evidence that COVID-19 image features can be detected with the deep learning approach, specifically with MobileNet v2. Moreover, it was demonstrated that MobileNet (v2) is an effective CNN for automatic COVID-19 detection, which could even be embedded in portable diagnostic systems due to its inherent low computational cost and its ability to process a new image in less than a second, at least in this particular study. Finally, a staged classification approach is suggested for diagnosing COVID-19, which exhibits an accuracy of 89.89%.

**Supplementary Materials:** The following supporting information can be downloaded at https://www.mdpi.com/article/10.3390/reports5020020/s1, Figure S1: Confusion Matrix for the Multiclass dataset; Figure S2: Confusion Matrix for the Abnormality discrimination dataset; Table S1: MobileNet (v2) parameters and hyper-parameters.

**Author Contributions:** Conceptualization, D.J.A. and N.D.P.; methodology, D.J.A.; software, D.J.A.; validation, D.J.A., N.D.P. and I.D.A.; writing—original draft preparation, I.D.A.; writing—review and editing, D.J.A., N.D.P. and I.D.A.; supervision, I.D.A. All authors have read and agreed to the published version of the manuscript.

**Funding:** This research received no external funding.

**Institutional Review Board Statement:** Not applicable.

**Informed Consent Statement:** Not applicable.

**Data Availability Statement:** All relative datasets are publicly available.

**Conflicts of Interest:** The authors declare no conflict of interest.

## References

1. Sahiner, B.; Pezeshk, A.; Hadjiiski, L.M.; Wang, X.; Drukker, K.; Cha, K.H.; Summers, R.M.; Giger, M.L. Deep learning in medical imaging and radiation therapy. *Med. Phys.* **2019**, *46*, e1–e36. [CrossRef] [PubMed]
2. Sedik, A.; Iliyasu, A.M.; El-Rahiem, A.; Abdel Samea, M.E.; Abdel-Raheem, A.; Hammad, M.; Peng, J.; El-Samie, A.; Fathi, E.; El-Latif, A.A.A.; et al. Deploying machine and deep learning models for efficient data-augmented detection of COVID-19 infections. *Viruses* **2020**, *12*, 769. [CrossRef] [PubMed]
3. Kovács, A.; Palásti, P.; Veréb, D.; Bozsik, B.; Palkó, A.; Kincses, Z.T. The Sensitivity and Specificity of Chest CT in the Diagnosis of COVID-19. *Eur. Radiol.* **2021**, *31*, 2819–2824. [CrossRef] [PubMed]
4. Brunese, L.; Mercaldo, F.; Reginelli, A.; Santone, A. Explainable deep learning for pulmonary disease and coronavirus COVID-19 detection from X-rays. *Comput. Methods Progr. Biomed.* **2020**, *196*, 105608. [CrossRef]
5. Apostolopoulos, I.D.; Mpesiana, T.A. COVID-19: Automatic Detection from X-Ray Images Utilizing Transfer Learning with Convolutional Neural Networks. *Phys. Eng. Sci. Med.* **2020**, *43*, 635–640. [CrossRef]
6. Das, N.N.; Kumar, N.; Kaur, M.; Kumar, V.; Singh, D. Automated deep transfer learning-based approach for detection of COVID-19 infection in chest X-rays. *IRBM* **2020**, *43*, 114–119.
7. Gozes, O.; Frid-Adar, M.; Greenspan, H.; Browning, P.D.; Zhang, H.; Ji, W.; Bernheim, A.; Siegel, E. Rapid ai development cycle for the coronavirus (COVID-19) pandemic: Initial results for automated detection & patient monitoring using deep learning ct image analysis. *arXiv* **2020**, arXiv:2003.05037.
8. Afshar, P.; Heidarian, S.; Naderkhani, F.; Oikonomou, A.; Plataniotis, K.N.; Mohammadi, A. Covid-caps: A capsule network-based framework for identification of COVID-19 cases from X-ray images. *arXiv* **2020**, arXiv:2004.02696. [CrossRef]
9. Apostolopoulos, I.D.; Aznaouridis, S.I.; Tzani, M.A. Extracting Possibly Representative COVID-19 Biomarkers from X-ray Images with Deep Learning Approach and Image Data Related to Pulmonary Diseases. *J. Med. Biol. Eng.* **2020**, *40*, 462–469. [CrossRef]
10. Ozturk, T.; Talo, M.; Yildirim, E.A.; Baloglu, U.B.; Yildirim, O.; Acharya, U.R. Automated detection of COVID-19 cases using deep neural networks with X-ray images. *Comput. Biol. Med.* **2020**, *121*, 103792. [CrossRef]
11. Selvaraju, R.R.; Cogswell, M.; Das, A.; Vedantam, R.; Parikh, D.; Batra, D. Grad-CAM: Visual Explanations from Deep Networks via Gradient-Based Localization. *Int. J. Comput. Vis.* **2020**, *128*, 336–359. [CrossRef]
12. Hou, J.; Gao, T. Explainable DCNN Based Chest X-ray Image Analysis and Classification for COVID-19 Pneumonia Detection. *Sci. Rep.* **2021**, *11*, 16071. [CrossRef] [PubMed]
13. Ahsan, M.M.; Nazim, R.; Siddique, Z.; Huebner, P. Detection of COVID-19 Patients from CT Scan and Chest X-ray Data Using Modified MobileNetV2 and LIME. *Healthcare* **2021**, *9*, 1099. [CrossRef] [PubMed]
14. Palatnik de Sousa, I.; Maria Bernardes Rebuzzi Vellasco, M.; Costa da Silva, E. Local Interpretable Model-Agnostic Explanations for Classification of Lymph Node Metastases. *Sensors* **2019**, *19*, 2969. [CrossRef]
15. Wang, L.; Lin, Z.Q.; Wong, A. COVID-Net: A Tailored Deep Convolutional Neural Network Design for Detection of COVID-19 Cases from Chest X-ray Images. *Sci. Rep.* **2020**, *10*, 19549. [CrossRef] [PubMed]
16. Lin, Z.Q.; Shafiee, M.J.; Bochkarev, S.; Jules, M.S.; Wang, X.Y.; Wong, A. Do Explanations Reflect Decisions? A Machine-Centric Strategy to Quantify the Performance of Explainability Algorithms. *arXiv* **2019**, arXiv:1910.07387.
17. van Ginneken, B. Fifty years of computer analysis in chest imaging: Rule-based, machine learning, deep learning. *Radiol. Phys. Technol.* **2017**, *10*, 23–32. [CrossRef] [PubMed]
18. LeCun, Y.; Bengio, Y.; Hinton, G. Deep Learning. *Nature* **2015**, *521*, 436–444. [CrossRef]
19. Huh, M.; Agrawal, P.; Efros, A.A. What makes ImageNet good for transfer learning? *arXiv* **2016**, arXiv:1608.08614.
20. Chlap, P.; Min, H.; Vandenberg, N.; Dowling, J.; Holloway, L.; Haworth, A. A Review of Medical Image Data Augmentation Techniques for Deep Learning Applications. *J. Med. Imaging Radiat. Oncol.* **2021**, *65*, 545–563. [CrossRef]
21. Howard, A.G.; Zhu, M.; Chen, B.; Kalenichenko, D.; Wang, W.; Weyand, T.; Andreetto, M.; Adam, H. MobileNets: Efficient Convolutional Neural Networks for Mobile Vision Applications. *arXiv* **2017**, arXiv:1704.04861.
22. Szegedy, C.; Ioffe, S.; Vanhoucke, V.; Alemi, A.A. Inception-v4, inception-resnet and the impact of residual connections on learning. In Proceedings of the Thirty-First AAAI Conference on Artificial Intelligence, San Francisco, CA, USA, 4–9 February 2017.
23. Chollet, F. Xception: Deep learning with depthwise separable convolutions. In Proceedings of the IEEE Conference on Computer Vision and Pattern Recognition, Honolulu, HI, USA, 21–26 July 2017; pp. 1251–1258.
24. Deng, J.; Dong, W.; Socher, R.; Li, L.-J.; Li, K.; Fei-Fei, L. Imagenet: A large-scale hierarchical image database. In Proceedings of the 2009 IEEE Conference on Computer Vision and Pattern Recognition, Miami, FL, USA; 2009; pp. 248–255.

25. Lin, M.; Chen, Q.; Yan, S. Network in Network. *arXiv* **2013**, arXiv:1312.4400.
26. Sait, U. *Curated Dataset for COVID-19 Posterior-Anterior Chest Radiography Images (X-rays)*; Mendeley Data: London, UK, 2020.
27. Wang, X.; Peng, Y.; Lu, L.; Lu, Z.; Bagheri, M.; Summers, R.M. Chestx-ray8: Hospital-scale chest x-ray database and benchmarks on weakly-supervised classification and localization of common thorax diseases. In Proceedings of the IEEE Conference on Computer Vision and Pattern Recognition, Honolulu, HI, USA, 21–26 July 2017; pp. 2097–2106.
28. Wang, J.; Perez, L. The effectiveness of data augmentation in image classification using deep learning. *arXiv* **2017**, arXiv:1712.04621.
29. Shorten, C.; Khoshgoftaar, T.M. A survey on image data augmentation for deep learning. *J. Big Data* **2019**, *6*, 60. [CrossRef]
30. Tartaglione, E.; Barbano, C.A.; Berzovini, C.; Calandri, M.; Grangetto, M. Unveiling COVID-19 from CHEST X-ray with Deep Learning: A Hurdles Race with Small Data. *Int. J. Environ. Res. Public Health* **2020**, *17*, 6933. [CrossRef]
31. Adebayo, J.; Gilmer, J.; Muelly, M.; Goodfellow, I.; Hardt, M.; Kim, B. Sanity Checks for Saliency Maps. *Adv. Neural Inf. Process. Syst.* **2018**, *31*, 9505–9515.
32. Binder, A.; Montavon, G.; Lapuschkin, S.; Müller, K.-R.; Samek, W. Layer-Wise Relevance Propagation for Neural Networks with Local Renormalization Layers. In Proceedings of the International Conference on Artificial Neural Networks, Barcelona, Spain, 6–9 September 2016; Springer: Cham, Switzerland, 2016; pp. 63–71.

reports

Communication

# Comparison of Allplex™ 2019-nCoV and TaqPath™ COVID-19 Assays

**Manuela Colosimo [1,†], Pasquale Minchella [1,†], Rossana Tallerico [1], Ilenia Talotta [1], Cinzia Peronace [1], Luca Gallelli [2,3], Giulio Di Mizio [4,*] and Erika Cione [5]**

1 Microbiology and Virology Unit, Pugliese-Ciaccio Hospital, 88100 Catanzaro, Italy; manuelacolosimo@hotmail.it (M.C.); pminchella@aocz.it (P.M.); rossana.tallerico@gmail.com (R.T.); ilenia.talotta@gmail.com (I.T.); cinziaperonace@hotmail.it (C.P.)
2 Operative Unit of Clinical Pharmacology, Mater Domini University Hospital, 88100 Catanzaro, Italy; gallelli@unicz.it
3 Research Center FAS@UMG, Department of Health Science, School of Medicine, University of Catanzaro, 88100 Catanzaro, Italy
4 Forensic Medicine, Department of Law, Magna Graecia University of Catanzaro, 88100 Catanzaro, Italy
5 Department of Pharmacy, Health and Nutritional Sciences, University of Calabria, 87036 Rende, Italy; erika.cione@unical.it
* Correspondence: giulio.dimizio@unicz.it; Tel.: +39-0961-3691111
† These authors contributed equally to this work.

**Abstract:** The clinical presentation of COVID-19 is non-specific, and to improve and limit the spread of the SARS-CoV-2 virus, an accurate diagnosis with a robust method is needed. A total of 500 nasopharyngeal swab specimens were tested for SARS-CoV-2. Of these, 184 samples were found to be positive with Allplex™ 2019-nCoV Assay, which is fully automated. All the positive samples were retested with TaqPath™ COVID-19 CE-IVD RT-PCR Kit (after this, referred to as TaqPath™ COVID-19), semi-automated. The comparison of RT-qPCR for SARS-CoV-2 genes target points shows only one target point in common, the N gene. Therefore, the N gene was used to compare both assays. We noticed different Ct values between the tests. Therefore, samples were divided into four groups depending to the Ct value results: (1) Ct < 25, (2) Ct 25–30, (3) Ct 30–35, (4) Ct > 35. TaqPath™ COVID-19 Kit reconfirmed the results obtained from Allplex™ 2019-nCoV Assay. In conclusion, both the Allplex™ 2019-nCoV assay and TaqPath™ COVID-19 tests accurately confirm the diagnosis of SARS-CoV-2 infection. Even if TaqPath™ COVID-19 has a semi-automated workflow, it does not introduce bias in the diagnostic screening of SARS-CoV-2, and it supports the indirect identification of variants of concern to undergo sequencing.

**Keywords:** COVID-19; RNA; Allplex™ 2019-nCoV; TaqPath™ COVID-19; safety of care



**Citation:** Colosimo, M.; Minchella, P.; Tallerico, R.; Talotta, I.; Peronace, C.; Gallelli, L.; Di Mizio, G.; Cione, E. Comparison of Allplex™ 2019-nCoV and TaqPath™ COVID-19 Assays. *Reports* **2022**, *5*, 14. http://doi.org/10.3390/reports5020014

Academic Editors: Toshio Hattori and Yugo Ashino

Received: 3 March 2022
Accepted: 22 April 2022
Published: 26 April 2022



## 1. Introduction

Two years have passed since the first coronavirus disease 2019 (COVID-19) case in December 2019. According to the exponential progression in the number of infections globally, COVID-19 has become one of the most significant pandemics in modern history. The clinical relationship between COVID-19 and symptoms is non-specific, and to improve and limit the spread of the SARS-CoV-2 virus, an accurate diagnosis through a robust method is mandatory [1,2]. Molecular epidemiology of SARS-CoV-2 offers new avenues to investigate associations between genetic and environmental factors of the disease [3]. Real-time reverse-transcription polymerase chain reaction (RT-qPCR) tests are performed on respiratory samples. Therefore, nasopharyngeal, nasal, oropharyngeal, and/or, when hospitalized, bronchoalveolar lavage, are analyzed. RT-qPCR represents the gold standard, and viral presence could appear earlier, even before clinical symptoms [4,5]. The viral genome consists of several genes encoding non-structural, structural, and accessory proteins. In the viral genome, genes for four structural proteins (spike surface glycoprotein S, envelope

E, membrane M, and nucleocapsid N) and several accessory proteins are located [6]. For diagnostic and screening monitoring, ORF1ab/RdRp, E, N, and S genes are the targets most frequently used by the RT-qPCR method [6]. However, according to Coronavirus COVID-19 Global Cases by the Center for Systems Science and Engineering (CSSE) at Johns Hopkins University (JHU), virus variants of COVID-19 are originating, even in our region (Figure 1) (accessed on 22 January 2022) [7]. Therefore, in the present study, we compared two commercial Reverse Transcriptase (RT) polymerase chain reaction (PCR) kits for COVID-19 diagnosis, all having the N gene in common. Therefore, the N gene was used to compared both kits, the Allplex™ 2019-nCoV assay, and TaqPath™ COVID-19 tests. By this latter, a peculiar drop-off of the S gene was evidenced and indicative of a possible variant of concern (VOC) that was sequenced by whole-genome-based next-generation sequencing (NGS) [8,9].

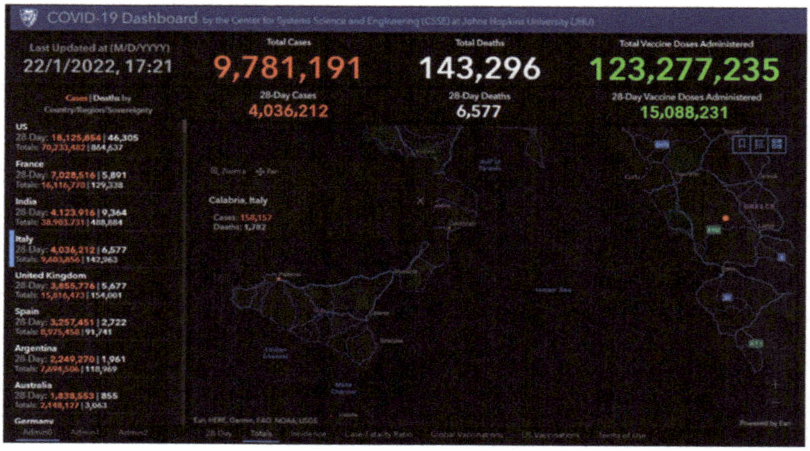


**Figure 1.** Adapted from COVID-19 Map–Johns Hopkins Coronavirus Resource Center (accessed on 22 January 2022).

## 2. Materials and Methods

We performed a prospective study on specimens referred to the Department of Microbiology and Virology of Pugliese Ciaccio's Hospital in Catanzaro from 4 to 24 December 2021. All study participants underwent a nasopharyngeal swab and real-time reverse-transcription polymerase chain reaction (RT-PCR) analysis for SARS-CoV-2. This study is part of the clinical trial recorded in clinicaltrial.gov (accessed on 25 October 2021) (NCT04322513) and was conducted in compliance with the Institutional Review Board/Human Subjects Research Committee requirements.

Experimental protocol

At the time of the study, for each patient, samples were collected in Universal Transport Media (UTM), opened in biosafety cabinet class-II, and then 600 µL of the UTM were further processed for viral nucleic acid extraction.

The viral nucleic acid extracted was evaluated through 2 RT-PCR kits specific for COVID-19:

(i). 200 µL of UTM was extracted for Allplex™ 2019-nCoV Assay (Seegene-Seoul, South Korea) with the fully Automated Liquid Handling Workstations NIMBUS which also arrange the PCR plate and the Real-Time PCR System from Bio-Rad CFX96™ Dx (Bio-Rad, Hercules, CA, USA);

(ii). TaqPath™ COVID-19 CE-IVD RT-PCR Kit (after this referred to as TaqPath™ COVID-19) with semi-automatic KingFisher Duo Prime by Thermofisher. Briefly, by extracting a 200 µL aliquot of specimen in UTM using the MagMAX™ Viral/Pathogen Nucleic

Acid isolation kit on the KingFisher Flex Purification system (Thermo Fisher Scientific, Waltham, MA, USA). Before RNA extraction, 10 µL of Proteinase K was added to each well in the KingFisher™ Deep 96-well Plate. In addition, 10 µL of the MS2 Phage Control was added to all specimens together with 10 µL of magnetic beads.

Elution volumes from the two workstations were different, at 100 µL and 50 µL for the Automated Liquid Handling Workstations NIMBUS and KingFisher Duo Prime, respectively. For both kits, a final volume of 25 µL was used in the reaction master mix and dispended as follows: Allplex™ 2019-nCoV Assay 17 µL of its master mix plus 8 µL of RNA-extracted sample; TaqPath™ COVID-19 15 µL of its master mix and 10 µL of RNA extracted sample.

### 2.1. *Allplex™ 2019-nCoV Assay*

All the samples included in the study were tested using Allplex™ 2019-nCoV Assay, following the manufacturer's manual (Ref: RV10284X Lot: RVA321D04). Accordingly, a sample is considered positive if at least N or RdRp targets amplify with cycle threshold (Ct) Ct $\leq$ 40. If only the E gene target is amplified with Ct $\leq$ 40, the sample is considered "presumptive positive" [9]. The range of Ct, only for the N gene, is reported in Table 1.

**Table 1.** Gene target points similarity.

| Developer | Commercial Name | Gene | | | | | Regulatory |
|---|---|---|---|---|---|---|---|
| | | ORF1ab | RdRP | E | N | S | |
| Seegene, Inc. | Allplex™ 2019-nCoV | | | | | | USA EUA; CE-IVD |
| Thermo Fisher | TaqPath™ COVID-19 | | | | | | CE-IVD |

### 2.2. *TaqPath™ COVID-19*

All the samples included in the study were tested using TaqPath™ COVID-19 CE-IVD RT-PCR Kit, following the manufacturer's manual (Ref: A48099 Lot: 2101036). Accordingly, a sample is considered positive if any of the targets (either ORF1ab, N or S) amplify with Ct $\leq$ 37, or the internal control MS2 (Bacteriophage MS2) with amplifying Ct value $\leq$ 32 [10]. The range of Ct, for the N gene and MS2, is reported in Table 2.

**Table 2.** N gene Ct value tested with Allplex™ 2019-nCoV Assay and TaqPath™ COVID-19.

| Commercial Name | N Gene Target | | | | Range Ct |
|---|---|---|---|---|---|
| | Ct < 25 | Ct 25–30 | Ct 30–35 | Ct > 35 | |
| Allplex™ 2019-nCoV | 22.79 ± 2.66 ($n$ = 31) | 28.18 ± 1.45 ($n$ = 55) | 33.05 ± 1.54 ($n$ = 42) | 37.90 ± 1.43 ($n$ = 56) | $\leq$40 |
| TaqPath™ COVID-19 | 21.61 ± 2.83 ($n$ = 87) | 27.98 ± 1.47 ($n$ = 61) | 32.99 ± 1.51 ($n$ = 17) | 37.01 ± 0.51 ($n$ = 19) | $\leq$37 with MS2 $\leq$ 32 |

### 2.3. *Sequencing SARS-CoV-2*

The NGS approach by MiSeq System (Illumina, San Diego, CA, USA), provided 2 × 250 bp read data. The SOPHIA DDM Platform analyzed FASTQ reads. Clade analysis was performed by ICOGEN Platform. Then, lineage information was described using the Pangolin nomenclatures [11,12].

### 2.4. *Statistical Analysis*

All data were analyzed using the GraphPad 5.0 statistical program (GraphPad Software Inc., San Diego, CA, USA) by evaluating the standard deviation (SD). Data were analyzed by one-way ANOVA analysis of variance followed by Tukey's multiple comparison test; HSD (honestly significant difference) was used to estimate difference amongst groups. The online free software from GraphPad Software Inc., CA-USA, was used (https://www.graphpad.com/quickcalcs/kappa1/, accessed on 25 January 2022) for the Cohen's kappa determination in order to obtain a value of the inter-observer agreement.

### 3. Results and Discussion

A total of 500 nasopharyngeal swab specimens were tested for SARS-CoV-2. Of these, 184 samples were positive with Allplex™ 2019-nCoV Assay (36.8%), and 316 were negative (63.2%). Positive samples from Allplex™ 2019-nCoV Assay were re-tested with TaqPath™ COVID-19 and 50 negative pooled samples (coming from 10 of each specimen), which were negative. The comparison of RT-qPCR for SARS-CoV-2 gene target points is presented in Table 1 (updated 29 December 2021, online sources) [13,14]. The common gene was the N gene (Table 1). Therefore, it was used to compare both assays.

The TaqPath™ COVID-19 Kit reconfirmed the results obtained from Allplex™ 2019-nCoV Assay, but we noticed a different distribution of Ct values. Therefore, samples were divided into four groups depending on the cycle threshold (Ct) value results: (1) Ct < 25, (2) Ct 25–30, (3) Ct 30–35, (4) Ct > 35 (Figure 2A,B).

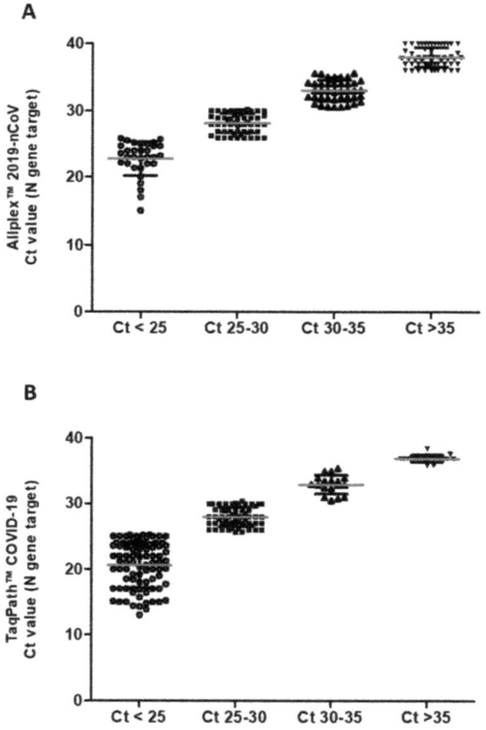


**Figure 2.** (**A**) Allplex™ 2019-nCoV Assay and (**B**) TaqPath™ COVID-19. In red, the average value is indicated for each group.

Samples that display the N gene with a Ct < 25 (Group 1) are almost three times greater with TaqPath™ COVID-19 compared to Allplex™ 2019-nCoV Assay, and any significant difference is highlighted between them (see Figure 3). Both TaqPath™ COVID-19 and Allplex™ 2019-nCoV Assay have similar samples at Ct 25–30 (Group 2). In contrast, samples with Ct values > 30 (Groups 3 and 4) were reached with Allplex™ 2019-nCoV Assay (Table 2). These results are consistent with the difference in elution volume used in the two workstations: 50 µL in TaqPath™ COVID-19 and 100 µL in Allplex™ 2019-nCoV. This difference could result in more diluted nucleic acids in the second kit (Allplex™ 2019-nCoV). Another reason could be the different complementarity of the primers' probe, crucial for PCR, where mismatch can give up to 7 Ct of difference [15].

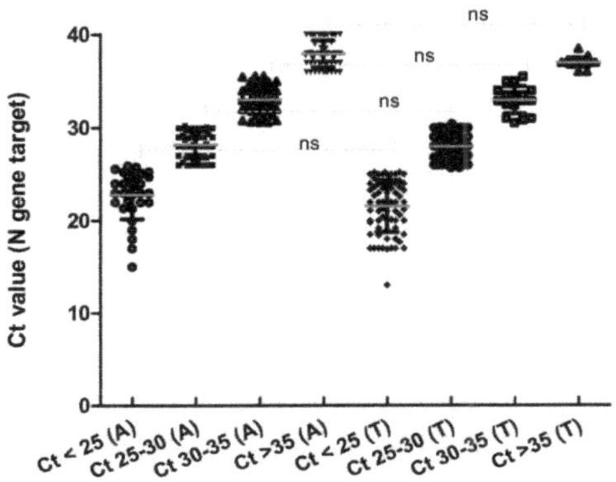


**Figure 3.** Comparison of Ct groups data from Allplex™ 2019-nCoV (A) TaqPath™ COVID-19 (T).

Tukey's multiple comparison test HSD statistical analysis was performed to evaluate the differences amongst the groups. No difference was highlighted between groups and the two analytical tests (see Figure 2).

Both Allplex™ 2019-nCoV Assay and TaqPath™ COVID-19 show similar agreement for the N genes. Kappa Cohen calculation for both Allplex™ 2019-nCoV Assay and TaqPath™ COVID-19 displays the following data. Number of observed agreements: 500 (100.00% of the observations) and number of agreements expected by chance: 267.4 (53.48% of the observations), Kappa = 1.000 and SE of Kappa = 0.000, 95% confidence interval from 1.000 to 1.000. Besides that, the diagnosis made by the infectious disease specialist shows an overall agreement of 100% and a Kappa value of 1 for both tests. Furthermore, in the 184 positive samples re-tested with TaqPath™ COVID-19, drop off of the S gene (indicative of VOC) was observed in four samples. Normally in routine practice, the samples that underwent sequencing are chosen randomly considering only that the Ct value must be lower than 25. By including TaqPath™ COVID-19 in our clinical laboratory setting, we were facilitated in this choice. In fact, the four samples with the drop-off S gene underwent genomic characterization by NGS sequencing, resulting in four Omicron VOC, as reported in Table 3.

Although the N gene in VOC Omicron presents several mutations, the amplification curve for this gene was not different between Allplex™ 2019-nCoV Assay and TaqPath™ COVID-19 (data not shown).

It is worth noting that real-time reverse-transcription polymerase chain reaction (RT-PCR) assays for SARS-CoV-2 RNA detection in clinical specimens are widely used in COVID-19 diagnostic laboratories as the standard-gold method. Although the Allplex™ 2019-nCoV Assay amplifies up to 40 cycles and states that any gene with Ct < 40 is a positive result, there is increasing appreciation that Ct 30–35 is considered borderline [16–18]. This issue is almost overcome by TaqPath™ COVID-19, as shown here. On the other hand, it was also reported that, in effect, the screening depends largely on frequency of testing and speed of reporting, and is only marginally improved by high test sensitivity, even in acute infection, therefore even specific biomarker is needed [18–21].

**Table 3.** NGS sequencing and amino acidic mutations.

| | Lineage | VOC | Clade | Gene | | |
|---|---|---|---|---|---|---|
| | | | | S | Orf1ab | N |
| 1 | BA.1 | OMICRON | 21k | A67V; IHV68I_del; T95I; GVYY142D_del; NL211I_del; D215EPED; G339D; S371L; S373P; S375F; K417N; N440K; G446S; T547K; D614G; H655Y; N679K; P681H; N764K; N856K; Q954H; N969K; D1146. | K38R; F106; A889; SL1265I_del; A1892T; T492I; P132H; LSGF105F_del; I189V; V57; P323L; N600; L749M. | P13L; ERS30G_del; R203K; G204R. |
| 2 | BA.1 | OMICRON | 21k | A67V; IHV68I_del; T95I; GVYY142D_del; NL211I_del; D215EPED; G339D; S371L; S373P; S375F; K417N; F456; T547K; D614G; H655Y; N679K; P681H; N764K; N856K; Q954H; N969K; D1146. | K38R; F106; D174; A889; V1069I; SL1265I_del; T492I; P132H; LSGF105F_del; I189V; V57; P323L; N600. | P13L; GERS30G_del; R203K; G204R. |
| 3 | BA.1 | OMICRON | 21k | A67V; IHV68I_del; T95I; GVYY142D_del; NL211I_del; D215EPED; G339D; S371L; S373P; S375F; K417N; Y449F; T547K; D614G; H655Y; N679K; P681H; N764K; N856K; Q954H; N969K; L981F; D1146. | K38R; F106; D174; A889; V1069I; SL1265I_del; T492I; P132H; LSGF105F_del; I189V; V57; P323L; N600. | P13L; GERS30G_del; R203K; G204R. |
| 4 | B.1.1.529 | OMICRON | 21k | T95I; V143; NL211I_del; D215EPED; G339D; K417N; Y449F; L452R; T547K; H655Y; P681R; N764K; G799D; N856K; N969K; L981F; D1146. | F106; D174; A889; V1069I; S1265; T492I; P132H; V57; P323L; A448G; I466L; N600; E204D; P429; A430S; L216. | P13L; ERS30G_del; D63G; R203K; 204R. |

## 4. Conclusions

The clinical presentation of COVID-19 is non-specific, and to improve and limit the spread of the SARS-CoV-2 virus, accurate diagnosis with a robust method is needed [16], even in light of reinfection [17]. Herein, we show that both, Allplex™ 2019-nCoV Assay and TaqPath™ COVID-19 tests are accurate enough to confirm the diagnosis of SARS-CoV-2 infection. The two methods tested are similar, with one substantial difference: TaqPath™ COVID-19 is performed in a semi-automated way. Despite this, TaqPath™ COVID-19 does not introduce bias in the diagnostic screening of SARS-CoV-2 and supports clinicians in the choice of VOC for NGS determination.

**Author Contributions:** Conceptualization, E.C., G.D.M. and P.M.; methodology, I.T.; E.C., R.T., C.P. and M.C.; software, E.C.; writing—original draft preparation, E.C. and M.C.; writing—review and editing, E.C., G.D.M. and L.G.; supervision, P.M. All authors have read and agreed to the published version of the manuscript.

**Funding:** This research received no external funding.

**Institutional Review Board Statement:** All the procedures followed the 1964 Helsinki Declaration and later amendments.

**Informed Consent Statement:** The study was conducted using residual, de-identified specimens, and no clinical or demographic information was collected. According to Italian health public law, this type of study did not require specific, informed consent and ethics committee approval.

**Data Availability Statement:** Data supporting reported results can be found at the Department of Microbiology and Virology, Pugliese Ciaccio's Hospital, Catanzaro, Italy.

**Conflicts of Interest:** The authors declare no conflict of interest.

## References


1. Clinical Characteristics of COVID-19. Available online: https://www.ecdc.europa.eu/en/covid-19/latest-evidence/clinical (accessed on 25 June 2021).
2. Yuen, K.S.; Ye, Z.W.; Fung, S.Y.; Chan, C.P.; Jin, D.Y. SARS-CoV-2 and COVID-19: The most important research questions. *Cell Biosci.* **2020**, *10*, 40. [CrossRef] [PubMed]
3. Recommendations for National SARS-CoV-2 Testing Strategies and Diagnostic Capacities. Available online: https://www.who.int/publications/i/item/WHO-2019-nCoV-Surveillance_Case_Definition-2020.2 (accessed on 7 September 2021).
4. Kostaki, E.G.; Pavlopoulos, G.A.; Verrou, K.M.; Ampatziadis-Michailidis, G.; Harokopos, V.; Hatzis, P.; Moulos, P.; Siafakas, N.; Pournaras, S.; Hadjichristodoulou, C.; et al. Molecular Epidemiology of SARS-CoV-2 in Greece Reveals Low Rates of Onward Virus Transmission after Lifting of Travel Restrictions Based on Risk Assessment during Summer 2020. *mSphere* **2021**, *6*, e0018021. [CrossRef] [PubMed]
5. Luciani, F.; Cione, E.; Caroleo, M.C.; Colosimo, M.; Zanolini, A.; Barca, A.; Cosimo, S.; Pasqua, P.; Gallelli, L. SARS-CoV-2 Translocate from Nasopharyngeal to Bronchoalveolar Site: A Case Presentation. *Reports* **2020**, *3*, 23. [CrossRef]
6. Kohmer, N.; Eckermann, L.; Böddinghaus, B.; Götsch, U.; Berger, A.; Herrmann, E.; Kortenbusch, M.; Tinnemann, P.; Gottschalk, R.; Hoehl, S.; et al. Self-Collected Samples to Detect SARS-CoV-2: Direct Comparison of Saliva, Tongue Swab, Nasal Swab, Chewed Cotton Pads and Gargle Lavage. *J. Clin. Med.* **2021**, *10*, 5751. [CrossRef] [PubMed]
7. Naqvi, A.A.T.; Fatima, K.; Mohammad, T.; Fatima, U.; Singh, I.K.; Singh, A.; Atif, S.M.; Hariprasad, G.; Hasan, G.M.; Hassan, M.I. Insights into SARS-CoV-2 genome, structure, evolution, pathogenesis and therapies: Structural genomics approach. *Biochim. Biophys. Acta Mol. Basis Dis.* **2020**, *1866*, 165878. [CrossRef] [PubMed]
8. Coronavirus COVID-19 Global Cases by Johns Hopkins. Available online: https://coronavirus.jhu.edu/map.html (accessed on 22 January 2022).
9. Rambaut, A.; Holmes, E.C.; O'Toole, Á.; Hill, V.; McCrone, J.T.; Ruis, C.; du Plessis, L.; Pybus, O.G. A dynamic nomenclature proposal for SARS-CoV-2 lineages to assist genomic epidemiology. *Nat. Microbiol.* **2020**, *5*, 1403–1407. [CrossRef] [PubMed]
10. Peronace, C.; Tallerico, R.; Colosimo, M.; De Fazio, M.; Pasceri, F.; Talotta, I.; Panduri, G.; Pintomalli, L.; Oteri, R.; Calantoni, V.; et al. BA.1 Omicron Variant of SARS-CoV-2: First Case Reported in Calabria Region, Italy. *COVID* **2022**, *2*, 211–215. [CrossRef]
11. Seegene. Allplex 2019-nCoV Assay (Version 2.2; 15 April 2021), Instruction for Use. Available online: https://www.fda.gov/media/137178/download (accessed on 4 December 2021).
12. TaqPath™ COVID-19 CE-IVD RT-PCR Kit MAN0019215, Revision F.0. Available online: https://assets.thermofisher.com/TFS-Assets/LSG/manuals/MAN0019215_TaqPathCOVID-19_CE-IVD_RT-PCR%20Kit_IFU.pdf (accessed on 4 December 2021).
13. Classification of Omicron (B.1.1.529): SARS-CoV-2 Variant of Concern. Available online: https://www.who.int/news/item/26-11-2021-classification-of-omicron-(b.1.1.529)-sars-cov-2-variant-of-concern (accessed on 1 January 2022).

14. COVID-19 Diagnostics Resource Centre. Available online: https://www.finddx.org/covid-19/ (accessed on 29 December 2021).
15. Stadhouders, R.; Pas, S.D.; Anber, J.; Voermans, J.; Mes, T.H.; Schutten, M. The effect of primer-template mismatches on the detection and quantification of nucleic acids using the 5′ nuclease assay. *J. Mol. Diagn.* **2010**, *12*, 109–117. [CrossRef] [PubMed]
16. Rabaan, A.A.; Tirupathi, R.; Sule, A.A.; Aldali, J.; Mutair, A.A.; Alhumaid, S.; Muzaheed Gupta, N.; Koritala, T.; Adhikari, R.; Bilal, M.; et al. Viral Dynamics and Real-Time RT-PCR Ct Values Correlation with Disease Severity in COVID-19. *Diagnostics* **2021**, *11*, 1091. [CrossRef] [PubMed]
17. Larremore, D.B.; Wilder, B.; Lester, E.; Shehata, S.; Burke, J.M.; Hay, J.A.; Tambe, M.; Mina, M.J.; Parker, R. Test sensitivity is secondary to frequency and turnaround time for COVID-19 screening. *Sci. Adv.* **2021**, *7*, eabd5393. [CrossRef] [PubMed]
18. Mina, M.J.; Parker, R.; Larremore, D.B. Rethinking Covid-19 Test Sensitivity—A Strategy for Containment. *N. Engl. J. Med.* **2020**, *383*, e120. [CrossRef] [PubMed]
19. Cione, E.; Siniscalchi, A.; Gangemi, P.; Cosco, L.; Colosimo, M.; Longhini, F.; Luciani, F.; De Sarro, G.; G&SPWorking Group Berrino, L.; D'Agostino, B.; et al. Neuron-specific enolase serum levels in COVID-19 are related to the severity of lung injury. *PLoS ONE* **2021**, *16*, e0251819. [CrossRef] [PubMed]
20. Bentivegna, E.; Sentimentale, A.; Luciani, M.; Speranza, M.L.; Guerritore, L.; Martelletti, P. New IgM seroconversion and positive RT-PCR test after exposure to the virus in recovered COVID-19 patient. *J. Med. Virol.* **2021**, *93*, 97–98. [CrossRef] [PubMed]
21. Smith, R.L.; Gibson, L.L.; Martinez, P.P.; Ke, R.; Mirza, A.; Conte, M.; Gallagher, N.; Conte, A.; Wang, L.; Fredrickson, R.; et al. Longitudinal Assessment of Diagnostic Test Performance Over the Course of Acute SARS-CoV-2 Infection. *J. Infect. Dis.* **2021**, *224*, 976–982. [CrossRef] [PubMed]

reports

MDPI

Case Report

# A Case of COVID-19 with Acute Exacerbation after Anti-Inflammatory Treatment

**Yugo Ashino [1,*], Yoichi Shirato [1], Masahiro Yaegashiwa [1], Satoshi Yamanouchi [2], Noriko Miyakawa [2], Kokichi Ando [3], Yumiko Sakurada [3], Haorile Chagan Yasutan [4,5] and Toshio Hattori [5,*]**

1 Department of Respiratory Medicine, Sendai City Hospital, Miyagi 982-8502, Japan; youichi0520@icloud.com (Y.S.); yaesan@k2.dion.ne.jp (M.Y.)
2 Department of Emergency, Sendai City Hospital, Miyagi 982-8502, Japan; manta3104@gmail.com (S.Y.); m-noriko@hosp.tohoku.ac.jp (N.M.)
3 Department of Anesthesiology, Sendai City Hospital, Miyagi 982-8502, Japan; Ko.andoh@gmail.com (K.A.); sakura@kjc.biglobe.ne.jp (Y.S.)
4 Mongolian Psychosomatic Medicine Department, International Mongolian Medicine Hospital of Inner Mongolia, Hohhot 010065, China; haorile@gjmyemail.gjmyy.cn
5 Research Institute of Health and Welfare, Kibi International University, Takahashi 716-8508, Japan
* Correspondence: ashino-yug@hospital.city.sendai.jp (Y.A.); hattorit@kiui.ac.jp (T.H.); Tel.: +81-22-308-7111 (Y.A.); +81-866-22-9469 (T.H.); Fax: +81-22-308-9921 (Y.A.); +81-866-22-9469 (T.H.)

**Abstract:** A COVID-19 patient (53-year-old woman from Japan) was admitted to our hospital. She had a high fever (38.3 °C), cough, fatigue, and loss of appetite. She was a smoker and took migraine medication. A thoracic computed tomography (CT) scan showed no evidence of pneumonia. She was treated with antibiotics, protease inhibitors, inhalant corticosteroids, and antivirals. Anti-interleukin-6 receptor antibody tocilizumab (TCZ 400 mg) was added on day 2. On day 4, her temperature decreased, but her vital signs suddenly worsened, with an $SpO_2$ of 70% in ambient air, a blood pressure of 70 mmHg (systolic), loss of consciousness, and tachypnea. Her CT showed bilateral lung consolidation and no pulmonary embolism. She was connected to the ventilator. On day 11, her respiratory condition improved ($PaO_2/FIO_2$ 400), and she was able to withdraw from the ventilator. Her laboratory data (white cell count, ferritin, d-Dimer, C-reactive protein, and $\beta_2$-microglobulin) did not increase even at the time of exacerbation, except for Galectin-9 (Gal-9). The plasma Gal-9 levels increased 2.3 times from before the administration of TCZ, followed by a swift decrease associated with improvements in respiratory status. She was discharged on day 16. Patients with TCZ-treated COVID-19 require careful observation.

**Keywords:** COVID-19; Galectin-9; SARS-CoV-2; acute exacerbation; tocilizumab (TCZ); acute respiratory distress (ARDS); tissue destruction; recover; ADE

check for updates

**Citation:** Ashino, Y.; Shirato, Y.; Yaegashiwa, M.; Yamanouchi, S.; Miyakawa, N.; Ando, K.; Sakurada, Y.; Yasutan, H.C.; Hattori, T. A Case of COVID-19 with Acute Exacerbation after Anti-Inflammatory Treatment. *Reports* **2022**, 5, 24. https://doi.org/10.3390/reports5020024

Academic Editor: Ivana Kholová

Received: 16 May 2022
Accepted: 16 June 2022
Published: 20 June 2022



## 1. Introduction

The severe acute respiratory syndrome coronavirus 2 (SARS-CoV-2) has spread rapidly worldwide since 2019. SARS-CoV-2 infection is known as coronavirus 2019 (COVID-19) and causes varying degrees of illness [1]. Today, pandemics do not end since there are repeated mutations of the virus genome [2]. This also makes the treatment of COVID-19 complex. For example, the loss of a vaccine effect or elimination of the effects of antibody treatment has been observed [3].

As one of the characteristics of COVID-19, the sudden onset of lung damage is believed to be caused by thrombotic events and cytokine release.

A pulmonary embolism consists of immune-mediated thrombotic mechanisms, complement activation, macrophage activation syndrome, antiphospholipid antibody syndrome, hyperferritinemia, and renin–angiotensin system dysregulation [4]. On the other hand, the high severity of acute respiratory distress is dependent on a cytokine storm, most likely induced by the interleukin-6 (IL-6) amplifier, which is hyperactivation machinery that regulates the nuclear factor kappa B (NF-κB) pathway [5]. The administration of drugs for anticoagulants and anticytokines is recommended for COVID-19 treatment with these inferences. The anti-interleukin-6 receptor antibody tocilizumab (TCZ) appears to be an effective treatment option in COVID-19 patients with a risk of cytokine storms [6]. Furthermore, patients with COVID-19 and pneumonia showed that TCZ reduced the risk of death by 45% [7]. We have proposed that the early administration of TCZ ameliorated pneumonia and kidney caused by hyperinflammation syndrome in a patient with COVID-19 [8].

However, the exact mechanism by which TCZ improves COVID-19 pneumonia has yet to be clarified. In addition, the biomarkers of COVID-19 pneumonia are in the middle of research. We have already reported that the levels of cleavage forms of plasma osteopontin (OPN) and Galectin-9 (Gal-9) are elevated in COVID-19 patients, and their levels decrease after TCZ administration. These might be used as an indicator of the therapeutic effect and the severity of pathological inflammation [9]. They had a significant association with laboratory markers for lung function, inflammation, coagulopathy, and kidney function in COVID-19 Pneumonia (CP) patients.

New therapeutic strategies recommend the administration of antibodies, which can block the interaction of the RBD (receptor-binding domain) and its ACE2 receptor or neutralize the SARS-CoV-2. However, the patients who were recommended for this treatment were the ones who did not need additional oxygen and were at high risk of progressing to severe COVID-19 [10]. The benefit-risk profile for patients requiring high-flow oxygen or mechanical ventilation was considered unfavorable [10]. This means these agents seemed ineffective in advanced cases, and sole virus control cannot save lives in severe cases. For instance, there was no observed benefit in those on high-flow oxygen, NIV (non-invasive ventilation), MV (mechanical ventilation), or ECMO (extracorporeal membrane oxygenation) in a placebo-controlled, double-blind RCT of Remdesivir in hospitalized patients with COVID-19 [10]. Although the mortality was lower in the TCZ arm than in the usual care arm on day 28, the effect was not marked [10]. It was speculated that lung disease had already progressed in the patients treated with TCZ, and it may have been used too late in previously reported cases. There has been little reporting of the effects of anti-inflammatories before lung damage.

To find an effective treatment for COVID-19, we need to find a novel biomarker that accurately reflects the heterogeneous host responses after the administration of TCZ. As a new method of treatment, the change in the ventral position is usually accompanied by a marked improvement in the arterial blood gases of both spontaneously breathing and mechanically vented patients [11,12]. Although the survival rate of patients in prone positions tends to have a growing trend, the effects of this procedure on outcomes are still uncertain.

This report describes a case of acute pulmonary exacerbation related to COVID-19 despite the preadministration of anticytokine, anticoagulants, and antiviral therapy drugs during hospitalization. A patient developed lung damage suddenly during treatment and did not show an elevation in inflammatory markers other than the plasma Gal-9 level. The patient was improved by pressurizing mechanical ventilation with dexamethasone and repositioning.

## 2. Case Presentation

A middle-aged woman with COVID-19 was hospitalized on 9 December 2020.

She had nine days of a history of high fever, arthralgia, anorexia, and dysgeusia before admission. A SARS-CoV-2 infection was confirmed by a PCR assay obtained from the patient's nasopharyngeal swab as described by us [8].

She had a history of migraine, myasthenia gravis, syringoencephalomyelia, and smoking one pack of cigarettes per day. The patient was not routinely taking any drugs, because she had no symptoms of these diseases. The patient's lab data showed neutrophilia and lymphopenia. It also showed elevated levels of LDH (342 U/mL), C-reactive protein (CRP; 3.65 mg/dL), fibrinogen (509 mg/dL), and urinary β2-microglobulin (B2M) (510 mg/mL) (Table 1).

**Table 1.** Laboratory data from the patient during hospitalization.

| Laboratory Data | Reference Range | Day 0 | Day 2 | Day 5 | Day 6 | Day 7 | Day 8 | Day 9 | Day 12 |
|---|---|---|---|---|---|---|---|---|---|
| Complete Blood Cell count and differential | | | | | | | | | |
| White cell unit (/μL) | 3700–8500 | 7400 | 5300 | 5700 | 5400 | 4400 | 3900 | 5500 | 6700 |
| Neutrophils (%) | 44.0–68.0 | **76.6** # | 67.2 | **73** | **70.5** | 62.5 | 55 | 61 | 65 |
| Lymphocytes (%)) | 27.0–44.0 | **16** | **23.5** | **13** | **22.5** | 29.5 | 33 | 31.5 | 28 |
| Monocytes (%) | 3.0–12.0 | 6.3 | 7.6 | 4 | 3.5 | 5.5 | 5.5 | 5.5 | 6 |
| Eosinophils (%) | 0.0–10.0 | 0.3 | 1.3 | 4 | 0.5 | 1.5 | 2 | 1.5 | 0 |
| Basophils (%) | 0.0–3.0 | 0.8 | 0.4 | 1 | 0.5 | 1 | 1 | 0 | 0 |
| Hematocrit (%) | 42.0–53 | 43.8 | **38.6** | **39.1** | **34.1** | **30.7** | **31.1** | **33.4** | **37.2** |
| Hemoglobin (g/dL) | 13.5–17.5 | 14.4 | **13** | **13.1** | **11.6** | **10** | **10.2** | **11.1** | **12.2** |
| Platelet count × $10^3$ (/μL) | 150–355 | 268 | 21.8 | 219 | 263 | 251 | 251 | 308 | **381** |
| Red cell count × $10^6$ (/μL) | 3.90–5.30 | 5.01 | 4.55 | 4.56 | 4.04 | **3.55** | **3.55** | **3.83** | 4.33 |
| Biochemical test | | | | | | | | | |
| Urea nitrogen (mg/dL) | 8–20 | 15 | 9 | 7 | 8 | 12 | 12 | 9 | 14 |
| Creatinine (mg/dL) | 0.42–1.07 | 0.64 | 0.6 | 0.53 | 0.45 | 0.47 | 0.48 | 0.42 | **0.41** |
| ALT (U/L) | 3–40 | 23 | 18 | 16 | 14 | 17 | **65** | **70** | **129** |
| AST (U/L) | 8–35 | 25 | 21 | 20 | 19 | 22 | **64** | **109** | **53** |
| LDH (U/L) | 124–222 | **342** | 201 | **295** | **346** | **296** | **302** | 331 | **275** |
| Ferritin (ng/mL) | 14–304 | 104 | 102 | 147 | 158 | 185 | **273** | 298 | 265 |
| CRP (mg/dL) | 0.00–0.3 | **3.67** | **7.33** | **1.64** | **0.88** | **0.48** | **0.31** | 0.25 | 0.09 |
| Total protein (g/dL) | 6.6–8.4 | 7.7 | 6.5 | 6.3 | **5.5** | **5** | **4.9** | **5.5** | **6.2** |
| Albumin (g/dL) | 3.8–5.2 | 4.4 | **3.4** | **3.3** | **2.9** | **2.7** | **2.7** | **3.0** | **3.4** |
| Coagulation test | | | | | | | | | |
| PT (s) | 10.0–13.5 | 11.4 | 11.8 | 12.1 | 12.6 | **13.6** | **13.7** | 13.2 | 11.3 |
| PT(%) | 80.0–120.0 | 100.6 | 98.7 | 89.7 | 82.4 | **71.8** | **70.7** | **75.9** | 102.4 |
| APTT (s) | 24.0–39.0 | 33.6 | 37.8 | 33.5 | **41** | **83.1** | **57.5** | **53.6** | 37.9 |
| D-dimer (μg/mL) | 0.00–1.00 | 0.6 | 0.75 | 0.65 | **1.8** | 0.94 | 0.93 | **1.06** | 0.78 |
| Fibrinogen (mg/dL) | 200–400 | **509** | **554** | 389 | 304 | 289 | 253 | 278 | **329** |
| Urine test | | | | | | | | | |
| β2-microglobulin (μg/L) | 30–340 | **510** | **2249** | **404** | **510** | 296 | **363** | **570** | 313 |

# Bold indicates the data is not within normal range.

A chest computed tomography (CT) scan on admission did not show ground-glass opacities (GGOs) in her lungs (Figure 1a). The vital signs of the patient included a heart rate of 108 beats/min, a respiratory rate of 20 breaths/min, an axillary temperature of 38.3 °C, oxygen saturation ($SpO_2$) in ambient air of 94% (Figure 2), and blood pressure of 120/79 mmHg. These were considered only mild diseases. Azithromycin (500 mg/day), ciclesonide (200 μg inhaler; 2 inhalations per day), nafamostat mesylate (40 mg/day), and favipiravir (3600 mg on the first day, 1600 mg thereafter) were administered. Despite these treatments, the patient's clinical status was not improved on day 2. Specifically, her high fever and exhaustion persisted. Furthermore, the CRP and urinary B2M levels were elevated. Because of the lack of improvement in clinical outcomes, 400 mg of TCZ was given intravenously. The fever disappeared. However, on day 4, a disturbance of consciousness, associated with tachypnea, appeared suddenly. Her vital signs worsened to an $SpO_2$ of 70% in ambient air and blood pressure of 70 mmHg (systolic). Her enhanced chest CT image showed consolidations in both lower lobes of her lungs and GGOs around the consolidation at this point (Figure 1(b1)). There was no proof of a pulmonary embolism (Figure 1(b2)). The patient was immediately brought to the ICU with the administration of adrenalin for endotracheal intubation and mechanical ventilation. In addition, the drugs already given were modified as follows: levofloxacin at 500 mg (for 4 days), heparin sodium at 15,000 units (for 4 days), dexamethasone at 6.6 mg (for 10 days), and remdesivir (200 mg loading dose on day 1 followed by 100 mg daily for up to 3 additional days). The ventilator was set to positive airway pressure (initial positive inspiratory pressure of 22 cm $H_2O$ and an expiratory positive airway pressure of 5 cm $H_2O$) under the condition of the fraction of inspiratory oxygen ($FIO_2$) of 0.6. Arterial blood gas analysis reported an arterial $O_2$ tension ($PaO_2$) of 74.1 Torr and an arterial $CO_2$ tension ($PaCO_2$) of 46.3 Torr.

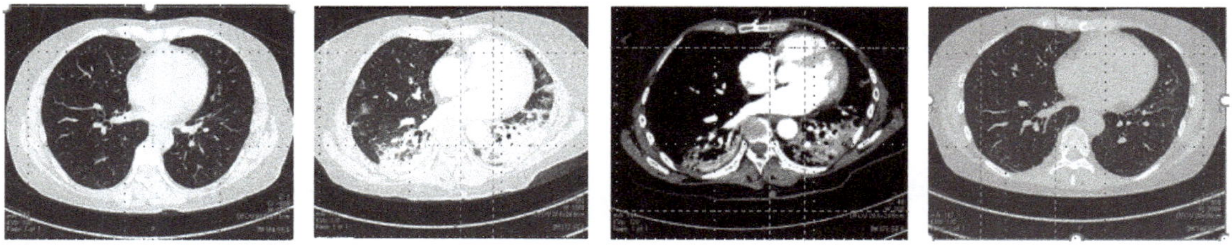

(**a**) (**b1**) (**b2**) (**c**)

**Figure 1.** Computed tomography (CT) images of the patient's lungs on day 0 (**a**), day 5 (**b1**,**b2**), and day 16 (**c**) with a: no abnormality; (**b1**): indicates consolidation and GGOs in bilateral lungs; (**b2**): indicates pulmonary artery contrast-enhanced findings without defect; and (**c**): indicates the disappearance of consolidation and GGOs.

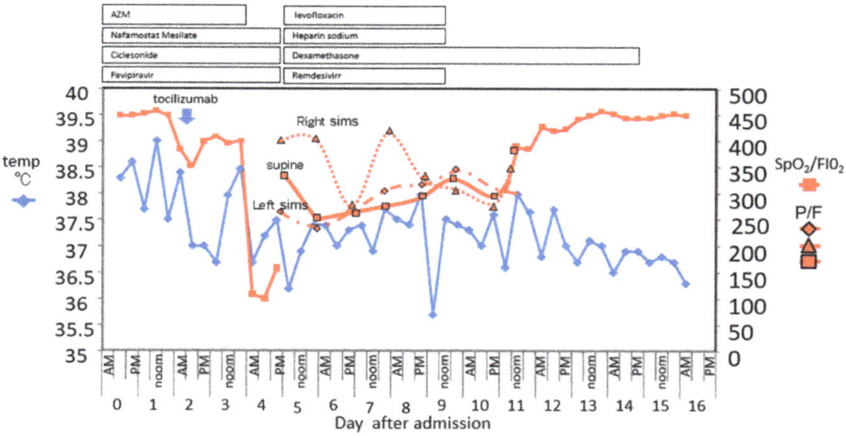


**Figure 2.** Fluctuations in the patient's body temperature and the $SpO_2/FIO_2$ and P/F ratio during hospitalization. The drug dosing period is shown at the top of the figure. From day 5 to day 10, the data are from an artificial ventilator in the ICU. The black bordered red square is the $SpaO_2/FIO_2$ or P/F in the supine position. The right sims' position is indicated by the black bordered red triangle. Left sims' position is indicated by the black bordered red diamond.

Lung compliance was greatly decreased at 24 mL/cm $H_2O$ (Figure 3).

The change in the right-hand sims' position was accompanied by a significant improvement in $PaO_2/FIO_2$ 407, but the left-hand $PaO_2/FIO_2$ was 267 (Figure 2). Differences in the respiration status were observed depending on the position. After being placed on a respirator, her respiratory condition had a lasting improvement from day to day. On day 10, $PaO_2$ and $PaCO_2$ were 90.6 and 48.3 Torr, respectively, after adjusting the ventilation to the CPAP mode (5 m $H_2O$ $FIO_2$ 0.3 setting) in the supine position. Then, she withdrew from the ventilator. Lung compliance just prior to intubation removal was 96 mL/cm $H_2O$ (Figure 3).

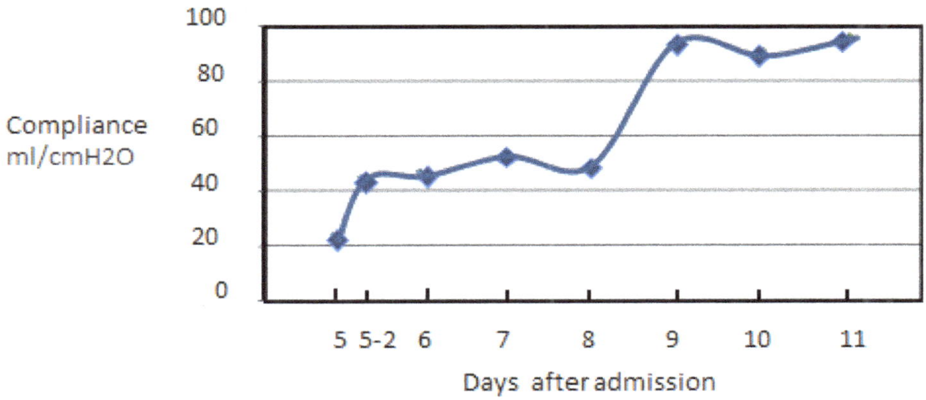


**Figure 3.** Lung compliance from the artificial ventilator vita XL (Dräger, Lübec, Germany). The x axis is days after admission. The label 5-2 means the afternoon of day 5.

The consolidation disappeared on the CT after extubation (Figure 1c). The patient's LDH, CRP, and urinary B2M decreased. The patient's ferritin and D-dimer levels were not extremely in excess of the normal range in the hospital (Table 1). Only Gal-9 was increased two days (day 2 and 6) after exacerbation. Gal-9 was measured using a human Gal-9 ELISA kit (GalPharma Co., Ltd., Takamatsu, Japan) as described [9]. It was also on the rise when admitted and had a second increase on day 6 (Figure 4). Gal-9 decreased with the improvement in the clinical outcomes. On day 16, the patient was discharged.

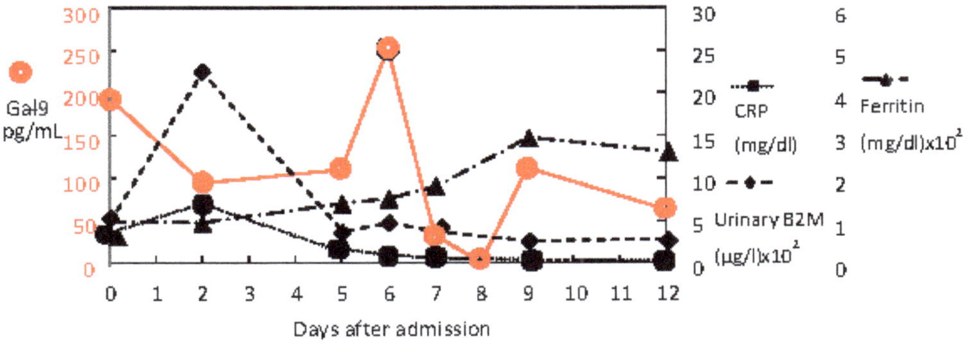


**Figure 4.** Changes in Galectin-9 (Gal-9) and other inflammatory biomarkers (CRP, urinary B2M, ferritin) during hospitalization.

### 3. Discussion

A 53-year-old Japanese COVID-19 patient woman was admitted and given four kinds of drugs (antibiotics, protease inhibitors, inhalant corticosteroids, and antivirals). However, there was no response in terms of symptom alleviation and high fever, cough, fatigue, and loss of appetite persisted. TCZ was administered to improve these clinical findings. Although TCZ demonstrated an antipyretic effect and an improvement in the patient's laboratory data, the consolidation shadow suddenly appeared in both lungs, and $SpO_2$ was lowered. This was consistent with COVID-19 pneumonia rather than a pulmonary embolism, because the contrast enhancement CT did not show pulmonary artery obstruction. Seven days after she was connected to the ventilator (11th day after hospitalization), her respiratory condition improved.

There are reports that COVID-19 can suddenly become severe [13,14]. The reasons why the case with mild COVID-19 suddenly worsened are not clear. Reports suggest it is more likely related to immune dysregulation or a cytokine storm after SRAS-CoV-2 infection [14], which leads to respiratory diseases. Moreover, interleukin-6 is regarded as the perpetrator of the COVID-19 cytokine storm [15]. In this case, we used TCZ to prevent this transition of COVID-19 to a cytokine storm. Unexpectedly, the onset of respiratory failure and worsening CT findings were observed, though most of the laboratory data did not change other than Gal-9. Since various adverse drug effects (ADEs) were reported in TCZ treatment of COVID-19, including respiratory disorders, it cannot be denied that this deterioration may be due to TCZ [16,17].

After being connected to a ventilator, her respiratory condition immediately recovered. In particular, the right sims' position resulted in dramatic improvements. The prone position can be used as adjuvant therapy for improving ventilation in patients with acute respiratory distress syndrome (ARDS). Lung damage from the novel coronavirus SRAS-CoV-2 resembles other causes of ARDS [18]. However, this case differed from ARDS caused by lung compliance reduced by vascular permeability. Her chest high-resolution computed tomography (HRCT) findings did not show the traction bronchiolectasis or bronchiectasis seen in COVID-19 ARDS [19]. Lung compliance was low. However, it rapidly recovered to the normal range immediately after intubation. Moreover, 7 days later, the consolidation had disappeared. Six-month follow-up CT showed fibrotic-like changes in the lung in more than one-third of patients who survived severe coronavirus disease 2019 pneumonia [20]. No fibrotic-like changes were observed in this case. After TCZ treatment in COVID-19 cases, the patients might have distinct ARDS, which might be different from COVID-19 ARDS. At least, cytokine storms cannot be positively recognized from a low CRP. It was considered that CRP levels decreased because TCZ blocks the IL-6 receptor. Biomarkers for this morbid condition are unknown. In our case, the levels of CRP, ferritin, D-dimer, and urinary B2M declined or did not increase when she worsened. Only the Gal-9 level was elevated with the deterioration in the respiratory condition and returned to a normal level with its improvement. We already reported that the plasma level of Gal-9 is a representative inflammatory biomarker in COVID-19, tuberculosis, and HIV infections [21]. In addition, Gal-9 may reflect the severity of acute and chronic infectious diseases. It has been discovered that Gal-9 has biological roles in innate and adaptive immune systems. Gal-9 is expressed in endothelial cells, the epithelium of the gastrointestinal tract, and several immune cells, including T cells, B cells, macrophages, mast cells, and dendritic cells. Gal-9 regulates the transduction of intra- and extracellular signals by interacting with several receptors [21]. While the inflammatory marker was not deregulated in this case, only Gal-9 was elevated followed by a decline associated with the deterioration and recovery of the respiratory conditions.

TCZ treatment was found to be associated with rapid, sustained, and significant clinical improvement [22]. However, there was an inconsistency between this fact and the changes in the CT image and $SpO_2$. The other reports indicated that fewer patients needed NIV or MV or died in the TCZ group than the usual-care-alone group [23]. These facts implicate the heterogenous host responses against TCZ. Additionally, a patient who is not COVID-19-infected but have CT findings with ground-glass opacities and clinical courses to this case was reported after TCZ administration [24].

It is of note that this patient recovered in 6 days after connection to a ventilator. Gal-9 can be an indicator for pulmonary regeneration [25,26]. Gal-9 has also been reported to regulate cell–cell and cell–matrix adhesion [27]. As SARS-CoV-2 targets various cell types of the proximal airways and the alveolar type 2 cells of the gas exchange region of the distal lung, the surfactant might be decreased in the lung. The decrease in the surfactant caused alveolar cell damage [28] and cell to cell adhesion was disabled. The increasing Gal-9 in our case indicates tissue destruction. Gal-9 was proposed to be one of the danger-associated molecules in dengue virus infection [29]. This tissue destruction was different from traditional ARDS caused by permeable pulmonary edema, because the immediate resuscitated lung conformance and CT after recovery showed no changes in fibrosis. TCZ terminates the IL-6-dependent inflammatory reaction. The released Gal-9 may modify the recovery process of COVID-19 pneumonia because this case recovered swiftly and there was no lung fibrosis as a sequela. A larger study is necessary for conclusions to be made regarding the clinical significance of Gal-9 in detecting ADEs in TCZ-treated COVID-19 patients.

In this case, the sims' position was useful for improving the respiratory state. Prone position pronation can also recruit the dorsal lung regions and drain airway secretions, improving gas exchange. The blowing of the decreasing area of the surfactant made the collapsed alveoli swell and encouraged surfactant secretion [30]. ATP secretion and [Ca(2+)] (i) oscillations induced by lung stretch could lead to tissue repair [31,32]. After virus infection, when the suppression of inflammation alone does not cure tissue destruction, etc., we may need to adopt another treatment method to recover from this destroyed lung damage.

This is a single-case report; to generate evidence, long-term follow-up studies with a large sample size will enlighten medical science about unknown ADEs associated with TCZ in COVID-19 patients.

### 3.1. Limitations

Since this is a rare case in which the condition of this COVID-19 case changed suddenly after TCZ administration, a systemic search with similar cases could not be performed.

### 3.2. Future Direction

It is necessary to also note the involvement of Gal-9 in cases of lung disorders other than patients with lung disorders related to COVID-19.

## 4. Conclusions

A 53-year-old COVID-19 patient without pneumonia was treated with TCZ. Her laboratory findings were improved, but acute exacerbation occurred on day 4. Gal-9 increased simultaneously with the appearance of symptoms; nevertheless, the other biomarkers did not increase. After positive pressure ventilation, the patient showed a remarkable recovery. We reported unexpected respiratory failure after TCZ treatment. Careful monitoring, including Gal-9, would be useful for identifying these patients.

**Author Contributions:** Conceptualization, Y.A. and T.H.; methodology, Y.A.; formal analysis, H.C.Y.; resources and data curation, Y.S. (Yoichi Shirato), M.Y., S.Y., N.M., K.A. and Y.S. (Yumiko Sakurada); writing—original draft preparation, Y.A.; writing—review and editing, H.C.Y. and T.H. All authors have read and agreed to the published version of the manuscript.

**Funding:** This work was partially supported by the Japan Society for the Promotion of Science (JSPS) Grants-in-Aid for Scientific Research (KAKENHI), Grant Number JP17H01690 and Sendai city hospital Medical Science Fund.

**Institutional Review Board Statement:** Not applicable.

**Informed Consent Statement:** Written informed consent was obtained from the patient to publish this paper.

**Acknowledgments:** We are grateful to T. Niki for measurement of plasma Gal-9 in this patient. All individuals included in this section have consented to the acknowledgement.

**Conflicts of Interest:** The authors declare no conflict of interest. The funders had no role in the design of the study; in the collection, analyses, or interpretation of data; in the writing of the manuscript, or in the decision to publish the results.

## References


1. Zhu, N.; Zhang, D.; Wang, W.; Li, X.; Yang, B.; Song, J.; Zhao, X.; Huang, B.; Shi, W.; Lu, R.; et al. A Novel Coronavirus from Patients with Pneumonia in China, 2019. *N. Engl. J. Med.* **2020**, *382*, 727–733. [CrossRef]
2. Mishra, S.K.; Tripathi, T. One year update on the COVID-19 pandemic: Where are we now? *Acta Trop.* **2021**, *214*, 105778. [CrossRef]
3. Haque, A.; Pant, A.B. Mitigating COVID-19 in the face of emerging virus variants, breakthrough infections and vaccine hesitancy. *J. Autoimmun.* **2022**, *127*, 102792. [CrossRef]
4. Hanff, T.C.; Mohareb, A.M.; Giri, J.; Cohen, J.B.; Chirinos, J.A. Thrombosis in COVID-19. *Am. J. Hematol.* **2020**, *95*, 1578–1589. [CrossRef]
5. Hojyo, S.; Uchida, M.; Tanaka, K.; Hasebe, R.; Tanaka, Y.; Murakami, M.; Hirano, T. How COVID-19 induces cytokine storm with high mortality. *Inflamm. Regen.* **2020**, *40*, 37. [CrossRef]
6. Luo, P.; Liu, Y.; Qiu, L.; Liu, X.; Liu, D.; Li, J. Tocilizumab treatment in COVID-19: A single center experience. *J. Med. Virol.* **2020**, *92*, 814–818. [CrossRef]
7. Kim, J.S.; Lee, J.Y.; Yang, J.W.; Lee, K.H.; Effenberger, M.; Szpirt, W.; Kronbichler, A.; Shin, J.I. Immunopathogenesis and treatment of cytokine storm in COVID-19. *Theranostics* **2021**, *11*, 316–329. [CrossRef]
8. Ashino, Y.; Chagan-Yasutan, H.; Hatta, M.; Shirato, Y.; Kyogoku, Y.; Komuro, H.; Hattori, T. Successful Treatment of a COVID-19 Case with Pneumonia and Renal Injury Using Tocilizumab. *Reports* **2020**, *3*, 29. [CrossRef]
9. Bai, G.; Furushima, D.; Niki, T.; Matsuba, T.; Maeda, Y.; Takahashi, A.; Hattori, T.; Ashino, Y. High Levels of the Cleaved Form of Galectin-9 and Osteopontin in the Plasma Are Associated with Inflammatory Markers That Reflect the Severity of COVID-19 Pneumonia. *Int. J. Mol. Sci.* **2021**, *22*, 4978. [CrossRef]
10. Coronavirus Disease 2019 (COVID-19) Treatment Guidelines. Available online: https://www.covid19treatmentguidelines.nih.gov (accessed on 2 March 2022).
11. Kharat, A.; Simon, M.; Guérin, C. Prone position in COVID 19-associated acute respiratory failure. *Curr. Opin.* **2022**, *28*, 57–65. [CrossRef]
12. Bahloul, M.; Kharrat, S.; Hafdhi, M.; Maalla, A.; Turki, O.; Chtara, K.; Ammar, R.; Suissi, B.; Hamida, C.B.; Chelly, H.; et al. Bouaziz M Impact of prone position on outcomes of COVID-19 patients with spontaneous breathing. *Acute Crit. Care* **2021**, *36*, 208–214. [CrossRef]
13. Nakamura, K.; Ide, S.; Saito, S.; Kinoshita, N.; Kutsuna, S.; Moriyama, Y.; Suzuki, T.; Ota, M.; Nomoto, H.; Mizoue, T.; et al. COVID-19 can suddenly become severe: A case series from Tokyo, Japan. *Glob. Health Med.* **2020**, *2*, 174–177. [CrossRef]
14. Ye, Q.; Wang, B.; Mao, J. The pathogenesis and treatment of the 'Cytokine Storm' in COVID-19. *J. Infect.* **2020**, *80*, 607–613. [CrossRef]
15. Copaescu, A.; Smibert, O.; Gibson, A.; Phillips, E.J.; Trubiano, J.A.J. The role of IL-6 and other mediators in the cytokine storm associated with SARS-CoV-2 infection. *Allergy Clin. Immunol.* **2020**, *146*, 518–534. [CrossRef]
16. Gatti, M.; Fusaroli, M.; Caraceni, P.; Poluzzi, E.; Ponti, D.F.; Raschi, E. Serious adverse events with tocilizumab: Pharmacovigilance asana aid to prioritize monitoring in COVID-19. *Br. J. Clin. Pharmacol.* **2021**, *87*, 1533–1540. [CrossRef]
17. Charan, J.; Dutta, S.; Kaur, R.; Bhardwaj, P.; Sharma, P.; Ambwani, S.; Jahan, I.; Abubakar, A.; Islam, S.; Hardcastle, C.T.; et al. Tocilizumab in COVID-19: A study of adverse drug events reported in the WHO database. *Expert Opin. Drug Saf.* **2021**, *20*, 1125–1136. [CrossRef]
18. Batah, S.S.; Fabro, A.T. Pulmonary pathology of ARDS in COVID-19: A pathological review for clinicians. *Respir. Med.* **2021**, *176*, 106239. [CrossRef]
19. Zeng, Z.; Xiang, M.; Guan, H.; Liu, Y.; Zhang, H.; Xia, L.; Zhan, J.; Hu, Q. Early fibroproliferative signs on high-resolution CT are associated with mortality in COVID-19 pneumonia patients with ARDS: A retrospective study. *Ther. Adv. Chronic Dis.* **2021**, *12*, 2040622320982171. [CrossRef]
20. Han, X.; Fan, Y.; Alwalid, O.; Li, N.; Jia, X.; Yuan, M.; Li, Y.; Cao, Y.; Gu, J.; Wu, H.; et al. Six-month Follow-up Chest CT Findings after Severe COVID-19 Pneumonia. *Radiology* **2021**, *299*, E177–E186. [CrossRef]
21. Iwasaki-Hozumi, H.; Chagan-Yasutan, H.; Ashino, Y.; Hattori, T. Blood Levels of Galectin-9, an Immuno-Regulating Molecule, Reflect the Severity for the Acute and Chronic Infectious. *Dis. Biomol.* **2021**, *11*, 430. [CrossRef]
22. Toniatia, P.; Pivab, S.; Cattalinid, M.; Garrafaf, E.; Regolaa, F.; Castellie, F.; Franceschinia, F.; Airòa, P.; Bazzania, C.; Beindorfi, E.-A.; et al. Tocilizumab for the treatment of severe COVID-19 pneumonia with hyperinflammatory syndrome and acute respiratory failure: A single center study of 100 patients in Brescia, Italy. *Nicola Latronicob Autoimmun. Rev.* **2020**, *19*, 102568. [CrossRef]
23. Hermine, O.; Mariette, X.; Tharaux, P.L.; Resche-Rigon, M.; Porcher, R.; Ravaud, P. Effect of Tocilizumab vs. Usual Care in Adults Hospitalized With COVID-19 and Moderate or Severe Pneumonia: A Randomized Clinical Trial. CORIMUNO-19 Collaborative Group. *JAMA Intern. Med.* **2021**, *181*, 32–40. [CrossRef]
24. Oliveira, A.L.; Ruano, C.; Riso, N.; Ribeiro, J.C.; Moraes-Fontes, M.F. Paradoxical pulmonary event under tocilizumab treatment for systemic sclerosis-associated usualinterstitial pneumonia. *Ann. Rheum. Dis.* **2020**, *79*, e22. [CrossRef]
25. Robinson, B.S.; Saeedi, B.; Arthur, C.M.; Owens, J.; Naudin, C.; Ahmed, N.; Luo, L.; Jones, R.; Neish, A.; Stowell, S.R. Galectin-9 Is a Novel Regulator of Epithelial Restitution. *Am. J. Pathol.* **2020**, *190*, 1657–1666. [CrossRef]

26. Arikawa, T.; Matsukawa, A.; Watanabe, K.; Sakata, K.M.; Seki, M.; Nagayama, M.; Takeshita, K.; Ito, K.; Niki, T.; Oomizu, S.; et al. Galectin-9 accelerates transforming growth factor beta3-induced differentiation of human mesenchymal stem cells to chondrocytes. *Bone* **2009**, *44*, 849–857. [CrossRef]
27. Hughes, R.C. Galectins as modulators of cell adhesion. *Biochimie* **2001**, *83*, 667–676. [CrossRef]
28. Calkovska, A.; Kolomaznik, M.; Calkovsky, V. Alveolar type II cells and pulmonary surfactant in COVID-19 era. *Physiol. Res.* **2021**, *70*, S195–S208. [CrossRef]
29. Dapat, I.C.; Pascapurnama, D.N.; Iwasaki, H.; Labayo, H.K.; Chagan-Yasutan, H.; Egawa, S.; Hattori, T. Secretion of Galectin-9 as a DAMP during Dengue Virus Infection in THP-1. *Cell Int. J. Mol. Sci.* **2017**, *18*, 1644. [CrossRef]
30. Ashino, Y.; Ying, X.; Dobbs, L.G.; Bhattacharya, J. $[Ca^{2+}]_i$ oscillations regulate type II cell exocytosis in the pulmonary alveolus. *Am. J. Physiol. Lung Cell Mol. Physiol.* **2000**, *279*, L5–L13. [CrossRef]
31. Takada, H.; Furuya, K.; Sokabe, M. Mechanosensitive ATP release from hemichannels and $Ca^{2+}$ influx through TRPC6 accelerate wound closure in keratinocytes. *J. Cell Sci.* **2014**, *127*, 4159–4171. [CrossRef]
32. Grygorczyk, R.; Furuya, K.; Sokabe, M. Imaging and characterization of stretch-induced ATP release from alveolar A549 cells. *J. Physiol.* **2013**, *591*, 1195–1215. [CrossRef]

*reports*

*Perspective*

# Neuronal and Non-Neuronal GABA in COVID-19: Relevance for Psychiatry

**Adonis Sfera [1,2,*], Karina G. Thomas [1], Sarvin Sasannia [3], Jonathan J. Anton [1,4], Christina V. Andronescu [5], Michael Garcia [2], Dan O. Sfera [1], Michael A. Cummings [1] and Zisis Kozlakidis [6]**

[1] Patton State Hospital, University of California, Riverside, CA 92521, USA; karina.thomas@dsh.ca.gov (K.G.T.); jonathan.anton@dsh.ca.gov (J.J.A.); dan.sfera@dsh.ca.gov (D.O.S.); cummings.michael@dsh.ca.gov (M.A.C.)
[2] Department of Psychiatry, University of California, Riverside, CA 92521, USA; michael.garcia@dsh.ca.gov
[3] Department of Medicine, Shiraz University of Medical Sciences, Shiraz 14336-71348, Iran; sasannia.sarvin@gmail.com
[4] College of Health Science, California Baptist University, Riverside, CA 92504, USA
[5] Medical Anthropology Department, Stanford University, Stanford, CA 94305, USA; christina.andronescu@dsh.ca.gov
[6] International Agency for Research on Cancer (IARC), 69372 Lyon, France; kozlakidisz@iarc.fr
* Correspondence: adonis.sfera@dsh.ca.gov

**Abstract:** Infection with SARS-CoV-2, the causative agent of the COVID-19 pandemic, originated in China and quickly spread across the globe. Despite tremendous economic and healthcare devastation, research on this virus has contributed to a better understanding of numerous molecular pathways, including those involving $\gamma$-aminobutyric acid (GABA), that will positively impact medical science, including neuropsychiatry, in the post-pandemic era. SARS-CoV-2 primarily enters the host cells through the renin–angiotensin system's component named angiotensin-converting enzyme-2 (ACE-2). Among its many functions, this protein upregulates GABA, protecting not only the central nervous system but also the endothelia, the pancreas, and the gut microbiota. SARS-CoV-2 binding to ACE-2 usurps the neuronal and non-neuronal GABAergic systems, contributing to the high comorbidity of neuropsychiatric illness with gut dysbiosis and endothelial and metabolic dysfunctions. In this perspective article, we take a closer look at the pathology emerging from the viral hijacking of non-neuronal GABA and summarize potential interventions for restoring these systems.

**Keywords:** GABA; SARS-CoV-2; renin–angiotensin system; microbiome; neuropsychiatric disorders



**Citation:** Sfera, A.; Thomas, K.G.; Sasannia, S.; Anton, J.J.; Andronescu, C.V.; Garcia, M.; Sfera, D.O.; Cummings, M.A.; Kozlakidis, Z. Neuronal and Non-Neuronal GABA in COVID-19: Relevance for Psychiatry. *Reports* **2022**, *5*, 22. https://doi.org/10.3390/reports5020022

Academic Editors: Toshio Hattori and Yugo Ashino

Received: 20 May 2022
Accepted: 6 June 2022
Published: 8 June 2022



## 1. Introduction

The infection with SARS-CoV-2 became a pandemic on 11 March 2020, ushering in immeasurable economic and healthcare catastrophes. Up until 14 May 2022, more than 517 million people had been afflicted by COVID-19, and more than 6 million had died (https://covid19.who.int/ (26 May 2022)). However, the extensive research conducted on this virus in a short period of time has broadened our understanding of its numerous pathogenetic mechanisms, leading to novel paradigms that will likely bear fruit in the post-pandemic era. For example, local renin–angiotensin systems (RAS) expressed in the brain and gastro-intestinal (GI) tract, although previously acknowledged, were poorly defined prior to the COVID-19 pandemic. Likewise, the crosstalk between host RAS and microbial $\gamma$-aminobutyric acid (mGABA) was seldom considered when explaining the high comorbidity of inflammatory bowel disease (IBD) and neuropsychiatric conditions, including anxiety, depression, psychosis, and seizure disorder [1–4]. By the same token, endothelial GABA (eGABA) and its role in blood pressure homeostasis and neuropsychiatric pathology began to be examined only after the appearance of COVID-19 [5].

Although neuronal GABA (nGABA) has been studied for several decades, also within the context of viral infections, its non-neurotransmitter functions were poorly understood until very recently [6,7]. For example, the antiviral and anti-inflammatory properties of GABA were highlighted by recent preclinical studies showing that GABA supplementation decreased COVID-19 death rates [8–10]. Along this line, a novel study has demonstrated that *Limosilactobacillus fermentum*, a GABA-producing gut microbe, thwarts Norovirus infection, further attesting to the antiviral actions of this biomolecule [11]. In addition, mGABA was demonstrated to augment host autophagy, including that of pathogen-infected cells, indicating participation in antimicrobial defenses [12]. Interestingly, gut angiotensin-converting enzyme-2 (ACE-2), the SARS-CoV-2 entry portal, upregulates mGABA by increasing its release from the gut flora [13]. This is significant, as earlier studies have demonstrated that angiotensin receptor blockers (ARBs) possess antiepileptic, anti-depressant, and anti-anxiety properties, suggesting that the functions of RAS and GABA are highly intertwined [14–16]. Indeed, blood–brain barrier (BBB)-crossing ARBs were reported to lower CNS inflammation, highlighting the role of RAS in neuropsychiatric pathology and placing this system on an equal footing with serotonin (5-HT) and dopamine (DA) [17,18]. Furthermore, in the CNS and pancreas, ACE2–GABA crosstalk was reported to optimize glucose metabolism, probably accounting for the anti-diabetic properties of ARBs [19,20]. As many psychotropic drugs are associated with metabolic dysfunction, using centrally acting ARBs, such as candesartan, for hypertension may bring additional benefits to psychiatric patients [21].

SARS-CoV-2 depletes host GABA by several mechanisms:

1. The viral spike (S) protein contains a GABA-mimicking sequence or short linear motif that can directly usurp host GABAergic signaling [22,23].
2. The SARS-CoV-2 proteins nonstructural protein 6 (NSP6), open reading frame 8 (ORF8), and open reading frame 3 (ORF3a) interact directly with host mammalian target of rapamycin complex 1 (mTORC-1), interleukin 17 (IL-17), and transmembrane protein 16F (TMEM16F), inducing premature EC senescence, a phenotype characterized by low GABA [24–29] (Figure 1).
3. SARS-CoV-2/ACE-2 binding disrupts the function of the protective renin–angiotensin system (RAS) branch, including Mas receptor (MasR) signaling, lowering GABA [14,30].
4. The viral protein ORF3a interacts with toll-like receptor 4(TLR4), triggering EC senescence and lowering GABA [31].
5. The SARS-CoV-2 viral proteins nonstructural protein 4 (NSP4), nonstructural protein 8 (NSP8), and open reading frame 9c (ORF9c) decrease GABA by disrupting the mitochondria, triggering vascular senescence [32] (Figure 1).

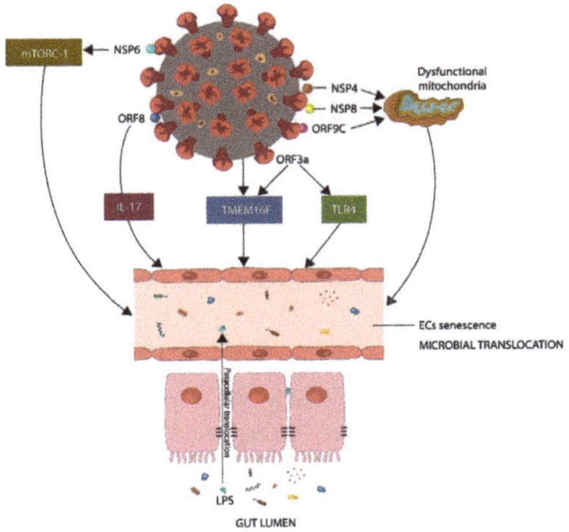


**Figure 1.** SARS-CoV-2 downregulates GABA by inducing endothelial senescence directly (by protein

–protein interactions) and indirectly (via mitochondrial dysfunction and ANG II upregulation). A dysfunctional endothelial barrier facilitates microbial translocation from the GI tract, where the flora is immunologically tolerated, into the systemic circulation, where it evokes inflammation and immunogenicity. Legend: NSP6, nonstructural protein 6, ORF8, open reading frame 8, IL-17, interleukin 17, TMEM16F, transmembrane protein 16F, TLR4, toll-like receptor 4, NSP4, nonstructural protein 4, NSP8, nonstructural protein 8, ORF9C, open reading frame 9C, ORF3a, open reading frame 3a, LPS, lipopolysaccharide.

SARS-CoV-2-mediated GABA depletion likely explains the neuropsychiatric manifestations of COVID-19, including anxiety, depression, posttraumatic stress disorder (PTSD), cognitive impairment, and seizure disorder [33–37].

In this perspective article, we take a closer look at the viral hijacking of endothelial, pancreatic, and gut GABA and the associated pathology. We also discuss potential interventions for GABAergic system restoration.

## 2. Two Senescence Mechanisms in SARS-CoV-2 Infection

SARS-CoV-2 is a single-stranded, enveloped RNA virus that contains four structural proteins: spike (S), nucleocapsid (N), membrane (M), and envelope (E). The S protein is composed of two subunits, S1 and S2. The former engages ACE-2, while the latter (FCS) interacts with furin, merging viral envelope and host plasma membrane as well as cells, thus forming syncytia [38]. The viral attachment to ACE-2 disrupts the physiological function of this protein, leading to the unchecked accumulation of angiotensin II (ANG II), a mitochondrial toxin linked to premature EC senescence [39,40].

### *2.1. S1/ACE-2 Attachment and ANG II-Induced Senescence*

The SARS-CoV-2 envelope protein S1 binds ACE-2, contributing to the loss of this enzyme's biological function as well as to the shutting down of the anti-inflammatory/antioxidant (protective) RAS (Figure 2). The unchecked accumulation of ANG II enhances the proinflammatory/prooxidative RAS branch, which, under normal circumstances is counterbalanced by the protective axis. The imbalance between the two RAS arms results in ANG II-driven hyperinflammation or "cytokine storm" [41,42] (Figure 2). Depletion of ACE-2 and loss of anti-inflammatory/antioxidant RAS induce premature cellular senescence, lowering eGABA, which in return may trigger a neuropsychiatric pathology [43–46].

### *2.2. S2/Furin Attachment and Syncytia-Induced Senescence*

Enveloped viruses are known for generating multinuclear giant cells by inducing cell–cell fusion or syncytia formation. Cell–cell fusion is a physiological or pathological process in which neighboring cells merge their plasma membranes, sharing intracellular organelles, including cytoplasm and nuclei [47,48].

SARS-CoV-2 entry into host cells requires furin cleavage of the S antigen at the S1/S2 site to initiate membrane fusion [49]. The insertion of the polybasic PRRAR motif at FCS is crucial for fusing viral envelopes with host plasma membrane, as well as the host cells with each other [50]. PRRAR is a triple-arginine motif that forms cell membrane pores via its guanidinium side chains, compelling the cells to fuse for protection [51,52].

Taken together, the SARS-CoV-2 virus induces cellular senescence via ANG II and/or syncytia formation, downregulating the antiviral amino acid GABA [53,54].

### *2.3. Molecular Mechanisms of Syncytia Formation*

The subunit β3 of GABA-A receptors contains a triple-arginine motif (RRR) that interacts with the endocytic pathway (EP) protein AP2, likely disrupting SARS-CoV-2 endocytosis [55]. On the other hand, the triple arginine (PRRAR) in the S antigen of SARS-CoV-2 may counteract this GABA action, usurping the EP and opening it for viral ingress.

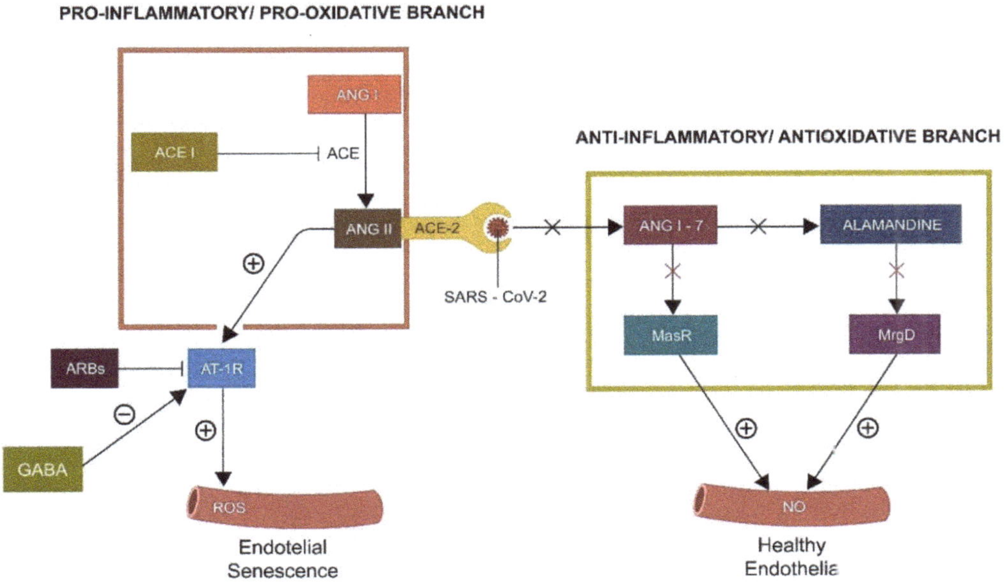


**Figure 2.** Human RAS consists of two opposing branches, the proinflammatory/prooxidative (driven by ANG II) branch and the anti-inflammatory/antioxidant (driven by ANG 1-7) one. ANG II, acting via AT-1Rs, induces EC senescence. ARBs and GABA negatively regulate AT-1Rs, opposing ANG II. The protective RAS branch, comprised of ANG 1-7, alamandine, and their respective receptors Mas and MrgD, inhibit inflammation and oxidative stress. SARS-CoV-2 engagement with ACE-2 disrupts the entire anti-inflammatory/antioxidant branch, leading to unchecked ANG II accumulation and premature EC senescence. Legend: ANG I, angiotensin I, ACEi, angiotensin-converting enzyme inhibitors, ANG II, angiotensin II, ARBs, angiotensin receptor blockers, AT-1r, angiotensin receptor type 1, ROS, reactive oxygen species, ANG1-7, angiotensin 1-7, MasR, Mas receptor, MrgD, MrgD receptor, NO, nitric oxide.

A human endogenous retrovirus W (HERV-W) was identified in the regulatory region of GABA-B receptor subunit 1 gene, suggesting that this ancestral retrovirus can be activated by exogenous viruses, including SARS-CoV-2 [56]. HERV-W activation and increased GABA-B expression likely depresses the antiviral GABA-A, facilitating SARS-CoV-2 replication [57]. We surmise that the triple-arginine FCS of SARS-CoV-2 has retrovirus-activating properties, switching on HERVs and human immunodeficiency virus-1 (HIV-1) [58,59] (please see section Ancient and modern viruses disrupt GABAergic signaling).

The SARS-CoV-2 proteins ORF3a and S activate TMEM16F, a calcium-dependent phospholipid scramblase that executes the fusion of both viral envelope with plasma membrane and host cells with each other [60]. In addition, SARS-CoV-2 can deplete GABA by disrupting the mitochondria, which in turn activate the cellular senescence program [24,61] (Figure 1). Furthermore, ORF3a stimulation of TLR4 can induce EC senescence and TMEM16F activation, forming syncytia [31,60,62].

### 2.4. Biological Barrier Dysfunction

Senescent endothelia may disrupt the BBB and the gut barrier, facilitating the translocation of GI tract microbes and/or their molecules, including LPS, into the systemic circulation, as reported in COVID-19 critically ill patients [63,64] (Figure 1). In addition, the S protein of SARS-CoV-2 can bind directly to circulating LPS, triggering a hyperinflammatory pathology [65]. Interestingly, ANG II upregulates TLR4, the main LPS sensor, augmenting inflammation and neuropsychiatric pathology [43,66–68]. As GABA is a negative regulator of TLR4, it likely inhibits both cell–cell fusion and premature senescence, counteracting not only the "cytokine storm" but also neuroinflammation [62,69]. Indeed, low GABA and elevated LPS were demonstrated in the brains of patients with Alzheimer's disease (AD), suggesting BBB dysfunction and poor LPS suppression [70,71]. Moreover, several studies have demonstrated that LPS can induce pathology by fusing cells into multinuclear structures [72]. For example, brain cells can merge, forming physiological or pathological syncytia that alter both neuronal networks and information processing [73,74] (Figure 3). For example, neuron–neuron fusion occurs during normal aging as well as in the presence of viral infections, multiple sclerosis (MS), AD, and following radiation exposure and chemotherapy [75].

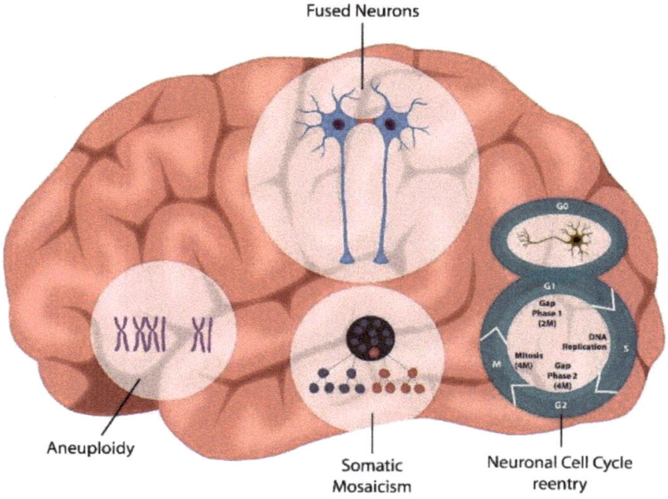


**Figure 3.** Neuronal cell–cell fusion occurs physiologically, in normal aging, or pathologically, in various conditions, including viral infections, Alzheimer's disease (AD), multiple sclerosis (MS), radiation exposure, or chemotherapy [76] Neuronal syncytia formation likely accounts for previously unexplained phenomena, such as aneuploidy, somatic mosaicism, and neuronal cell cycle reactivation, documented in various neuropsychiatric conditions.

Cell–cell fusion is a major cause of genome destabilization and generation of aneuploidy, somatic mosaicism, and reactivation of the cell cycle in postmitotic cells [61,75–78] (Figure 3).

Taken together, SARS-CoV-2 may precipitate premature vascular aging via ACE-2 depletion and syncytia formation. Senescent ECs downregulate eGABA, predisposing to neuropsychiatric disorders.

### 3. Cellular Senescence in Psychopathology

Psychiatric disorders have been associated with shorter-than-average patient lifespan and high comorbidity with age-related diseases, suggesting that premature cellular senescence plays a major role in the pathogenesis of these conditions [79,80]. SARS-CoV-2, like many other viruses, induces premature tissue aging, a phenomenon also demonstrated in depression, anxiety, schizophrenia, and seizure disorder, indicating that GABA depletion may be the common denominator of these pathologies [81–84]. On the other hand, GABA supplementation was associated with less inflammaging and improved sleep and mood, pointing to a potential therapeutic modality [85,86]. In addition, as GABA promotes autophagic elimination of damaged and virus-infected cells, GABA supplementation may benefit not only COVID-19-affected patients but also those with age-related diseases [5,12].

*Adult Neurogenesis and SARS-CoV-2 Infection*

The COVID-19 pandemic has highlighted the role of RAS dysfunction, especially ANG II, in the pathogenesis of neuropsychiatric disorders [87]. On the other hand, ARBs and ACEi showed promising results in the treatment of these conditions, emphasizing the pathological role of dysregulated ANG II [88,89]. Moreover, recent epidemiological studies found that COVID-19 survivors may be at increased risk of several neuropsychiatric disorders, further emphasizing the role of RAS in this pathology [30,90,91].

COVID-19-induced premature cellular senescence may engender neuropathology by suppressing adult neurogenesis in the hippocampal subgranular zone (SGZ) and cerebral subventricular zone (SVZ) [92,93]. Unlike in the adult CNS, GABA is an excitatory neurotransmitter in immature neurons; therefore, the loss of GABAergic signaling may disrupt adult neurogenesis [92,94–96]. Interestingly, TLR4 was reported to play a key role in the conversion of immature into mature neuronal cells, linking viral exploitation of this protein to dysfunctional neurogenesis [97,98].

Taken together, virus-induced senescence lowers eGABA, contributing to neuropsychiatric pathology by precipitating premature vascular aging and disrupting neurogenesis.

## 4. GABA, Neuronal and Non-Neuronal Information Processing

GABA is a non-protein amino acid present in almost all life forms, including plants, bacteria, and gut microbes. In the central nervous system (CNS), GABA, signaling via inotropic (GABA-A) and metabotropic (GABA-B) receptors, functions as an inhibitory neurotransmitter and participates in numerous physiological processes, including cognition, wakefulness, and self-awareness [99–101].

Neuronal and non-neuronal GABA are synthesized from glutamate via glutamic acid decarboxylase (GAD), an enzyme located in all GABA-generating cells, including the gut microbes [102,103]. This is significant, as autoantibodies against GAD were documented in COVID-19 patients, suggesting molecular mimicry between this enzyme and SARS-CoV-2 proteins [104,105]. Dysfunctional GABAergic systems were associated with neuropsychiatric illness and disorders of consciousness [106–111]. For example, the GABAergic system was linked to gamma oscillations on electroencephalogram (EEG), a self-awareness pattern, disrupted in many neuropsychiatric disorders, including epilepsy, schizophrenia, autism, anxiety, and depression [112–114]. The EEG gamma-band (25–90 Hz) was positively correlated with resting GABA concentration as well as with the cerebral blood flow, emphasizing the potential of eGABA as a biomarker [115,116].

During development and early life, GABA is an excitatory neurotransmitter that matures gradually throughout childhood and early adolescence [117]. During this time, the partial or total loss of GABA causes circulatory abnormalities and inhibits the migration and placement of cortical interneurons [118]. In adolescence, GABA reaches sufficient levels to initiate microglia-mediated synapse elimination and axonal pruning, characteristic of mature cognition [119]. Indeed, recent studies have shown that GABA-sensing microglia are required for synapse remodeling in adolescence and the installment of adult information processing [120]. On the other hand, dysfunctional GABA signaling may contribute to the pathological reactivation of microglia known to eliminate healthy neurons and synapses, a phenomenon documented in both psychopathology and neurodegeneration [121]. These microglial functions can be hijacked by intracellular pathogens, especially those linked to mental illness [122–124].

### 4.1. Non-Neuronal Information Processing

Recent studies have shown that EC can form cellular networks and communicate via Ca2+ waves, suggesting that information processing may take place at the vascular level [125,126]. Likewise, astrocytes form physiological syncytia, a finding consistent with the Ca2+ wave hypothesis of information processing [127]. In addition, the dysfunctional eGABA association with altered cortical circuits and behavior likely highlights the role of ECs in cognition [118]. Indeed, ECs communicate with and shadow neurons throughout the brain, likely participating in cognitive processes mediated by Ca2+. Moreover, as Ca2+ drives the rudimentary memory of plants and unicellular organisms, an ancient modality of non-neuronal information processing is emphasized [128–130]. Along this line, the antidepressant action of ketamine, based, at least in part, on its impact on calcium/calmodulin-dependent protein kinase II (CaMKII), likely implicates Ca2+ in emotional intelligence and cognition [131]. This is important, as virtual screening studies documented the existence of a CaMKII system in the S protein of SARS-CoV-2, linking this pathogen to affective disorders [132]. Moreover, non-neuronal information processing was reported in skeletal muscle, heart, and fascia, indicating that neuronal cells do not hold the exclusive monopoly on cognitive processes [133,134]. Along this line, the acquisition of donor personality characteristics following heart transplantation, documented by numerous studies, may reflect EC-mediated cognition [135–137]. This is in line with the hemo-neural hypothesis that connects information processing to endothelial blood flow [138].

In the following sections, we take a closer look at the COVID-19 influence on non-neuronal GABAergic systems, especially the endothelial, microbial, and pancreatic pathways, emphasizing their potential participation in neuropsychiatric pathology.

### 4.2. *eGABA*

ECs line the inner layer of the circulatory system and regulate the vascular function via membrane-bound receptors that interact with various neurotransmitters, hormones, and metabolites. While previously conceptualized as passive components of membranes and biological barriers, ECs are now known to play an essential role in vascular homeostasis and the pathogenesis of thrombosis and inflammation [139]. Under normal circumstances, ECs synthesize and secrete eGABA, a molecule depleted in the virus-induced cellular senescence phenotype [118,140,141]. Aside from viral infections, EC senescence and low eGABA were associated with PTSD, anxiety, depression, autism, schizophrenia, and epilepsy, suggesting that the viral manipulation of this neurotransmitter may initiate or exacerbate neuropsychiatric pathology [35,142–146]. Moreover, as human ECs express abundant ACE-2, a positive regulator of eGABA, SARS-CoV-2 could disrupt the GABAergic signaling directly [20]. Indeed, ACE-2 variants with depleted GABA were linked to major depressive disorder, schizophrenia, bipolar disorder, and epilepsy, emphasizing the importance of RAS/GABA crosstalk for central nervous system (CNS) homeostasis [14,87,91,147].

### 4.3. *pGABA*

Recent studies have identified another GABA pool in pancreatic β cells that may be altered by SARS-CoV-2 infection, promoting metabolic dysfunction [148,149]. On the other hand, the administration of exogenous GABA was demonstrated to improve glucose tolerance in rodents, indicating that this biomolecule may play a key role in β cell homeostasis [150,151].

Excessive ANG II was associated with diabetes mellitus type 2 (DMT2), indicating that SARS-CoV-2 can trigger dysmetabolism by disrupting RAS [152]. In addition, the S and ORF3a antigens of SARS-CoV-2 were shown to activate TMEM16F, promoting cell–cell fusion, a phenotype associated with premature cellular senescence and low GABA [53,54,153]. Moreover, premature senescence of β cells and depleted pGABA may drive DMT2 and the neuropsychiatric pathology-linked dysmetabolism [154,155]. So far, several neuropsychiatric disorders and psychotropic drugs have been associated with impaired metabolism, suggesting that exogenous GABA may benefit individuals with these conditions [82]. Indeed, in a previous article, we discussed the relationship between obesity and impulsivity in psychiatric patients, emphasizing that attaining optimal results requires the concomitant treatment of both conditions [156].

### 4.4. *mGABA*

SARS-CoV-2 affinity for ACE-2 suggests that tissues with high expression of this protein, such as intestinal epithelial cells (IECs), are more vulnerable to infection [157]. As

ACE-2 protects the beneficial GI tract microbes, many of which generate mGABA, the viral exploitation of this protein may trigger intestinal dysbiosis [158,159]. Interestingly, gut ACE-2 is co-expressed with L-dopa decarboxylase (DDC), an enzyme required for microbial DA generation; thus, the viral exploitation of ACE-2 likely affects the brain dopaminergic system (DAS) [160]. As elevated DDC was demonstrated in patients with schizophrenia, the importance of RAS and DAS crosstalk is further emphasized [161].

In the GI tract, ACE-2 heterodimerizes with broad neutral amino acid transporter 1 (B0AT1) that participates in tryptophan (Trp) absorption, indicating that SARS-CoV-2 infection may deplete this amino acid [162] (Figure 4). For example, ACE2-deficient mice display low Trp blood levels, emphasizing the role of this protein in Trp homeostasis [163,164]. As Trp is crucial for serotonin biosynthesis, the viral exploitation of this essential amino acid may trigger neuropsychiatric symptoms, including depression [165]. Moreover, the gut microbes involved in tryptophan (Trp) metabolism are also implicated in adult neurogenesis via aryl hydrocarbon receptor (Ahr), a protein usurped by COVID-19 [166,167]. Ahr is a cytoplasmic ligand and xenobiotic sensor that regulates the microbiota population and the host–microbe crosstalk [168,169]. In our earlier work, we discussed the role of Ahr in psychotropic drugs-induced metabolic dysfunction and suggested that various microbial products, including indole-3-propionic acid, could ameliorate glucose tolerance [170]. As recent studies have linked Ahr to cellular senescence, it is likely that impaired Trp absorption may predispose to this low mGABA phenotype [171,172]. Moreover, mGABA enhances the expression of T helper 17 cells (Th17) characterized by the release of IL-17, an mTORC1-activating antiviral biomolecule [173–175]. Interestingly, SARS-CoV-2 exploits mTORC-1 and IL-17, disrupting both host antiviral defenses and the gut barrier [176,177] (Figure 1).

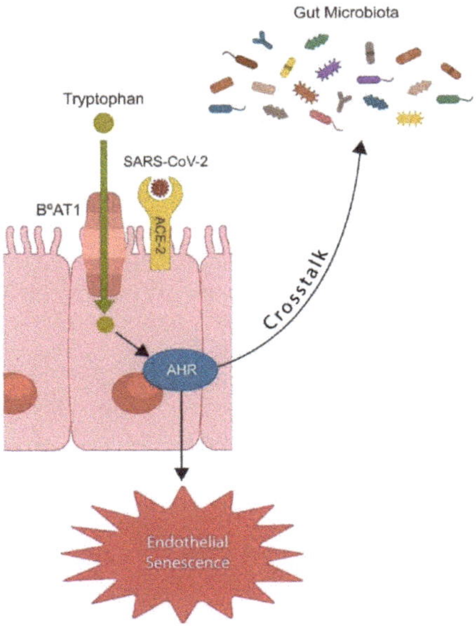


**Figure 4.** In the GI tract, ACE-2 dimerizes with the neutral amino acid transporter B0AT1 involved in Trp absorption. Trp, an Ahr ligand, coordinates host–microbiota interaction and local metabolism. Dysfunctional Trp absorption and defective Ahr may contribute to barrier disruption and microbial translocation into the systemic circulation. Legend: Trp, tryptophan, B0AT1, neutral amino acid transporter, AHR, aryl hydrocarbon receptor.

## 5. Ancient and Modern Viruses Disrupt GABAergic Signaling

The syncytia-forming S2 protein of SARS-CoV-2 is crucial for infectivity, as highlighted by its presence in several highly contagious viruses [178,179]. Indeed, FCS, absent in other SARS-linked coronaviruses, usurps host furin, enhancing COVID-19 transmissibility [180]. On the other hand, loss of FCS was shown to attenuate SARS-CoV-2 virulence and pathogenicity, emphasizing the utmost importance of S2 for the pandemic spread of this viral infection [181].

Aside from SARS-CoV-2, arginine-rich FCSs were identified in HIV-1 protein GP160 ENV, as well as in syncytin-1, a physiological placental fusogen encoded by HERV-W, suggesting that COVID-19 can activate dormant viral fossils [58,182,183]. This is significant, as it connects COVID-19 to retroviruses as well as to the reproductive pathology [184,185].

HERVs are ancient viruses, comprising about 8% of the human DNA, that under normal circumstances are not transcribed. However, various pathologies, including exogenous viral infections, can reactivate HERVs, and translate their DNA into proteins, such as syncytin-1, a molecule that generates trophoblast syncytia during placentation [186]. Pathologically, syncytin-1 promotes cell–cell fusion, hyperinflammation, and autoimmunity, as well as the psychopathology linked to defective GABA [187].

Posttranslational cleavage of syncytin-1 is executed by furin, a host protein usurped by viral FCS, disrupting both CNS and placental GABA [188]. Indeed, a recent meta-analysis connected SARS-CoV-2 infection during pregnancy to preeclampsia, linking this condition to usurped syncytin-1 [189]. Dysregulated GABA was previously reported in patients with preeclampsia, implicating the furin–syncytin-1 axis in reproductive pathologies [190,191]. Moreover, in the first trimester of pregnancy, GABA upregulates human chorionic gonadotropin (hCG), a key hormone for prenatal brain development, suggesting that the viral exploitation of GABA may trigger a developmental pathology [192,193].

### 5.1. Syncytia Inhibitors

Over the past decade, a considerable effort was devoted to the development of syncytia-blocking agents, including furin inhibitors [194]. The finding that arginine repeats play a major role in virus-induced cell–cell fusion, contributed to the development of FCS-attached arginine mimetics, including phenylacetyl-Arg-Val-Arg-4-amidinobenzylamide, to inhibit the formation of syncytia [195,196]. As furin is highly expressed in ECs and involved in vascular aging and dysmetabolism, furin inhibitors may be capable of averting premature EC senescence and disrupt viral replication [197,198] (Table 1).

Aside from inhibiting furin, syncytia formation can be blocked by lowering the expression of TMEM16F. TMEM16F is a Ca2+-driven phospholipid scramblase that maintains phosphatidylserine (PS) in the inner leaflet of the cell membrane, allowing its externalization only when the cell is ready for apoptosis or fusion [199,200]. Since externalized PS (ePS) is indispensable for syncytia formation, TMEM16F inhibitors may block pathological cell–cell fusion [201]. For example, niclosamide, a TMEM16F-targeting drug, was reported to inhibit both SARS-CoV-2 syncytia and viral transmissibility [202]. Niclosamide is an anthelmintic compound with demonstrated antiviral properties that is currently being evaluated for the treatment of COVID-19 [203]. Several recent studies show that TMEM16F interacts with inositol 1,4,5-triphosphate receptor 1 (IP3R1) in many cell types, including the GABAergic interneurons, implicating this protein in cell–cell fusion [204,205]. Interestingly, IP3R1 was associated with psychopathology, including schizophrenia, neurodegenerative disorders, and epilepsy, suggesting that niclosamide may have a therapeutic value in the treatment of these conditions [206–208]. Indeed, lithium and valproic acid, drugs routinely utilized in the treatment of bipolar disorder, alter IP3R1 expression, indicating that TMEM16F inhibitors could have a place in neuropsychiatry [209]. As lithium, valproate, and niclosamide alter the Wnt/β-catenin signaling, the latter may possess mood-stabilizing properties. Interestingly, a valproic acid/niclosamide combination was found therapeutic in some cancers, emphasizing the pleotropic role of the Wnt/β-catenin pathway [210,211]. Furthermore, dysfunctional TMEM16F–IP3R1–GABA signaling was found to pathologically activate the microglia, probably leading to aberrant phagocytosis of healthy neurons and synapses, documented in neuropsychiatric pathologies [212].

It has been known for several decades that diazepam displays anti-syncytial properties, as it inhibits the fusion of myoblasts during musculoskeletal system development [213]. In contrast, as arginine enhances myoblast fusion and abolishes the anxiolytic effects of diazepam, benzodiazepines may be able to counteract FCS-mediated cell–cell fusion [214,215]. Interestingly, ivermectin binds GABA-A receptors at the diazepam site, highlighting this drug's anti-syncytial mechanism of action [216].

Taken together, the TMEM16F–IP3R1–GABA axis comprises a signaling hub involved in viral infections, cancer, and neuropsychiatric illness. GABA upregulation may inhibit TMEM16F and the formation of pathological syncytia.

### 5.2. GABA, Autophagy, and Blood Pressure

The antiviral properties of GABA—the elimination of virus-infected cells—highlight the autophagy-activating role of this amino acid [217,218]. Indeed, GABA interferes with host EP that many viruses, including SARS-CoV-2, exploit to enter host cells [12,219]. Viral FCS usurps GABA-mediated autophagy by inhibiting subunit β3 interaction with the clathrin endocytosis AP2 protein [55].

Autophagy modulation may account for the other beneficial properties of GABA, including anti-hypertension, anti-diabetes, antioxidant, and anti-inflammatory actions, suggesting that supplementation with this amino acid may be salutary for patients with these disorders [220,221]. Exogenous GABA may or may not cross the BBB, as conflicting results were reported by different studies. However, CNS-reaching GABA ligands are routinely utilized for the treatment of neuropsychiatric diseases [222,223]. For example, GABA-enhancing anticonvulsants, including tiagabine, gabapentin, and topiramate not only increase neuronal GABA but also augment the non-neuronal GABAergic pathways [224]. For example, gabapentin and tiagabine lower blood pressure in patients with hypertension, while topiramate decreases intracranial pressure, connecting eGABA to the homeostasis of extracellular compartments [225,226]. Interestingly, diazepam displays both antihypertensive and antiretroviral properties (against HIV-1), further emphasizing the beneficial effects of GABA signaling [227,228]. Furthermore, due to their antiretroviral function, benzodiazepines may suppress HERV activation by exogenous viral infections, including SARS-CoV-2 [228,229].

**Table 1.** Potential syncytia-inhibiting drugs and mechanisms of action.

| Drug | Mechanism | References |
|---|---|---|
| Arginine mimetics | Furin inhibition | [195,196] |
| Niclosamide | TMEM16F inhibition | [202] |
| Ivermectin | GABA upregulation | [36,37] |
| ARBs/ACEi | GABA upregulation | [14–16] |
| Benzodiazepines | GABA upregulation | [213] |

Taken together, the syncytia-inducing FCS of SARS-CoV-2 activates HERV-W and lowers retrovirus-inhibiting GABA. GABA and its agonists likely inhibit S2-mediated HERV activation.

## 6. Conclusions

The COVID-19 pandemic has stimulated research highlighting numerous molecular pathways that were poorly defined prior to the arrival of this virus. The viral predilection for ACE-2 has shed light on RAS and the importance of balancing its two branches to prevent pathology, including neuropsychiatric diseases. As SARS-CoV-2 has been extensively studied in a relatively short period of time, several cellular mechanisms relevant for psychiatry have been highlighted, including:

1. ACE-2 is protective for the GABAergic signaling in both neuronal and non-neuronal pathways.

2. Inhibition of protective RAS promotes cellular senescence, lowering neuronal and non-neuronal GABA.
3. Virus-induced syncytia formation is a major trigger of premature cellular senescence and related pathology.
4. Aside from functioning as a neurotransmitter, GABA displays anti-hypertension, anti-senescence, anti-diabetes, antioxidant, and anti-inflammatory properties.
5. ARBs and ACEi upregulate GABA, promoting adult neurogenesis that prevents senescence-mediated psychopathologies.
6. The S2 protein of SARS-CoV-2 contains a triple-arginine insert that activates HERVs, promoting hyperinflammatory pathologies.
7. SARS-CoV-2 alters Trp catabolism and the GABA-producing gut flora, facilitating microbial translocation from the GI tract into various tissues and organs, including the brain.
8. Furin and TMEM16F inhibitors suppress syncytia formation, while ARBs and ACEi upregulate GABA, lowering ANG II-induced senescence.

**Author Contributions:** Conceptualization, A.S.; Methodology, K.G.T.; Formal analysis, investigation, S.S.; data curation, J.J.A.; writing, M.G.; original draft preparation, C.V.A.; review and editing, M.A.C.; supervision, Z.K.; project administration, D.O.S. All authors have read and agreed to the published version of the manuscript.

**Funding:** This research received no external funding.

**Institutional Review Board Statement:** Not applicable.

**Informed Consent Statement:** Not applicable.

**Data Availability Statement:** The study did not report any data.

**Conflicts of Interest:** The authors declare no conflict of interest.

**Disclaimer:** Where authors are identified as personnel of the International Agency for Research on Cancer/WHO, the authors alone are responsible for the views expressed in this article and they do not necessarily represent the decisions, policy or views of the International Agency for Research on Cancer/WHO.

## Abbreviations

| | |
|---|---|
| eGABA | endothelial GABA |
| mGABA | microbial GABA |
| pGABA | pancreatic GABA |
| nGABA | neuronal GABA |
| TLR4 | toll-like receptor 4 |
| ANG II | angiotensin converting enzyme 2 |

## References

1. Benavente, L.; Morís, G. Neurologic disorders associated with inflammatory bowel disease. *Eur. J. Neurol.* **2010**, *18*, 138–143. [CrossRef] [PubMed]
2. Abautret-Daly, Á.; Dempsey, E.; Parra-Blanco, A.; Medina, C.; Harkin, A. Gut–brain actions underlying comorbid anxiety and depression associated with inflammatory bowel disease. *Acta Neuropsychiatr.* **2017**, *30*, 275–296. [CrossRef] [PubMed]
3. Nowakowski, J.; Chrobak, A.; Dudek, D. Psychiatry Illness in Inflammatory Bowel Diseases-Psychiatric Comorbidity and Biological Underpinnings. *Psychiatr. Polska* **2016**, *50*, 1157–1166. [CrossRef] [PubMed]
4. Fernández-Rodríguez, E.; Camarero-González, E. Paciente con enfermedad de Crohn y convulsiones por hipomagnesemia [Patient with Crohn's disease and seizures due to hypomagnesemia]. *Nutr. Hosp.* **2007**, *22*, 720–722.
5. Ma, P.; Li, T.; Ji, F.; Wang, H.; Pang, J. Effect of GABA on blood pressure and blood dynamics of anesthetic rats. *Int. J. Clin. Exp. Med.* **2015**, *8*, 14296–14302. [PubMed]
6. Buzhdygan, T.; Lisinicchia, J.; Patel, V.; Johnson, K.; Neugebauer, V.; Paessler, S.; Jennings, K.; Gelman, B. Neuropsychological, Neurovirological and Neuroimmune Aspects of Abnormal GABAergic Transmission in HIV Infection. *J. Neuroimmune Pharmacol.* **2016**, *11*, 279–293. [CrossRef]

7. Jehmlich, U.; Ritzer, J.; Grosche, J.; Härtig, W.; Liebert, U.G. Experimental measles encephalitis in Lewis rats: Dissemination of infected neuronal cell subtypes. *J. Neurovirol.* **2013**, *19*, 461–470. [CrossRef]
8. Tian, J.; Middleton, B.; Kaufman, D.L. GABA administration prevents severe illness and death following coronavirus infection in mice. *bioRxiv* 2020, *Preprint*. [CrossRef]
9. Bhat, R.; Axtell, R.; Mitra, A.; Miranda, M.; Lock, C.; Tsien, R.W.; Steinman, L. Inhibitory role for GABA in autoimmune inflammation. *Proc. Natl. Acad. Sci. USA* **2010**, *107*, 2580–2585. [CrossRef]
10. Prud'Homme, G.J.; Glinka, Y.; Wang, Q. Immunological GABAergic interactions and therapeutic applications in autoimmune diseases. *Autoimmun. Rev.* **2015**, *14*, 1048–1056. [CrossRef]
11. Li, Y.; Gao, J.; Xue, L.; Shang, Y.; Cai, W.; Xie, X.; Jiang, T.; Chen, H.; Zhang, J.; Wang, J.; et al. Determination of Antiviral Mechanism of Centenarian Gut-Derived Limosilactobacillus fermentum Against Norovirus. *Front. Nutr.* **2022**, *9*, 812623. [CrossRef] [PubMed]
12. Kim, J.K.; Kim, Y.S.; Lee, H.-M.; Jin, H.S.; Neupane, C.; Kim, S.; Lee, S.-H.; Min, J.-J.; Sasai, M.; Jeong, J.-H.; et al. GABAergic signaling linked to autophagy enhances host protection against intracellular bacterial infections. *Nat. Commun.* **2018**, *9*, 4184. [CrossRef] [PubMed]
13. Otaru, N.; Ye, K.; Mujezinovic, D.; Berchtold, L.; Constancias, F.; Cornejo, F.A.; Krzystek, A.; de Wouters, T.; Braegger, C.; Lacroix, C.; et al. GABA Production by Human Intestinal Bacteroides spp.: Prevalence, Regulation, and Role in Acid Stress Tolerance. *Front. Microbiol.* **2021**, *12*, 656895. [CrossRef]
14. Krasniqi, S.; Daci, A. Role of the Angiotensin Pathway and its Target Therapy in Epilepsy Management. *Int. J. Mol. Sci.* **2019**, *20*, 726. [CrossRef] [PubMed]
15. Liu, F.; Havens, J.; Yu, Q.; Wang, G.; Davisson, R.L.; Pickel, V.M.; Iadecola, C. The link between angiotensin II-mediated anxiety and mood disorders with NADPH oxi-dase-induced oxidative stress. *Int. J. Physiol. Pathophysiol. Pharmacol.* **2012**, *4*, 28–35. [PubMed]
16. Pereira, M.G.; Becari, C.; Oliveira, J.A.; Salgado, M.C.O.; Garcia-Cairasco, N.; Costa-Neto, C.M. Inhibition of the renin–angiotensin system prevents seizures in a rat model of epilepsy. *Clin. Sci.* **2010**, *119*, 477–482. [CrossRef]
17. Jo, Y.; Kim, S.; Ye, B.S.; Lee, E.; Yu, Y.M. Protective Effect of Renin-Angiotensin System Inhibitors on Parkinson's Disease: A Nationwide Cohort Study. *Front. Pharmacol.* **2022**, *13*, 837890. [CrossRef] [PubMed]
18. Saavedra, J.M. Angiotensin II AT1 receptor blockers as treatments for inflammatory brain disorders. *Clin. Sci.* **2012**, *123*, 567–590. [CrossRef]
19. Chang, C.-H.; Chang, Y.-C.; Wu, L.-C.; Lin, J.-W.; Chuang, L.-M.; Lai, M.-S. Different angiotensin receptor blockers and incidence of diabetes: A nationwide population-based cohort study. *Cardiovasc. Diabetol.* **2014**, *13*, 91. [CrossRef]
20. Ma, X.; Gao, F.; Chen, Q.; Xuan, X.; Wang, Y.; Deng, H.; Yang, F.; Yuan, L. ACE2 modulates glucose homeostasis through GABA signaling during metabolic stress. *J. Endocrinol.* **2020**, *246*, 223–236. [CrossRef]
21. Sánchez-Lemus, E.; Honda, M.; Saavedra, J.M. Angiotensin II AT1 receptor blocker candesartan prevents the fast up-regulation of cerebrocortical benzodiazepine-1 receptors induced by acute inflammatory and restraint stress. *Behav. Brain Res.* **2012**, *232*, 84–92. [CrossRef] [PubMed]
22. Beaudoin, C.A.; Jamasb, A.R.; Alsulami, A.F.; Copoiu, L.; van Tonder, A.J.; Hala, S.; Bannerman, B.P.; Thomas, S.E.; Vedithi, S.C.; Torres, P.H.; et al. Predicted structural mimicry of spike receptor-binding motifs from highly pathogenic human coronaviruses. *Comput. Struct. Biotechnol. J.* **2021**, *19*, 3938–3953. [CrossRef] [PubMed]
23. Yapici-Eser, H.; Koroglu, Y.E.; Oztop-Cakmak, O.; Keskin, O.; Gursoy, A.; Gursoy-Ozdemir, Y. Neuropsychiatric Symptoms of COVID-19 Explained by SARS-CoV-2 Proteins' Mimicry of Human Protein Interactions. *Front. Hum. Neurosci.* **2021**, *15*, 656313. [CrossRef]
24. Porges, E.C.; Jensen, G.; Foster, B.; Edden, R.A.; Puts, N.A. The trajectory of cortical GABA across the lifespan, an individual participant data meta-analysis of edited MRS studies. *eLife* **2021**, *10*, e62575. [CrossRef] [PubMed]
25. Ethiraj, J.; Palpagama, T.H.; Turner, C.; van der Werf, B.; Waldvogel, H.J.; Faull, R.L.M.; Kwakowsky, A. The effect of age and sex on the expression of GABA signaling components in the human hippocampus and entorhinal cortex. *Sci. Rep.* **2021**, *11*, 21470. [CrossRef] [PubMed]
26. Lin, L.; Li, Q.; Wang, Y.; Shi, Y. Syncytia formation during SARS-CoV-2 lung infection: A disastrous unity to eliminate lymphocytes. *Cell Death Differ.* **2021**, *28*, 2019–2021. [CrossRef] [PubMed]
27. Gordon, D.E.; Jang, G.M.; Bouhaddou, M.; Xu, J.; Obernier, K.; White, K.M.; O'Meara, M.J.; Rezelj, V.V.; Guo, J.Z.; Swaney, D.L.; et al. A SARS-CoV-2 protein interaction map reveals targets for drug repurposing. *Nature* **2020**, *583*, 459–468. [CrossRef]
28. Mao, L.-Y.; Ding, J.; Peng, W.-F.; Ma, Y.; Zhang, Y.-H.; Fan, W.; Wang, X. Interictal interleukin-17A levels are elevated and correlate with seizure severity of epilepsy patients. *Epilepsia* **2013**, *54*, e142–e145. [CrossRef]
29. Griffith, J.L.; Wong, M. The mTOR pathway in treatment of epilepsy: A clinical update. *Futur. Neurol.* **2018**, *13*, 49–58. [CrossRef]
30. Wang, L.; de Kloet, A.; Pati, D.; Hiller, H.; Smith, J.A.; Pioquinto, D.J.; Ludin, J.A.; Oh, S.P.; Katovich, M.J.; Frazier, C.J.; et al. Increasing brain angiotensin converting enzyme 2 activity decreases anxiety-like behavior in male mice by activating central Mas receptors. *Neuropharmacology* **2016**, *105*, 114–123. [CrossRef]
31. Zhang, J.; Li, Q.; Cosme, R.S.C.; Gerzanich, V.; Tang, Q.; Simard, J.M.; Zhao, R.Y. Genome-Wide Characterization of SARS-CoV-2 Cytopathogenic Proteins in the Search of Antiviral Targets. *mBio* **2022**, *13*. [CrossRef] [PubMed]

32. Targhetta, V.P.; Amaral, M.A.; Camara, N.O.S. Through DNA sensors and hidden mitochondrial effects of SARS-CoV-2. *J. Venom. Anim. Toxins Incl. Trop. Dis.* **2021**, *27*, e20200183. [CrossRef] [PubMed]
33. Han, Y.; Yuan, K.; Wang, Z.; Liu, W.-J.; Lu, Z.-A.; Liu, L.; Shi, L.; Yan, W.; Yuan, J.-L.; Li, J.-L.; et al. Neuropsychiatric manifestations of COVID-19, potential neurotropic mechanisms, and therapeutic interventions. *Transl. Psychiatry* **2021**, *11*, 499. [CrossRef] [PubMed]
34. Emami, A.; Fadakar, N.; Akbari, A.; Lotfi, M.; Farazdaghi, M.; Javanmardi, F.; Rezaei, T.; Asadi-Pooya, A.A. Seizure in patients with COVID-19. *Neurol. Sci.* **2020**, *41*, 3057–3061. [CrossRef] [PubMed]
35. Sfera, A.; Osorio, C.; Rahman, L.; del Campo, C.M.Z.-M.; Maldonado, J.C.; Jafri, N.; Cummings, M.A.; Maurer, S.; Kozlakidis, Z. PTSD as an Endothelial Disease: Insights from COVID-19. *Front. Cell. Neurosci.* **2021**, *15*, 770387. [CrossRef] [PubMed]
36. Krusek, J.; Zemkova´, H. Effect of ivermectin on γ-aminobutyric acid-induced chloride currents in mouse hippocampal embryonic neurones. *Eur. J. Pharmacol.* **1994**, *259*, 121–128. [CrossRef]
37. Li, M.P.; Eaton, M.M.M.; Steinbach, J.H.; Akk, G. The Benzodiazepine Diazepam Potentiates Responses of $\alpha 1\beta 2\gamma 2L$ γ-Aminobutyric Acid Type A Receptors Activated by either γ-Aminobutyric Acid or Allosteric Agonists. *Anesthesiology* **2013**, *118*, 1417–1425. [CrossRef]
38. Chan, Y.A.; Zhan, S.H. The Emergence of the Spike Furin Cleavage Site in SARS-CoV-2. *Mol. Biol. Evol.* **2021**, *39*, msab327. [CrossRef]
39. Hu, Y.; Liu, L.; Lu, X. Regulation of Angiotensin-Converting Enzyme 2: A Potential Target to Prevent COVID-19? *Front. Endocrinol.* **2021**, *12*, 725967. [CrossRef]
40. Doughan, A.K.; Harrison, D.G.; Dikalov, S.I. Molecular Mechanisms of Angiotensin II–Mediated Mitochondrial Dysfunction. *Circ. Res.* **2008**, *102*, 488–496. [CrossRef]
41. Bobkova, N.V. The Balance between Two Branches of RAS Can Protect from Severe COVID-19 Course. *Biochem. (Moscow) Suppl. Ser. A Membr. Cell Biol.* **2021**, *15*, 36–51. [CrossRef] [PubMed]
42. Mahmudpour, M.; Roozbeh, J.; Keshavarz, M.; Farrokhi, S.; Nabipour, I. COVID-19 cytokine storm: The anger of inflammation. *Cytokine* **2020**, *133*, 155151. [CrossRef] [PubMed]
43. Romero, E.; Guaza, C.; Castellano, B.; I Borrell, J. Ontogeny of sensorimotor gating and immune impairment induced by prenatal immune challenge in rats: Implications for the etiopathology of schizophrenia. *Mol. Psychiatry* **2008**, *15*, 372–383. [CrossRef] [PubMed]
44. Sen, S.; Roy, S.; Bandyopadhyay, G.; Scott, B.; Xiao, D.; Ramadoss, S.; Mahata, S.K.; Chaudhuri, G. γ-Aminobutyric Acid Is Synthesized and Released by the Endothelium. *Circ. Res.* **2016**, *119*, 621–634. [CrossRef] [PubMed]
45. Chen, Y.; Wang, J.; Liu, C.; Su, L.; Zhang, D.; Fan, J.; Yang, Y.; Xiao, M.; Xie, J.; Xu, Y.; et al. IP-10 and MCP-1 as biomarkers associated with disease severity of COVID-19. *Mol. Med.* **2020**, *26*, 97. [CrossRef] [PubMed]
46. Stragier, B.; Hristova, I.; Sarre, S.; Ebinger, G.; Michotte, Y. In vivo characterization of the angiotensin-(1-7)-induced dopamine and γ-aminobutyric acid release in the striatum of the rat. *Eur. J. Neurosci.* **2005**, *22*, 658–664. [CrossRef]
47. Brukman, N.G.; Uygur, B.; Podbilewicz, B.; Chernomordik, L.V. How cells fuse. *J. Cell Biol.* **2019**, *218*, 1436–1451. [CrossRef]
48. Zhang, Y.; Le, T.; Grabau, R.; Mohseni, Z.; Kim, H.; Natale, D.R.; Feng, L.; Pan, H.; Yang, H. TMEM16F phospholipid scramblase mediates trophoblast fusion and placental development. *Sci. Adv.* **2020**, *6*, eaba0310. [CrossRef]
49. Peacock, T.P.; Goldhill, D.H.; Zhou, J.; Baillon, L.; Frise, R.; Swann, O.C.; Kugathasan, R.; Penn, R.; Brown, J.C.; Sanchez-David, R.Y.; et al. The furin cleavage site in the SARS-CoV-2 spike protein is required for transmission in ferrets. *Nat. Microbiol.* **2021**, *6*, 899–909. [CrossRef]
50. Leroy, H.; Han, M.; Woottum, M.; Bracq, L.; Bouchet, J.; Xie, M.; Benichou, S. Virus-Mediated Cell-Cell Fusion. *Int. J. Mol. Sci.* **2020**, *21*, 9644. [CrossRef]
51. Armstrong, C.T.; Mason, P.; Anderson, R.; Dempsey, C.E. Arginine side chain interactions and the role of arginine as a gating charge carrier in voltage sensitive ion channels. *Sci. Rep.* **2016**, *6*, 21759. [CrossRef] [PubMed]
52. Osorio, C.; Sfera, A.; Anton, J.J.; Thomas, K.G.; Andronescu, C.V.; Li, E.; Yahia, R.W.; Avalos, A.G.; Kozlakidis, Z. Virus-Induced Membrane Fusion in Neurodegenerative Disorders. *Front. Cell. Infect. Microbiol.* **2022**, *12*, 845580. [CrossRef] [PubMed]
53. Chuprin, A.; Gal, H.; Biron-Shental, T.; Biran, A.; Amiel, A.; Rozenblatt, S.; Krizhanovsky, V. Cell fusion induced by ERVWE1 or measles virus causes cellular senescence. *Genes Dev.* **2013**, *27*, 2356–2366. [CrossRef] [PubMed]
54. Berndt, B.; Zanker, K.S.; Dittmar, T. Cell fusion is a potent inducer of aneuploidy and drug resistance in tumor cell/ normal cell hybrids. *Crit. Rev. Oncog.* **2013**, *18*, 97–113. [CrossRef] [PubMed]
55. Smith, K.R.; Muir, J.; Rao, Y.; Browarski, M.; Gruenig, M.C.; Sheehan, D.F.; Haucke, V.; Kittler, J.T. Stabilization of GABAA Receptors at Endocytic Zones Is Mediated by an AP2 Binding Motif within the GABAA Receptor β3 Subunit. *J. Neurosci.* **2012**, *32*, 2485–2498. [CrossRef] [PubMed]
56. Hegyi, H. GABBR1 has a HERV-W LTR in its regulatory region—A possible implication for schizophrenia. *Biol. Direct* **2013**, *8*, 5. [CrossRef] [PubMed]
57. Obrietan, K.; Pol, A.N.V.D. GABAB receptor-mediated inhibition of GABAA receptor calcium elevations in developing hypothalamic neurons. *J. Neurophysiol.* **1998**, *79*, 1360–1370. [CrossRef]
58. Hallenberger, S.; Bosch, V.; Angliker, H.; Shaw, E.; Klenk, H.-D.; Garten, W. Inhibition of furin-mediated cleavage activation of HIV-1 glycoprotein gpl60. *Nature* **1992**, *360*, 358–361. [CrossRef]

59. Charvet, B.; Brunel, J.; Pierquin, J.; Iampietro, M.; Decimo, D.; Queruel, N.; Lucas, A.; Encabo-Berzosa, M.d.M.; Arenaz, I.; Marmolejo, T.P.; et al. SARS-CoV-2 induces human endogenous retrovirus type W envelope protein expression in blood lymphocytes and in tissues of COVID-19 patients. *medRxiv* **2022**. Available online: https://www.medrxiv.org/content/10.1101/2022.01.18.21266111v2 (accessed on 15 May 2022). [CrossRef]
60. Schleiss, M.R. Letermovir and HCT: Too much of a good thing? *Blood* **2021**, *138*, 1–2. [CrossRef]
61. Sikora, E.; Bielak-Zmijewska, A.; Dudkowska, M.; Krzystyniak, A.; Mosieniak, G.; Wesierska, M.; Wlodarczyk, J. Cellular Senescence in Brain Aging. *Front. Aging Neurosci.* **2021**, *13*, 646924. [CrossRef] [PubMed]
62. Kim, S.; Shan, P.; Hwangbo, C.; Zhang, Y.; Min, J.; Zhang, X.; Ardito, T.; Li, A.; Peng, T.; Sauler, M.; et al. Endothelial toll-like receptor 4 maintains lung integrity via epigenetic suppression of p16 $^{INK4a}$. *Aging Cell* **2019**, *18*, e12914. [CrossRef] [PubMed]
63. Sun, Z.; Song, Z.-G.; Liu, C.; Tan, S.; Lin, S.; Zhu, J.; Dai, F.-H.; Gao, J.; She, J.-L.; Mei, Z.; et al. Gut microbiome alterations and gut barrier dysfunction are associated with host immune homeostasis in COVID-19 patients. *BMC Med.* **2022**, *20*, 24. [CrossRef] [PubMed]
64. Peerapornratana, S.; Sirivongrangson, P.; Tungsanga, S.; Tiankanon, K.; Kulvichit, W.; Putcharoen, O.; Kellum, J.A.; Srisawat, N. Endotoxin Adsorbent Therapy in Severe COVID-19 Pneumonia. *Blood Purif.* **2021**, *51*, 47–54. [CrossRef]
65. Petruk, G.; Puthia, M.; Petrlova, J.; Samsudin, F.; Strömdahl, A.-C.; Cerps, S.; Uller, L.; Kjellström, S.; Bond, P.J.; Schmidtchen, A. SARS-CoV-2 Spike protein binds to bacterial lipopolysaccharide and boosts proinflammatory activity. *J. Mol. Cell Biol.* **2020**, *12*, 916–932. [CrossRef]
66. Wolf, G.; Bohlender, J.; Bondeva, T.; Roger, T.; Thaiss, F.; Wenzel, U.O. Angiotensin II Upregulates Toll-Like Receptor 4 on Mesangial Cells. *J. Am. Soc. Nephrol.* **2006**, *17*, 1585–1593. [CrossRef]
67. Lu, Y.-C.; Yeh, W.-C.; Ohashi, P.S. LPS/TLR4 signal transduction pathway. *Cytokine* **2008**, *42*, 145–151. [CrossRef]
68. O'Connor, J.C.; A Lawson, M.; André, C.; Moreau, M.; Lestage, J.; Castanon, N.; Kelley, K.W.; Dantzer, R. Lipopolysaccharide-induced depressive-like behavior is mediated by indoleamine 2,3-dioxygenase activation in mice. *Mol. Psychiatry* **2008**, *14*, 511–522. [CrossRef]
69. Wang, Y.-Y.; Sun, S.-P.; Zhu, H.-S.; Jiao, X.-Q.; Zhong, K.; Guo, Y.-J.; Zha, G.-M.; Han, L.-Q.; Yang, G.-Y.; Li, H.-P. GABA regulates the proliferation and apoptosis of MAC-T cells through the LPS-induced TLR4 signaling pathway. *Res. Veter. Sci.* **2018**, *118*, 395–402. [CrossRef]
70. Zhao, Y.; Cong, L.; Lukiw, W.J. Lipopolysaccharide (LPS) Accumulates in Neocortical Neurons of Alzheimer's Disease (AD) Brain and Impairs Transcription in Human Neuronal-Glial Primary Co-cultures. *Front. Aging Neurosci.* **2017**, *9*, 407. [CrossRef]
71. Solas, M.; Puerta, E.; Ramirez, M. Treatment Options in Alzheimer´s Disease: The GABA Story. *Curr. Pharm. Des.* **2015**, *21*, 4960–4971. [CrossRef] [PubMed]
72. Nakanishi-Matsui, M.; Yano, S.; Matsumoto, N.; Futai, M. Lipopolysaccharide induces multinuclear cell from RAW264.7 line with increased phagocytosis activity. *Biochem. Biophys. Res. Commun.* **2012**, *425*, 144–149. [CrossRef] [PubMed]
73. Giordano-Santini, R.; Kaulich, E.; Galbraith, K.M.; Ritchie, F.K.; Wang, W.; Li, Z.; Hilliard, M.A. Fusogen-mediated neuron–neuron fusion disrupts neural circuit connectivity and alters animal behavior. *Proc. Natl. Acad. Sci. USA* **2020**, *117*, 23054–23065. [CrossRef] [PubMed]
74. Kemp, K.; Wilkins, A.; Scolding, N. Cell fusion in the brain: Two cells forward, one cell back. *Acta Neuropathol.* **2014**, *128*, 629–638. [CrossRef]
75. Arendt, T.; Mosch, B.; Morawski, M. Neuronal Aneuploidy in Health and Disease:A Cytomic Approach to Understand the Molecular Individuality of Neurons. *Int. J. Mol. Sci.* **2009**, *10*, 1609–1627. [CrossRef]
76. Kemp, K.; Gray, E.; Wilkins, A.; Scolding, N. Purkinje cell fusion and binucleate heterokaryon formation in multiple sclerosis cerebellum. *Brain* **2012**, *135*, 2962–2972. [CrossRef]
77. Potter, H.; Chial, H.J.; Caneus, J.; Elos, M.; Elder, N.; Borysov, S.; Granic, A. Chromosome Instability and Mosaic Aneuploidy in Neurodegenerative and Neurodevelopmental Disorders. *Front. Genet.* **2019**, *10*, 1092. [CrossRef]
78. Paquola, A.C.; Erwin, J.; Gage, F.H. Insights into the role of somatic mosaicism in the brain. *Curr. Opin. Syst. Biol.* **2016**, *1*, 90–94. [CrossRef]
79. Lindqvist, D.; Epel, E.S.; Mellon, S.H.; Penninx, B.W.; Révész, D.; Verhoeven, J.E.; Reus, V.I.; Lin, J.; Mahan, L.; Hough, C.M.; et al. Psychiatric disorders and leukocyte telomere length: Underlying mechanisms linking mental illness with cellular aging. *Neurosci. Biobehav. Rev.* **2015**, *55*, 333–364. [CrossRef]
80. Pousa, P.; Souza, R.; Melo, P.; Correa, B.; Mendonça, T.; Simões-E-Silva, A.; Miranda, D. Telomere Shortening and Psychiatric Disorders: A Systematic Review. *Cells* **2021**, *10*, 1423. [CrossRef]
81. E Verhoeven, J.; Révész, D.; Epel, E.S.; Lin, J.; Wolkowitz, O.M.; Penninx, B.W.J.H. Major depressive disorder and accelerated cellular aging: Results from a large psychiatric cohort study. *Mol. Psychiatry* **2013**, *19*, 895–901. [CrossRef] [PubMed]
82. Papanastasiou, E.; Gaughran, F.; Smith, S. Schizophrenia as segmental progeria. *J. R. Soc. Med.* **2011**, *104*, 475–484. [CrossRef] [PubMed]
83. Huang, W.-Y.; Lai, Y.-L.; Liu, K.-H.; Lin, S.; Chen, H.-Y.; Liang, C.-H.; Wu, H.-M.; Hsu, K.-S. TNFα-mediated necroptosis in brain endothelial cells as a potential mechanism of increased seizure susceptibility in mice following systemic inflammation. *J. Neuroinflammation* **2022**, *19*, 29. [CrossRef] [PubMed]

84. Ogrodnik, M.; Zhu, Y.; Langhi, L.G.; Tchkonia, T.; Krüger, P.; Fielder, E.; Victorelli, S.; Ruswhandi, R.A.; Giorgadze, N.; Pirtskhalava, T.; et al. Obesity-Induced Cellular Senescence Drives Anxiety and Impairs Neurogenesis. *Cell Metab.* **2019**, *29*, 1061–1077. [CrossRef] [PubMed]
85. Sekiguchi, F.; Tsubota, M.; Kawabata, A. Involvement of voltage-gated calcium channels in inflammation and inflam-matory pain. *Biol. Pharm. Bull.* **2018**, *41*, 1127–1134. [CrossRef] [PubMed]
86. Gilbert, N. The science of tea's mood-altering magic. *Nature* **2019**, *566*, S8. [CrossRef] [PubMed]
87. Sanches, M.; Colpo, G.D.; Cuellar, V.A.; Bockmann, T.; Rogith, D.; Soares, J.C.; Teixeira, A.L. Decreased Plasma Levels of Angiotensin-Converting Enzyme Among Patients with Bipolar Disorder. *Front. Neurosci.* **2021**, *15*, 617888. [CrossRef]
88. Colbourne, L.; Luciano, S.; Harrison, P.J. Onset and recurrence of psychiatric disorders associated with anti-hypertensive drug classes. *Transl. Psychiatry* **2021**, *11*, 319. [CrossRef]
89. Vian, J.; Pereira, C.; Chavarria, V.; Köhler, C.; Stubbs, B.; Quevedo, J.; Kim, S.-W.; Carvalho, A.F.; Berk, M.; Fernandes, B.S. The renin–angiotensin system: A possible new target for depression. *BMC Med.* **2017**, *15*, 144. [CrossRef]
90. Xie, Y.; Xu, E.; Al-Aly, Z. Risks of mental health outcomes in people with covid-19: Cohort study. *BMJ* **2022**, *376*, e068993. [CrossRef]
91. Firouzabadi, N.; Farshadfar, P.; Haghnegahdar, M.; Alavi-Shoushtari, A.; Ghanbarinezhad, V. Impact of ACE2 genetic variant on antidepressant efficacy of SSRIs. *Acta Neuropsychiatr.* **2021**, *34*, 30–36. [CrossRef] [PubMed]
92. Apple, D.M.; Fonseca, R.S.; Kokovay, E. The role of adult neurogenesis in psychiatric and cognitive disorders. *Brain Res.* **2017**, *1655*, 270–276. [CrossRef] [PubMed]
93. Klein, R.; Soung, A.; Sissoko, C.; Nordvig, A.; Canoll, P.; Mariani, M.; Jiang, X.; Bricker, T.; Goldman, J.; Rosoklija, G.; et al. COVID-19 induces neuroinflammation and loss of hippocampal neurogenesis. *Preprint Res. Sq.* **2021**, *1*, rs.3.rs-1031824. [CrossRef]
94. Ge, S.; Pradhan, D.A.; Ming, G.-L.; Song, H. GABA sets the tempo for activity-dependent adult neurogenesis. *Trends Neurosci.* **2007**, *30*, 1–8. [CrossRef]
95. Mu, Y.; Lee, S.W.; Gage, F.H. Signaling in adult neurogenesis. *Curr. Opin. Neurobiol.* **2010**, *20*, 416–423. [CrossRef] [PubMed]
96. Owens, D.F.; Kriegstein, A.R. Is there more to GABA than synaptic inhibition? *Nat. Rev. Neurosci.* **2002**, *3*, 715–727. [CrossRef]
97. Grasselli, C.; Ferrari, D.; Zalfa, C.; Soncini, M.; Mazzoccoli, G.; Facchini, F.A.; Marongiu, L.; Granucci, F.; Copetti, M.; Vescovi, A.L.; et al. Toll-like receptor 4 modulation influences human neural stem cell proliferation and differentiation. *Cell Death Dis.* **2018**, *9*, 280. [CrossRef]
98. Kase, Y.; Okano, H. Expression of ACE2 and a viral virulence-regulating factor CCN family member 1 in human iPSC-derived neural cells: Implications for COVID-19-related CNS disorders. *Inflamm. Regen.* **2020**, *40*, 32. [CrossRef]
99. Yu, X.; Ye, Z.; Houston, C.M.; Zecharia, A.Y.; Ma, Y.; Zhang, Z.; Uygun, D.S.; Parker, S.; Vyssotski, A.L.; Yustos, R.; et al. Wakefulness Is Governed by GABA and Histamine Cotransmission. *Neuron* **2015**, *87*, 164–178. [CrossRef]
100. Möhler, H. Role of GABAA receptors in cognition. *Biochem. Soc. Trans.* **2009**, *37*, 1328–1333. [CrossRef]
101. Lou, H.C.; Thomsen, K.R.; Changeux, J.-P. The Molecular Organization of Self-awareness: Paralimbic Dopamine-GABA Interaction. *Front. Syst. Neurosci.* **2020**, *14*, 3. [CrossRef] [PubMed]
102. Lyu, C.; Zhao, W.; Peng, C.; Hu, S.; Fang, H.; Hua, Y.; Yao, S.; Huang, J.; Mei, L. Exploring the contributions of two glutamate decarboxylase isozymes in Lactobacillus brevis to acid resistance and $\gamma$-aminobutyric acid production. *Microb. Cell Fact.* **2018**, *17*, 180. [CrossRef] [PubMed]
103. Bak, L.K.; Schousboe, A.; Waagepetersen, H.S. The glutamate/GABA-glutamine cycle: Aspects of transport, neurotransmitter homeostasis and ammonia transfer. *J. Neurochem.* **2006**, *98*, 641–653. [CrossRef] [PubMed]
104. Omotosho, Y.B.; Ying, G.W.; Stolar, M.; Mallari, A.J.P. COVID-19-Induced Diabetic Ketoacidosis in an Adult with Latent Autoimmune Diabetes. *Cureus* **2021**, *13*, e12690. [CrossRef]
105. Emekli, A.S.; Parlak, A.; Göcen, N.Y.; Kürtüncü, M. Anti-GAD associated post-infectious cerebellitis after COVID-19 infection. *Neurol. Sci.* **2021**, *42*, 3995–4002. [CrossRef]
106. Jin, Z.; Mendu, S.K.; Birnir, B. GABA is an effective immunomodulatory molecule. *Amino Acids* **2013**, *45*, 87–94. [CrossRef]
107. Qin, P.; Wu, X.; Duncan, N.W.; Bao, W.; Tang, W.; Zhang, Z.; Hu, J.; Jin, Y.; Wu, X.; Gao, L.; et al. GABAA receptor deficits predict recovery in patients with disorders of consciousness: A preliminary multimodal [11C]Flumazenil PET and fMRI study. *Hum. Brain Mapp.* **2015**, *36*, 3867–3877. [CrossRef]
108. Fujimori, S.; Yoneda, Y. [Neuropsychiatric disorders and GABA]. *Nihon Shinkei Seishin Yakurigaku Zasshi* **2004**, *24*, 265–271. (In Japanese)
109. Clauss, R. Disorders of consciousness and pharmaceuticals that act on oxygen based amino acid and monoamine neuro-transmitter pathways of the brain. *Curr. Pharm. Des.* **2014**, *20*, 4053–4140.
110. Tsubomoto, M.; Kawabata, R.; Zhu, X.; Minabe, Y.; Chen, K.; A Lewis, D.; Hashimoto, T. Expression of Transcripts Selective for GABA Neuron Subpopulations across the Cortical Visuospatial Working Memory Network in the Healthy State and Schizophrenia. *Cereb. Cortex* **2018**, *29*, 3540–3550. [CrossRef]
111. Sakimoto, Y.; Oo, P.M.-T.; Goshima, M.; Kanehisa, I.; Tsukada, Y.; Mitsushima, D. Significance of $GABA_A$ Receptor for Cognitive Function and Hippocampal Pathology. *Int. J. Mol. Sci.* **2021**, *22*, 12456. [CrossRef] [PubMed]
112. Wyss, C.; Tse, D.H.Y.; Kometer, M.; Dammers, J.; Achermann, R.; Shah, N.J.; Kawohl, W.; Neuner, I. GABA metabolism and its role in gamma-band oscillatory activity during auditory processing: An MRS and EEG study. *Hum. Brain Mapp.* **2017**, *38*, 3975–3987. [CrossRef] [PubMed]

113. Herrmann, C.S.; Demiralp, T. Human EEG gamma oscillations in neuropsychiatric disorders. *Clin. Neurophysiol.* **2005**, *116*, 2719–2733. [CrossRef] [PubMed]
114. Coghlan, S.; Horder, J.; Inkster, B.; Mendez, M.A.; Murphy, D.; Nutt, D. GABA system dysfunction in autism and related disorders: From synapse to symptoms. *Neurosci. Biobehav. Rev.* **2012**, *36*, 2044–2055. [CrossRef]
115. Harris, S.; Ma, H.; Zhao, M.; Boorman, L.; Zheng, Y.; Kennerley, A.; Bruyns-Haylett, M.; Overton, P.G.; Berwick, J.; Schwartz, T.H. Coupling between gamma-band power and cerebral blood volume during recurrent acute neocortical seizures. *NeuroImage* **2014**, *97*, 62–70. [CrossRef]
116. Muthukumaraswamy, S.D.; Edden, R.A.; Jones, D.K.; Swettenham, J.B.; Singh, K.D. Resting GABA concentration predicts peak gamma frequency and fMRI amplitude in response to visual stimulation in humans. *Proc. Natl. Acad. Sci. USA* **2009**, *106*, 8356–8361. [CrossRef]
117. Kilb, W. Development of the GABAergic System from Birth to Adolescence. *Neuroscience* **2011**, *18*, 613–630. [CrossRef]
118. Li, S.; Kumar T, P.; Joshee, S.; Kirschstein, T.; Subburaju, S.; Khalili, J.S.; Kloepper, J.; Du, C.; Elkhal, A.; Szabó, G.; et al. Endothelial cell-derived GABA signaling modulates neuronal migration and postnatal behavior. *Cell Res.* **2017**, *28*, 221–248. [CrossRef]
119. Wu, X.; Fu, Y.; Knott, G.W.; Lu, J.; Di Cristo, G.; Huang, Z.J. GABA Signaling Promotes Synapse Elimination and Axon Pruning in Developing Cortical Inhibitory Interneurons. *J. Neurosci.* **2012**, *32*, 331–343. [CrossRef]
120. Favuzzi, E.; Huang, S.; Saldi, G.A.; Binan, L.; Ibrahim, L.A.; Fernández-Otero, M.; Cao, Y.; Zeine, A.; Sefah, A.; Zheng, K.; et al. GABA-receptive microglia selectively sculpt developing inhibitory circuits. *Cell* **2021**, *184*, 4048–4063.e32. [CrossRef]
121. Whitelaw, B. Microglia-mediated synaptic elimination in neuronal development and disease. *J. Neurophysiol.* **2018**, *119*, 1–4. [CrossRef] [PubMed]
122. Fuks, J.; Arrighi, R.B.G.; Weidner, J.M.; Mendu, S.K.; Jin, Z.; Wallin, R.P.A.; Rethi, B.; Birnir, B.; Barragan, A. GABAergic Signaling Is Linked to a Hypermigratory Phenotype in Dendritic Cells Infected by Toxoplasma gondii. *PLoS Pathog.* **2012**, *8*, e1003051. [CrossRef] [PubMed]
123. Fruntes, V.; Limosin, F. Schizophrenia and viral infection during neurodevelopment: A pathogenesis model? *Med. Sci. Monit.* **2008**, *14*, RA71–RA77. [PubMed]
124. Scordel, C.; Huttin, A.; Cochet-Bernoin, M.; Szelechowski, M.; Poulet, A.; Richardson, J.; Benchoua, A.; Gonzalez-Dunia, D.; Eloit, M.; Coulpier, M. Borna Disease Virus Phosphoprotein Impairs the Developmental Program Controlling Neurogenesis and Reduces Human GABAergic Neurogenesis. *PLoS Pathog.* **2015**, *11*, e1004859. [CrossRef] [PubMed]
125. McCarron, J.G.; Lee, M.D.; Wilson, C. The Endothelium Solves Problems That Endothelial Cells Do Not Know Exist. *Trends Pharmacol. Sci.* **2017**, *38*, 322–338. [CrossRef]
126. Lee, M.D.; Buckley, C.; Zhang, X.; Louhivuori, L.; Uhlén, P.; Wilson, C.; McCarron, J.G. Small-world connectivity dictates collective endothelial cell signaling. *Proc. Natl. Acad. Sci. USA* **2022**, *119*, e2118927119. [CrossRef] [PubMed]
127. Junior, A.P.; Dos Santos, R.P.; Barrros, R.F. The Calcium Wave Model of the Perception-Action Cycle: Evidence from Semantic Relevance in Memory Experiments. *Front. Psychol.* **2013**, *4*, 252. [CrossRef]
128. Carafoli, E.; Krebs, J. Why Calcium? How Calcium Became the Best Communicator. *J. Biol. Chem.* **2016**, *291*, 20849–20857. [CrossRef]
129. Knight, H.; Brandt, S.; Knight, M.R. A history of stress alters drought calcium signalling pathways in Arabidopsis. *Plant J.* **1998**, *16*, 681–687. [CrossRef]
130. Kawamoto, E.M.; Vivar, C.; Camandola, S. Physiology and Pathology of Calcium Signaling in the Brain. *Front. Pharmacol.* **2012**, *3*, 61. [CrossRef]
131. Adaikkan, C.; Taha, E.; Barrera, I.; David, O.; Rosenblum, K. Calcium/Calmodulin-Dependent Protein Kinase II and Eukaryotic Elongation Factor 2 Kinase Pathways Mediate the Antidepressant Action of Ketamine. *Biol. Psychiatry* **2018**, *84*, 65–75. [CrossRef] [PubMed]
132. Wenzhong, L.; Hualan, L. COVID-19: The CaMKII-like system of S protein drives membrane fusion and induces syncytial multinucleated giant cells. *Immunol. Res.* **2021**, *69*, 496–519. [CrossRef] [PubMed]
133. Baluška, F.; Levin, M. On Having No Head: Cognition throughout Biological Systems. *Front. Psychol.* **2016**, *7*, 902. [CrossRef] [PubMed]
134. Snijders, T.; Aussieker, T.; Holwerda, A.; Parise, G.; Van Loon, L.J.C.; Verdijk, L.B. The concept of skeletal muscle memory: Evidence from animal and human studies. *Acta Physiol.* **2020**, *229*, e13465. [CrossRef]
135. Pearsall, P.; Schwartz, G.E.; Russek, L.G. Changes in heart transplant recipients that parallel the personalities of their donors. *Integr. Med.* **2000**, *2*, 65–72. [CrossRef]
136. Bunzel, B.; Schmidl-Mohl, B.; Wollenek, G. Does changing the heart mean changing personality? A retrospective inquiry on 47 heart transplant patients. *Qual. Life Res.* **1992**, *1*, 251–256. [CrossRef]
137. Liester, M.B. Personality changes following heart transplantation: The role of cellular memory. *Med. Hypotheses* **2019**, *135*, 109468. [CrossRef]
138. Moore, C.I.; Cao, R. The Hemo-Neural Hypothesis: On The Role of Blood Flow in Information Processing. *J. Neurophysiol.* **2008**, *99*, 2035–2047. [CrossRef]
139. Cines, D.B.; Pollak, E.S.; A Buck, C.; Loscalzo, J.; A Zimmerman, G.; McEver, R.P.; Pober, J.S.; Wick, T.; A Konkle, B.; Schwartz, B.S.; et al. Endothelial cells in physiology and in the pathophysiology of vascular disorders. *Blood* **1998**, *91*, 3527–3561.

140. Datta, D.; Subburaju, S.; Kaye, S.; Baruah, J.; Choi, Y.K.; Nian, Y.; Khalili, J.S.; Chung, S.; Elkhal, A.; Vasudevan, A. Human forebrain endothelial cell therapy for psychiatric disorders. *Mol. Psychiatry* **2020**, *26*, 4864–4883. [CrossRef]
141. Choi, Y.K.; Vasudevan, A. Endothelial GABA signaling: A phoenix awakened. *Aging* **2018**, *10*, 859–860. [CrossRef] [PubMed]
142. Do, D.P.; Dowd, J.; Ranjit, N.; House, J.S.; Kaplan, G.A. Hopelessness, Depression, and Early Markers of Endothelial Dysfunction in U.S. Adults. *Psychosom. Med.* **2010**, *72*, 613–619. [CrossRef] [PubMed]
143. Vetter, M.W.; Martin, B.-J.; Fung, M.; Pajevic, M.; Anderson, T.J.; Raedler, T.J. Microvascular dysfunction in schizophrenia: A case–control study. *Schizophrenia* **2015**, *1*, 15023. [CrossRef] [PubMed]
144. Azmitia, E.C.; Saccomano, Z.T.; Alzoobaee, M.F.; Boldrini, M.; Whitakerazmitia, P.M. Persistent Angiogenesis in the Autism Brain: An Immunocytochemical Study of Postmortem Cortex, Brainstem and Cerebellum. *J. Autism Dev. Disord.* **2015**, *46*, 1307–1318. [CrossRef] [PubMed]
145. Sara, J.D.S.; Ahmad, A.; Toya, T.; Pardo, L.S.; Lerman, L.O.; Lerman, A. Anxiety Disorders Are Associated With Coronary Endothelial Dysfunction in Women With Chest Pain and Nonobstructive Coronary Artery Disease. *J. Am. Heart Assoc.* **2021**, *10*, e021722. [CrossRef]
146. Ogaki, A.; Ikegaya, Y.; Koyama, R. Vascular Abnormalities and the Role of Vascular Endothelial Growth Factor in the Epileptic Brain. *Front. Pharmacol.* **2020**, *11*, 20. [CrossRef]
147. Mohite, S.; de Campos-Carli, S.M.; Rocha, N.P.; Sharma, S.; Miranda, A.S.; Barbosa, I.G.; Salgado, J.V.; Simoes-E-Silva, A.C.; Teixeira, A.L. Lower circulating levels of angiotensin-converting enzyme (ACE) in patients with schizophrenia. *Schizophr. Res.* **2018**, *202*, 50–54. [CrossRef]
148. Braun, M.; Ramracheya, R.; Bengtsson, M.; Clark, A.; Walker, J.N.; Johnson, P.R.; Rorsman, P. $\gamma$-Aminobutyric Acid (GABA) Is an Autocrine Excitatory Transmitter in Human Pancreatic $\beta$-Cells. *Diabetes* **2010**, *59*, 1694–1701. [CrossRef]
149. Wu, C.-T.; Lidsky, P.V.; Xiao, Y.; Lee, I.T.; Cheng, R.; Nakayama, T.; Jiang, S.; Demeter, J.; Bevacqua, R.J.; Chang, C.A.; et al. SARS-CoV-2 infects human pancreatic $\beta$ cells and elicits $\beta$ cell impairment. *Cell Metab.* **2021**, *33*, 1565–1576.e5. [CrossRef]
150. Sohrabipour, S.; Sharifi, M.R.; Talebi, A.; Soltani, N. GABA dramatically improves glucose tolerance in streptozotocin-induced diabetic rats fed with high-fat diet. *Eur. J. Pharmacol.* **2018**, *826*, 75–84. [CrossRef]
151. Soltani, N.; Qiu, H.; Aleksic, M.; Glinka, Y.; Zhao, F.; Liu, R.; Li, Y.; Zhang, N.; Chakrabarti, R.; Ng, T.; et al. GABA exerts protective and regenerative effects on islet beta cells and reverses diabetes. *Proc. Natl. Acad. Sci. USA* **2011**, *108*, 11692–11697. [CrossRef] [PubMed]
152. Chu, K.Y.; Leung, P.S. Angiotensin II in Type 2 Diabetes Mellitus. *Curr. Protein Pept. Sci.* **2009**, *10*, 75–84. [CrossRef] [PubMed]
153. Gal, H.; Krizhanovsky, V. Cell fusion induced senescence. *Aging* **2014**, *6*, 353–354. [CrossRef] [PubMed]
154. Menegaz, D.; Hagan, D.W.; Almaça, J.; Cianciaruso, C.; Rodriguez-Diaz, R.; Molina, J.; Dolan, R.M.; Becker, M.W.; Schwalie, P.C.; Nano, R.; et al. Mechanism and effects of pulsatile GABA secretion from cytosolic pools in the human beta cell. *Nat. Metab.* **2019**, *1*, 1110–1126. [CrossRef] [PubMed]
155. Aguayo-Mazzucato, C.; Midha, A. $\beta$-cell senescence in type 2 diabetes. *Aging* **2019**, *11*, 9967–9968. [CrossRef] [PubMed]
156. Sfera, A.; Osorio, C.; Inderias, L.A.; Parker, V.; Price, A.I.; Cummings, M. The Obesity–Impulsivity Axis: Potential Metabolic Interventions in Chronic Psychiatric Patients. *Front. Psychiatry* **2017**, *8*, 20. [CrossRef] [PubMed]
157. Xu, J.; Chu, M.; Zhong, F.; Tan, X.; Tang, G.; Mai, J.; Lai, N.; Guan, C.; Liang, Y.; Liao, G. Digestive symptoms of COVID-19 and expression of ACE2 in digestive tract organs. *Cell Death Discov.* **2020**, *6*, 76. [CrossRef]
158. Yu, W.; Ou, X.; Liu, X.; Zhang, S.; Gao, X.; Cheng, H.; Zhu, B.; Yan, J. ACE2 contributes to the maintenance of mouse epithelial barrier function. *Biochem. Biophys. Res. Commun.* **2020**, *533*, 1276–1282. [CrossRef]
159. Koester, S.T.; Li, N.; Lachance, D.M.; Morella, N.M.; Dey, N. Variability in digestive and respiratory tract Ace2 expression is associated with the microbiome. *PLoS ONE* **2021**, *16*, e0248730. [CrossRef]
160. Mpekoulis, G.; Frakolaki, E.; Taka, S.; Ioannidis, A.; Vassiliou, A.G.; Kalliampakou, K.I.; Patas, K.; Karakasiliotis, I.; Aidinis, V.; Chatzipanagiotou, S.; et al. Alteration of L-Dopa decarboxylase expression in SARS-CoV-2 infection and its association with the interferon-inducible ACE2 isoform. *PLoS ONE* **2021**, *16*, e0253458. [CrossRef]
161. Reith, J.; Benkelfat, C.; Sherwin, A.; Yasuhara, Y.; Kuwabara, H.; Andermann, F.; Bachneff, S.; Cumming, P.; Diksic, M.; E Dyve, S. Elevated dopa decarboxylase activity in living brain of patients with psychosis. *Proc. Natl. Acad. Sci. USA* **1994**, *91*, 11651–11654. [CrossRef] [PubMed]
162. Stevens, B.R.; Ellory, J.C.; Preston, R.L. B0AT1 Amino Acid Transporter Complexed With SARS-CoV-2 Receptor ACE2 Forms a Heterodimer Functional Unit: In Situ Conformation Using Radiation Inactivation Analysis. *Function* **2021**, *2*, zqab027. [CrossRef] [PubMed]
163. Eroğlu, I.; Eroğlu, B.; Güven, G.S. Altered tryptophan absorption and metabolism could underlie long-term symptoms in survivors of coronavirus disease 2019 (COVID-19). *Nutrition* **2021**, *90*, 111308. [CrossRef] [PubMed]
164. Singer, D.; Camargo, S.; Ramadan, T.; Schäfer, M.; Mariotta, L.; Herzog, B.; Huggel, K.; Wolfer, D.; Werner, S.; Penninger, J.; et al. Defective intestinal amino acid absorption in Ace2 null mice. *Am. J. Physiol. Liver Physiol.* **2012**, *303*, G686–G695. [CrossRef]
165. Deng, J.; Zhou, F.; Hou, W.; Silver, Z.; Wong, C.Y.; Chang, O.; Huang, E.; Zuo, Q.K. The prevalence of depression, anxiety, and sleep disturbances in COVID-19 patients: A meta-analysis. *Ann. N. Y. Acad. Sci.* **2020**, *1486*, 90–111. [CrossRef]
166. Giovannoni, F.; Li, Z.; Remes-Lenicov, F.; Dávola, M.E.; Elizalde, M.; Paletta, A.; Ashkar, A.A.; Mossman, K.L.; Dugour, A.V.; Figueroa, J.M.; et al. AHR signaling is induced by infection with coronaviruses. *Nat. Commun.* **2021**, *12*, 5148. [CrossRef]

167. Wei, G.Z.; Martin, K.A.; Xing, P.Y.; Agrawal, R.; Whiley, L.; Wood, T.K.; Hejndorf, S.; Ng, Y.Z.; Low, J.Z.Y.; Rossant, J.; et al. Tryptophan-metabolizing gut microbes regulate adult neurogenesis via the aryl hydrocarbon receptor. *Proc. Natl. Acad. Sci. USA* **2021**, *118*, e2021091118. [CrossRef]
168. Ji, J.; Qu, H. Cross-regulatory Circuit Between AHR and Microbiota. *Curr. Drug Metab.* **2019**, *20*, 4–8. [CrossRef]
169. Lindén, J.; Lensu, S.; Tuomisto, J.; Pohjanvirta, R. Dioxins, the aryl hydrocarbon receptor and the central regulation of energy balance. *Front. Neuroendocr.* **2010**, *31*, 452–478. [CrossRef]
170. Sfera, A.; Osorio, C.; Diaz, E.L.; Maguire, G.; Cummings, M. The Other Obesity Epidemic—Of Drugs and Bugs. *Front. Endocrinol.* **2020**, *11*, 488. [CrossRef]
171. Sabbatinelli, J.; Prattichizzo, F.; Olivieri, F.; Procopio, A.D.; Rippo, M.R.; Giuliani, A. Where Metabolism Meets Senescence: Focus on Endothelial Cells. *Front. Physiol.* **2019**, *10*, 1523. [CrossRef] [PubMed]
172. Brinkmann, V.; Ale-Agha, N.; Haendeler, J.; Ventura, N. The Aryl Hydrocarbon Receptor (AhR) in the Aging Process: Another Puzzling Role for This Highly Conserved Transcription Factor. *Front. Physiol.* **2020**, *10*, 1561. [CrossRef] [PubMed]
173. Ren, W.; Liao, Y.; Ding, X.; Jiang, Y.; Yan, J.; Xia, Y.; Tan, B.; Lin, Z.; Duan, J.; Jia, X.; et al. Slc6a13 deficiency promotes Th17 responses during intestinal bacterial infection. *Mucosal Immunol.* **2018**, *12*, 531–544. [CrossRef] [PubMed]
174. Brevi, A.; Cogrossi, L.L.; Grazia, G.; Masciovecchio, D.; Impellizzieri, D.; Lacanfora, L.; Grioni, M.; Bellone, M. Much More Than IL-17A: Cytokines of the IL-17 Family Between Microbiota and Cancer. *Front. Immunol.* **2020**, *11*, 565470. [CrossRef]
175. Hamada, H.; Garcia-Hernandez, M.D.L.L.; Reome, J.B.; Misra, S.K.; Strutt, T.M.; McKinstry, K.K.; Cooper, A.; Swain, S.L.; Dutton, R.W. Tc17, a Unique Subset of CD8 T Cells That Can Protect against Lethal Influenza Challenge. *J. Immunol.* **2009**, *182*, 3469–3481. [CrossRef]
176. Zhang, L.; Liu, M.; Liu, W.; Hu, C.; Li, H.; Deng, J.; Cao, Q.; Wang, Y.; Hu, W.; Li, Q. Th17/IL-17 induces endothelial cell senescence via activation of NF-κB/p53/Rb signaling pathway. *Lab. Investig.* **2021**, *101*, 1418–1426. [CrossRef]
177. Ming, X.-F.; Montani, J.-P.; Yang, Z. Perspectives of Targeting mTORC1–S6K1 in Cardiovascular Aging. *Front. Physiol.* **2012**, *3*, 5. [CrossRef]
178. Fuentes-Prior, P. Priming of SARS-CoV-2 S protein by several membrane-bound serine proteinases could explain enhanced viral infectivity and systemic COVID-19 infection. *J. Biol. Chem.* **2021**, *296*, 100135. [CrossRef]
179. Zhang, Z.; Zheng, Y.; Niu, Z.; Zhang, B.; Wang, C.; Yao, X.; Peng, H.; Franca, D.N.; Wang, Y.; Zhu, Y.; et al. SARS-CoV-2 spike protein dictates syncytium-mediated lymphocyte elimination. *Cell Death Differ.* **2021**, *28*, 2765–2777. [CrossRef]
180. Winstone, H.; Lista, M.J.; Reid, A.C.; Bouton, C.; Pickering, S.; Galao, R.P.; Kerridge, C.; Doores, K.J.; Swanson, C.M.; Neil, S.J.D. The Polybasic Cleavage Site in SARS-CoV-2 Spike Modulates Viral Sensitivity to Type I Interferon and IFITM2. *J. Virol.* **2021**, *95*, e02422-20. [CrossRef]
181. Johnson, B.A.; Xie, X.; Bailey, A.L.; Kalveram, B.; Lokugamage, K.G.; Muruato, A.; Zou, J.; Zhang, X.; Juelich, T.; Smith, J.K.; et al. Loss of furin cleavage site attenuates SARS-CoV-2 pathogenesis. *Nature* **2021**, *591*, 293–299. [CrossRef] [PubMed]
182. Balestrieri, E.; Minutolo, A.; Petrone, V.; Fanelli, M.; Iannetta, M.; Malagnino, V.; Zordan, M.; Vitale, P.; Charvet, B.; Horvat, B.; et al. Evidence of the pathogenic HERV-W envelope expression in T lymphocytes in association with the respiratory outcome of COVID-19 patients. *EBioMedicine* **2021**, *66*, 103341. [CrossRef] [PubMed]
183. Chang, C.; Chen, P.-T.; Chang, G.-D.; Huang, C.-J.; Chen, H. Functional Characterization of the Placental Fusogenic Membrane Protein Syncytin1. *Biol. Reprod.* **2004**, *71*, 1956–1962. [CrossRef] [PubMed]
184. Huppertz, B. The Critical Role of Abnormal Trophoblast Development in the Etiology of Preeclampsia. *Curr. Pharm. Biotechnol.* **2018**, *19*, 771–780. [CrossRef]
185. Zhang, L.; Richards, A.; Barrasa, M.I.; Hughes, S.H.; Young, R.A.; Jaenisch, R. Reverse-transcribed SARS-CoV-2 RNA can integrate into the genome of cultured human cells and can be expressed in patient-derived tissues. *Proc. Natl. Acad. Sci. USA* **2021**, *118*, e2105968118. [CrossRef]
186. Mi, S.; Lee, X.; Li, X.-P.; Veldman, G.M.; Finnerty, H.; Racie, L.; LaVallie, E.; Tang, X.-Y.; Edouard, P.; Howes, S.; et al. Syncytin is a captive retroviral envelope protein involved in human placental morphogenesis. *Nature* **2000**, *403*, 785–789. [CrossRef]
187. Wang, X.; Huang, J.; Zhu, F. Human Endogenous Retroviral Envelope Protein Syncytin-1 and Inflammatory Abnormalities in Neuropsychological Diseases. *Front. Psychiatry* **2018**, *9*, 422. [CrossRef]
188. Chen, C.-P.; Chen, L.-F.; Yang, S.-R.; Chen, C.-Y.; Ko, C.-C.; Chang, G.-D.; Chen, H. Functional Characterization of the Human Placental Fusogenic Membrane Protein Syncytin 21. *Biol. Reprod.* **2008**, *79*, 815–823. [CrossRef]
189. Conde-Agudelo, A.; Romero, R. SARS-CoV-2 infection during pregnancy and risk of preeclampsia: A systematic review and meta-analysis. *Am. J. Obstet. Gynecol.* **2021**, *226*, 68–89.e3. [CrossRef]
190. Terán, Y.; Ponce, O.; Betancourt, L.; Hernández, L.; Rada, P. Amino acid profile of plasma and cerebrospinal fluid in preeclampsia. *Pregnancy Hypertens. Int. J. Women's Cardiovasc. Health* **2012**, *2*, 416–422. [CrossRef]
191. Lu, J.; Zhang, Q.; Tan, D.; Luo, W.; Zhao, H.; Ma, J.; Liang, H.; Tan, Y. GABA A receptor π subunit promotes apoptosis of HTR-8/SVneo trophoblastic cells: Implications in preeclampsia. *Int. J. Mol. Med.* **2016**, *38*, 105–112. [CrossRef] [PubMed]
192. Licht, P.; Harbarth, P.; E Merz, W. Evidence for a modulation of human chorionic gonadotropin (hCG) subunit messenger ribonucleic acid levels and hCG secretion by gamma-aminobutyric acid in human first trimester placenta in vitro. *Endocrinology* **1992**, *130*, 490–496. [CrossRef] [PubMed]

193. Vacher, C.-M.; Lacaille, H.; O'Reilly, J.J.; Salzbank, J.; Bakalar, D.; Sebaoui, S.; Liere, P.; Clarkson-Paredes, C.; Sasaki, T.; Sathyanesan, A.; et al. Placental endocrine function shapes cerebellar development and social behavior. *Nat. Neurosci.* **2021**, *24*, 1392–1401. [CrossRef] [PubMed]
194. Cheng, Y.-W.; Chao, T.-L.; Li, C.-L.; Chiu, M.-F.; Kao, H.-C.; Wang, S.-H.; Pang, Y.-H.; Lin, C.-H.; Tsai, Y.-M.; Lee, W.-H.; et al. Furin Inhibitors Block SARS-CoV-2 Spike Protein Cleavage to Suppress Virus Production and Cytopathic Effects. *Cell Rep.* **2020**, *33*, 108254. [CrossRef]
195. Becker, G.L.; Sielaff, F.; Than, M.E.; Lindberg, I.; Routhier, S.; Day, R.; Lu, Y.; Garten, W.; Steinmetzer, T. Potent Inhibitors of Furin and Furin-like Proprotein Convertases Containing Decarboxylated P1 Arginine Mimetics. *J. Med. Chem.* **2009**, *53*, 1067–1075. [CrossRef]
196. Devi, K.P.; Pourkarim, M.R.; Thijssen, M.; Sureda, A.; Khayatkashani, M.; Cismaru, C.A.; Neagoe, I.B.; Habtemariam, S.; Razmjouei, S.; Kashani, H.R.K. A perspective on the applications of furin inhibitors for the treatment of SARS-CoV-2. *Pharmacol. Rep.* **2022**, *74*, 425–430. [CrossRef]
197. Yakala, G.K.; Cabrera-Fuentes, H.A.; Crespo-Avilan, G.E.; Rattanasopa, C.; Burlacu, A.; George, B.L.; Anand, K.; Mayan, D.C.; Corlianò, M.; Hernández-Reséndiz, S.; et al. FURIN Inhibition Reduces Vascular Remodeling and Atherosclerotic Lesion Progression in Mice. *Arter. Thromb. Vasc. Biol.* **2019**, *39*, 387–401. [CrossRef]
198. AbdelMassih, A.F.; Ye, J.; Kamel, A.; Mishriky, F.; Ismail, H.-A.; Ragab, H.A.; El Qadi, L.; Malak, L.; Abdu, M.; El-Husseiny, M.; et al. A multicenter consensus: A role of furin in the endothelial tropism in obese patients with COVID-19 infection. *Obes. Med.* **2020**, *19*, 100281. [CrossRef]
199. Pomorski, T.G.; Menon, A.K. Lipid somersaults: Uncovering the mechanisms of protein-mediated lipid flipping. *Prog. Lipid Res.* **2016**, *64*, 69–84. [CrossRef]
200. Whitlock, J.M.; Chernomordik, L.V. Flagging fusion: Phosphatidylserine signaling in cell—Cell fusion. *J. Biol. Chem.* **2021**, *296*, 100411. [CrossRef]
201. Braga, L.; Ali, H.; Secco, I.; Chiavacci, E.; Neves, G.; Goldhill, D.; Penn, R.; Jimenez-Guardeño, J.M.; Ortega-Prieto, A.M.; Bussani, R.; et al. Drugs that inhibit TMEM16 proteins block SARS-CoV-2 spike-induced syncytia. *Nature* **2021**, *594*, 88–93. [CrossRef] [PubMed]
202. Cheng, Y.; Feng, S.; Puchades, C.; Ko, J.; Figueroa, E.; Chen, Y.; Wu, H.; Gu, S.; Han, T.; Li, J.; et al. Identification of a conserved drug binding pocket in TMEM16 proteins. *Preprint Res. Sq.* **2022**, *1*, rs.3.rs-1296933. [CrossRef]
203. Cairns, D.M.; Dulko, D.; Griffiths, J.K.; Golan, Y.; Cohen, T.; Trinquart, L.; Price, L.L.; Beaulac, K.R.; Selker, H.P. Efficacy of Niclosamide vs Placebo in SARS-CoV-2 Respiratory Viral Clearance, Viral Shedding, and Duration of Symptoms Among Patients with Mild to Moderate COVID-19. *JAMA Netw. Open* **2022**, *5*, e2144942. [CrossRef] [PubMed]
204. Pedemonte, N.; Galietta, L.J. Structure and Function of TMEM16 Proteins (Anoctamins). *Physiol. Rev.* **2014**, *94*, 419–459. [CrossRef]
205. Slawecki, M.L.; Carlson, G.C.; Keller, A. Differential distribution of inositol 1,4,5-triphosphate receptors in the rat olfactory bulb. *J. Comp. Neurol.* **1997**, *389*, 224–234. [CrossRef]
206. Egorova, P.A.; Bezprozvanny, I.B. Inositol 1,4,5-trisphosphate receptors and neurodegenerative disorders. *FEBS J.* **2018**, *285*, 3547–3565. [CrossRef]
207. Heuser, K.; Nome, C.G.; Pettersen, K.H.; Åbjørsbråten, K.S.; Jensen, V.; Tang, W.; Sprengel, R.; Taubøll, E.; A Nagelhus, E.; Enger, R. $Ca^{2+}$ Signals in Astrocytes Facilitate Spread of Epileptiform Activity. *Cereb. Cortex* **2018**, *28*, 4036–4048. [CrossRef]
208. Park, S.J.; Jeong, J.; Park, Y.-U.; Park, K.-S.; Lee, H.; Lee, N.; Kim, S.-M.; Kuroda, K.; Nguyen, M.D.; Kaibuchi, K.; et al. Disrupted-in-schizophrenia-1 (DISC1) Regulates Endoplasmic Reticulum Calcium Dynamics. *Sci. Rep.* **2015**, *5*, 8694. [CrossRef]
209. de Bartolomeis, A.; Tomasetti, C.; Cicale, M.; Yuan, P.-X.; Manji, H.K. Chronic treatment with lithium or valproate modulates the expression of Homer1b/c and its related genes Shank and Inositol 1,4,5-trisphosphate receptor. *Eur. Neuropsychopharmacol.* **2012**, *22*, 527–535. [CrossRef]
210. Khanim, F.; Ferretti, L.; Raffles, S.; Giles, H.; Jankute, M.; Merrick, B.; Bunce, C.; Drayson, M. Epilepsy doses of valproate combined with the anti-helminthic, niclosamide, synergistically kill myeloma cells: A potent new anti-myeloma drug combination. *Exp. Hematol.* **2014**, *42*, S26. [CrossRef]
211. Akgun, O.; Erkisa, M.; Ari, F. Effective and new potent drug combination: Histone deacetylase and Wnt/β-catenin pathway inhibitors in lung carcinoma cells. *J. Cell. Biochem.* **2019**, *120*, 15467–15482. [CrossRef] [PubMed]
212. Batti, L.; Sundukova, M.; Murana, E.; Pimpinella, S.; Reis, F.D.C.; Pagani, F.; Wang, H.; Pellegrino, E.; Perlas, E.; Di Angelantonio, S.; et al. TMEM16F Regulates Spinal Microglial Function in Neuropathic Pain States. *Cell Rep.* **2016**, *15*, 2608–2615. [CrossRef] [PubMed]
213. Bandman, E.; Walker, C.R.; Strohman, R.C. Diazepam Inhibits Myoblast Fusion and Expression of Muscle Specific Protein Synthesis. *Science* **1978**, *200*, 559–561. [CrossRef] [PubMed]
214. Volke, V.; Soosaar, A.; Koks, S.; Vasar, E.; Männistö, P. l-Arginine abolishes the anxiolytic-like effect of diazepam in the elevated plus-maze test in rats. *Eur. J. Pharmacol.* **1998**, *351*, 287–290. [CrossRef]
215. Gong, L.; Zhang, X.; Qiu, K.; He, L.; Wang, Y.; Yin, J. Arginine promotes myogenic differentiation and myotube formation through the elevation of cytoplasmic calcium concentration. *Anim. Nutr.* **2021**, *7*, 1115–1123. [CrossRef]
216. Williams, M.; Risley, E.A. Ivermectin Interactions with Benzodiazepine Receptors in Rat Cortex and Cerebellum In Vitro. *J. Neurochem.* **1984**, *42*, 745–753. [CrossRef]

217. Bhandage, A.K.; Olivera, G.C.; Kanatani, S.; Thompson, E.; Loré, K.; Varas-Godoy, M.; Barragan, A. A motogenic GABAergic system of mononuclear phagocytes facilitates dissemination of coccidian parasites. *eLife* **2020**, *9*, e60528. [CrossRef]
218. Tian, J.; Middleton, B.; Kaufman, D. $GABA_A$-Receptor Agonists Limit Pneumonitis and Death in Murine Coronavirus-Infected Mice. *Viruses* **2021**, *13*, 966. [CrossRef]
219. Kittler, J.T.; Delmas, P.; Jovanovic, J.N.; Brown, D.A.; Smart, T.G.; Moss, S.J. Constitutive Endocytosis of GABAA Receptors by an Association with the Adaptin AP2 Complex Modulates Inhibitory Synaptic Currents in Hippocampal Neurons. *J. Neurosci.* **2000**, *20*, 7972–7977. [CrossRef]
220. Ngo, D.-H.; Vo, T.S. An Updated Review on Pharmaceutical Properties of Gamma-Aminobutyric Acid. *Molecules* **2019**, *24*, 2678. [CrossRef]
221. Shimada, M.; Hasegawa, T.; Nishimura, C.; Kan, H.; Kanno, T.; Nakamura, T.; Matsubayashi, T. Anti-Hypertensive Effect of γ-Aminobutyric Acid (GABA)-Rich *Chlorella* on High-Normal Blood Pressure and Borderline Hypertension in Placebo-Controlled Double Blind Study. *Clin. Exp. Hypertens.* **2009**, *31*, 342–354. [CrossRef]
222. Shyamaladevi, N.; Jayakumar, A.; Sujatha, R.; Paul, V.; Subramanian, E. Evidence that nitric oxide production increases γ-amino butyric acid permeability of blood-brain barrier. *Brain Res. Bull.* **2002**, *57*, 231–236. [CrossRef]
223. Yoto, A.; Murao, S.; Motoki, M.; Yokoyama, Y.; Horie, N.; Takeshima, K.; Masuda, K.; Kim, M.; Yokogoshi, H. Oral intake of γ-aminobutyric acid affects mood and activities of central nervous system during stressed condition induced by mental tasks. *Amino Acids* **2011**, *43*, 1331–1337. [CrossRef] [PubMed]
224. Czuczwar, S.J.; Patsalos, P.N. The New Generation of GABA Enhancers. *CNS Drugs* **2001**, *15*, 339–350. [CrossRef] [PubMed]
225. Iaria, P.; Blacher, J.; Asplanato, M.; Edric, K.; Safar, M.; Girerd, X. Une nouvelle cause d'hypertension artérielle résistante: La co-prescription avec des traitements anticomitiaux [A new cause of resistant arterial hypertension: Coprescription with anti-convulsant treatments]. *Arch. Mal. Coeur. Vaiss.* **1999**, *92*, 1005–1008.
226. Chen, H.-H.; Li, Y.-D.; Cheng, P.-W.; Fang, Y.-C.; Lai, C.-C.; Tseng, C.-J.; Pan, J.-Y.; Yeh, T.-C. Gabapentin Reduces Blood Pressure and Heart Rate through the Nucleus Tractus Solitarii. *Acta Cardiol. Sin.* **2019**, *35*, 627–633. [CrossRef]
227. Kitajima, T.; Kanbayashi, T.; Saito, Y.; Takahashi, Y.; Ogawa, Y.; Sugiyama, T.; Kaneko, Y.; Aizawa, R.; Shimizu, T. Diazepam reduces both arterial blood pressure and muscle sympathetic nerve activity in human. *Neurosci. Lett.* **2004**, *355*, 77–80. [CrossRef]
228. Lokensgard, J.R.; Gekker, G.; Hu, S.; Arthur, A.F.; Chao, C.C.; Peterson, P.K. Diazepam-mediated inhibition of human immunodeficiency virus type 1 expression in human brain cells. *Antimicrob. Agents Chemother.* **1997**, *41*, 2566–2569. [CrossRef]
229. Lin, A.; Elbezanti, W.O.; Schirling, A.; Ahmed, A.; Van Duyne, R.; Cocklin, S.; Klase, Z. Alprazolam Prompts HIV-1 Transcriptional Reactivation and Enhances CTL Response Through RUNX1 Inhibition and STAT5 Activation. *Front. Neurol.* **2021**, *12*, 663793. [CrossRef]

reports

MDPI

Case Report

# Spontaneous Post-COVID-19 Pneumothorax in a Patient with No Prior Respiratory Tract Pathology: A Case Report

**Vladimir Grigorov [1,2], Mladen Grigorov [3], Evgeni Grigorov [4,*] and Hristina Nocheva [5]**

1 Arwyp Medical Center, Johannesburg 1620, South Africa; vladimir.grigorov@mu-pleven.bg
2 Faculty of Medicine, Medical University-Pleven, 5800 Pleven, Bulgaria
3 Department of Medicine, University of Louisville Hospital, Louisville, KY 40202, USA; mvgrig01@gmail.com
4 Faculty of Pharmacy, Medical University-Varna, 9000 Varna, Bulgaria
5 Pathophysiology Department, Faculty of Medicine, Medical University-Sofia, 1431 Sofia, Bulgaria; hndimitrova@medfac.mu-sofia.bg
* Correspondence: evgeni.grigorov@mu-varna.bg

**Abstract:** Spontaneous pneumothorax in the setting of coronavirus disease 19 (COVID-19) has been first described as an unlikely complication, mainly occurring in critically ill patients or as a consequence of mechanical ventilation. We report a case with COVID-19 pneumonia followed by a spontaneous pneumothorax in a young non-smoker without any predisposing pathology.

**Keywords:** COVID-19; pneumonia; spontaneous pneumothorax

check for updates

**Citation:** Grigorov, V.; Grigorov, M.; Grigorov, E.; Nocheva, H. Spontaneous Post-COVID-19 Pneumothorax in a Patient with No Prior Respiratory Tract Pathology: A Case Report. *Reports* **2022**, 5, 11. https://doi.org/10.3390/reports5010011

Academic Editors: Toshio Hattori and Yugo Ashino

Received: 25 December 2021
Accepted: 11 March 2022
Published: 21 March 2022



## 1. Introduction

The first cases of Coronavirus disease 2019 (COVID-19) were described in Wuhan, China, and quickly spread around the world to become a threat to public health, the economy, and other areas [1]. According to JHU CSSE COVID-19 data, since the outbreak of COVID-19, more than 136 million cases have been confirmed, with nearly 3 million fatal outcomes. The WHO declared the disease as a pandemic.

It seems that COVID-19 does not spare a system: Even though the disease mainly affects the respiratory tract, manifesting as viral pneumonia with common symptoms of dyspnea or respiratory failure. Additionally, the nervous, cardiovascular, gastrointestinal, and/or renal systems can be involved [2,3].

Most of the patients present with a mild course of the disease—the mortality ranges from less than 1% to 8% depending on the country [4,5]. Additionally, new variants have been reported showing differences in infection rate, severity, and mortality [5,6].

Most cases present with a relatively mild symptoms, yet severe complications have been observed, with even fatal outcomes—cytokine release syndrome, responsible for acute respiratory distress syndrome; acute kidney failure; or severe myocardial damage, as well as secondary infections with septic shock [7,8]. According to some literature data, approximately 20% of patients progressed to acute respiratory distress syndrome requiring mechanical ventilation [9,10]. Decreased pulmonary compliance and alveolar inflammation demand higher levels of airway pressure and fraction of inspired oxygen in order to achieve adequate ventilation and gas exchange. Higher levels of airway pressure are among the most probable causes for a number of pulmonary complications, including secondary spontaneous pneumothorax.

Pneumothorax or pneumomediastinum development during the course of COVID-19 disease was first described as a rather unlikely complication (1% of cases), usually affecting critically ill patients or those with mechanical ventilation [11–14]. However, recent data suggest that pneumothorax could also occur in patients without ventilation support [15–17].

We report on a case with COVID-19 pneumonia followed by a spontaneous pneumothorax in a young non-smoker, no alcohol abuse, and HIV-negative, without any predisposing pathology.

## 2. Case Report

A 35-year-old male patient presented with suspected COVID-19 pneumonia. He complained about fever (up to 38.5 °C), headache, cough, shortness of breath, and chest tightness for the last 2 days. No comorbidities were known, except for ulcerative colitis in remission. The patient denied smoking, as well as alcohol abuse; there were no data about other drug abuses(e.g., steroids, 5-ASA, etc.). No family history of respiratory tract diseases was available or other specific lung anomalies.

His vitals on admission were as follows: heart rate of 98/min, respiratory rate of 24/min, and peripheral oxygen saturation of 90%.

The laboratory results (Table 1) showed an elevation of the c-reactive protein (CRP: 106 mg/L; normal range: <5 mg/L) with a normal procalcitonin level (PCT: 0.08 ng/mL; normal range: <0.5 ng/mL). Creatinine was normal (Crea: 0.8 mg/dL; normal range 0.7–1.2 mg/dL), while lactate dehydrogenase was elevated (LDH: 367 U/L; normal range: <250 U/L). D-dimer was also elevated (d-dimer: 310 ng/mL; normal range: <250 ng/mL).

**Table 1.** Laboratory findings on admission.

| Laboratory Evaluation | Patient's Result | Normal Range |
|---|---|---|
| CRP | 106 mg/L | <5 mg/L |
| PCT | 0.08 ng/mL | <0.5 ng/mL |
| Crea | 0.8 mg/dL | 0.7–1.2 mg/dL |
| LDH | 367 U/L | <250 U/L |
| d-dimer | 310 ng/mL | <250 ng/mL |

Chest X-ray showed bilateral interstitial infiltrates (Figure 1). Positive reverse transcriptase polymerase chain reaction (RT-PCR) test with nasal swab (Genexpect system) confirmed COVID-19 infection. The patient was admitted to the isolation ward and received supportive treatment. Oxygen supplementation was also necessary—poly mask was applied (his $pO_2$ increased to 98%), with no mechanical ventilation. The patient was discharged in a stable condition at day +5 after admission. A chest CT was performed, revealing no bulla present at the time of discharge.

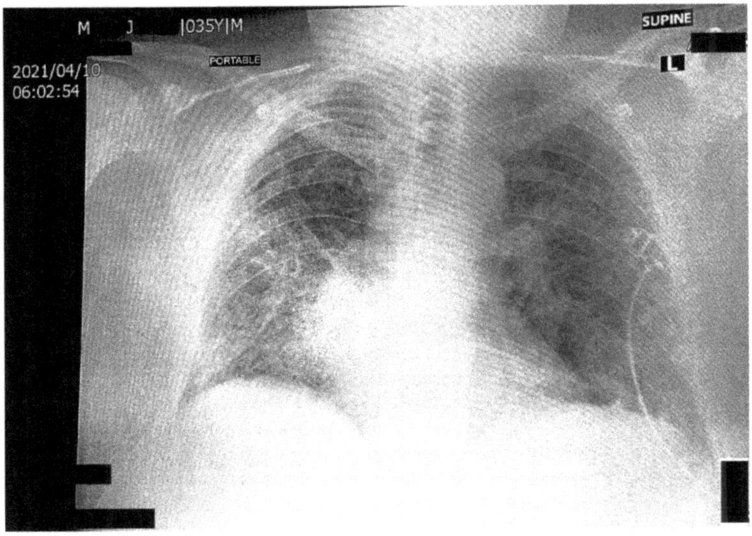


**Figure 1.** Chest X-ray on admission—showing bilateral interstitial infiltrates without blebs.

Twenty days after discharge, the patient presented again in the emergency department with severe chest pain and shortness of breath. CT chest revealed a significant pneumothorax on the right side (Figure 2). A chest tube was inserted with subsequent drainage, leading to a re-expansion of the right lung.

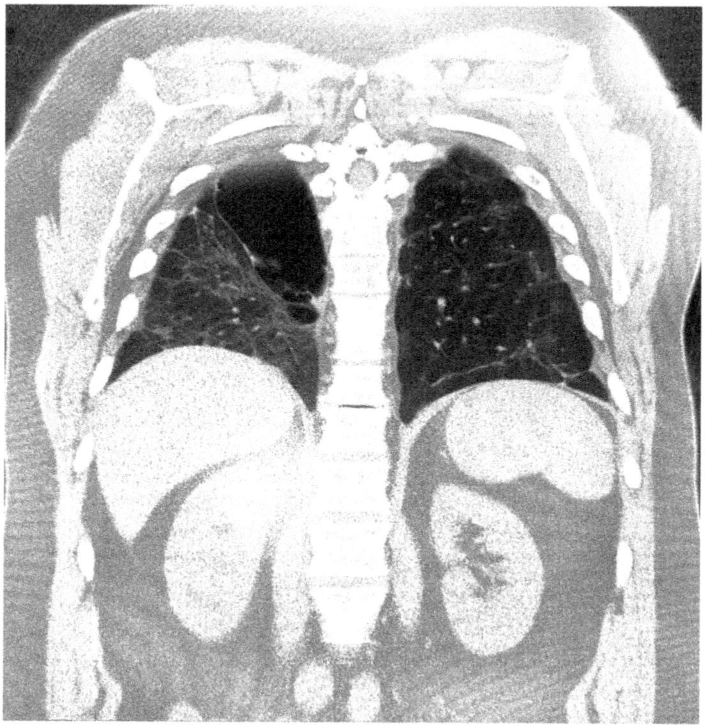

**Figure 2.** CT chest—showing pneumothorax on the right side.

The patient was followed-up once again a month later. He could walk a kilometer distance without getting breathless. Clinically, there was a normal expansion of the both lungs with normal percussion margins. There was no need for new X-rays as the patient was clinically stable, asymptomatic, and was feeling fine.

## 3. Discussion

Approximately 1% of patients with COVID-19 pneumonia develop pneumothorax, presumably due to the barotrauma caused by positive pressure ventilation [12,18].

In the case presented, no such trauma could be suspected. Other possible "culprits" (emphysema, cystic fibrosis, necrotizing pneumonia, severe asthma, lung inflammation/malignancy, as well as Marfan syndrome and alpha 1-antitrypsin deficiency) also cannot be taken in consideration [19,20]. The patient is a non-smoker and in good physical condition (could walk for 5 km prior to the COVID-19 infection); he was tested for alpha 1-antitripsin deficiency (negative). The control CT scan before the discharge did not show any bulla or emphysema. The patient denies having significant cough—thus, the so-called Maclin effect (occurs due to extensive cough in an area that the alveolar walls are weakened) should also be excluded.

There are a few possibilities to explain the complication described:

- Small (micro) sub pleural bleb formation in the course of the disease that broke later into the pleural space [20];

- Given the hypercoagulable state observed in COVID-19 patients, a microembolus leading to infection with subsequent alveolar wall damage and leakage in the pleural compartment could be suspected [21,22];
- Diffuse alveolar damage leading to alveolar rupture and air leak [17].

## 4. Conclusions

It is obvious that there is only a thin burden between the mild course of the disease and full-blown respiratory failure (with life-threatening consequences), as well as between the "really recovered" patient after the discharge and the patient with unsuspected risk for ulterior complications.

Increasing evidence of spontaneous pneumothorax in non-ventilated patients after COVID-19 should make clinicians aware of the "rare" possibility for a spontaneous pneumothorax to cause acute worsening dyspnea or acute clinical deterioration in patients with a recent COVID-19 history.

**Author Contributions:** Conceptualization, V.G. and H.N.; methodology, M.G., E.G. and H.N.; software, M.G. and E.G.; validation, M.G. and E.G.; formal analysis, M.G., E.G. and H.N.; investigation, V.G. and M.G.; resources, V.G., M.G., E.G. and H.N.; data curation, E.G.; writing—original draft preparation, M.G., E.G. and H.N.; writing—review and editing, V.G.; visualization, M.G., E.G. and H.N.; supervision, V.G. and H.N.; project administration, E.G.; All authors have read and agreed to the published version of the manuscript.

**Funding:** This research received no external funding.

**Institutional Review Board Statement:** Not applicable.

**Informed Consent Statement:** Not applicable.

**Conflicts of Interest:** The authors declare no conflict of interest.

## References

1. Zhu, N.; Zhang, D.; Wang, W.; Li, X.; Yang, B.; Song, J.; Zhao, X.; Huang, B.; Shi, W.; Lu, R.; et al. Novel coronavirus from patients with pneumonia in China, 2019. *N. Engl. J. Med.* **2020**, *382*, 727–733. [CrossRef] [PubMed]
2. Wang, D.; Hu, B.; Hu, C.; Zhu, F.; Liu, X.; Zhang, J.; Wang, B.; Xiang, H.; Cheng, Z.; Xiong, Y.; et al. Clinical Characteristics of 138 Hospitalized Patients with 2019 Novel Coronavirus-Infected Pneumonia in Wuhan, China. *JAMA* **2020**, *323*, 1061–1069. [CrossRef]
3. Zhou, F.; Yu, T.; Du, R.; Fan, G.; Liu, Y.; Liu, Z.; Xiang, J.; Wang, Y.; Song, B.; Gu, X.; et al. Clinical course and risk factors for mortality of adult in patients with COVID-19 in Wuhan, China: A retrospective cohort study. *Lancet* **2020**, *395*, 1054–1062. [CrossRef]
4. Grasselli, G.; Zangrillo, A.; Zanella, A.; Antonelli, M.; Cabrini, L.; Castelli, A.; Cereda, D.; Coluccello, A.; Foti, G.; Fumagalli, R.; et al. Baseline characteristics and outcomes of 1591 patients infected with SARS-CoV-2 admitted to ICUs of the Lombardy region, Italy. *JAMA* **2020**, *323*, 1574–1581. [CrossRef] [PubMed]
5. Da Silva, J.C.; Félix, V.B.; Leão, S.A.B.F.; Trindade-Filho, E.M.; Scorza, F.A. New Brazilian variant of the SARS-CoV-2 (P1/Gamma) of COVID-19 in Alagoas state. *Braz. J. Infect. Dis.* **2021**, *25*, 101588. [CrossRef]
6. Da Silva, S.J.R.; Pena, L. Collapse of the public health system and the emergence of new variants during the second wave of the COVID-19 pandemic in Brazil. *One Health* **2021**, *13*, 100287. [CrossRef]
7. Young, B.E.; Ong, S.W.X.; Kalimuddin, S.; Low, J.G.; Tan, S.Y.; Loh, J.; Ng, O.T.; Marimuthu, K.; Ang, L.W.; Mak, T.M.; et al. Epidemiologic Features and Clinical Course of Patients Infected With SARS-CoV-2 in Singapore. *JAMA* **2020**, *323*, 1488–1494. [CrossRef]
8. Baig, A.M.; Khaleeq, A.; Ali, U.; Syeda, H. Evidence of the COVID-19 Virus Targeting the CNS: Tissue Distribution, Host-Virus Interaction, and Proposed Neurotropic Mechanisms. *ACS Chem. Neurosci.* **2020**, *11*, 995–998. [CrossRef]
9. Ziehr, D.; Alladina, J.; Petri, C.A.; Maley, J.H.; Moskowitz, A.; Medoff, B.D.; Hibbert, K.A.; Thompson, B.T.; Hardin, C.C. Pathophysiology of mechanically ventilated patients with COVID 19 a Cohort study. *Am. J. Respir. Crit. Care Med.* **2020**, *201*, 1560–1564. [CrossRef]
10. Wu, Z.; McGoogan, J.M. Characteristics of and important lessons from the coronavirus disease 2019 (COVID-19) outbreak in China: Summary of a report of 72,314 cases from the Chinese Center for Disease Control and Prevention. *JAMA* **2020**, *323*, 1239–1242. [CrossRef]
11. Quincho-Lopez, A.; Quincho-Lopez, D.L.; Hurtado-Medina, F.D. Case Report: Pneumothorax and Pneumomediastinum as Uncommon Complications of COVID-19 Pneumonia-Literature Review. *Am. J. Trop. Med. Hyg.* **2020**, *103*, 1170–1176. [CrossRef]

12. Martinelli, A.W.; Ingle, T.; Newman, J.; Nadeem, I.; Jackson, K.; Lane, N.D.; Melhorn, J.; Davies, H.E.; Rostron, A.J.; Adeni, A.; et al. COVID-19 and pneumothorax: A multicentre retrospective case series. *Eur. Respir. J.* **2020**, *56*, 2002697. [CrossRef] [PubMed]
13. Yang, X.; Yu, Y.; Xu, J.; Shu, H.; Xia, J.; Liu, H.; Wu, Y.; Zhang, L.; Yu, Z.; Fang, M.; et al. Clinical course and outcomes of critically ill patients with SARS-CoV-2 pneumonia in Wuhan, China: A single-centered, retrospective, observational study. *Lancet Respir. Med.* **2020**, *8*, 475–481. [CrossRef]
14. Belletti, A.; Palumbo, D.; Zangrillo, A.; Fominskiy, E.V.; Franchini, S.; Dell'Acqua, A.; Marinosci, A.; Monti, G.; Vitali, G.; Colombo, S.; et al. Predictors of Pneumothorax/Pneumomediastinum in Mechanically Ventilated COVID-19 Patients. *J. Cardiothorac. Vasc. Anesth.* **2021**, *35*, 3642–3651. [CrossRef] [PubMed]
15. Schiller, M.; Wunsch, A.; Fisahn, J.; Gschwendtner, A.; Huebner, U.; Kick, W. Pneumothorax with bullous lesions as a late complication of COVID-19 pneumonia—A report on two clinical cases. *J. Emerg. Med.* **2021**, *61*, 581–586. [CrossRef]
16. Sun, R.; Liu, H.; Sang, X. Mediastinal emphysema, giant bulla and pneumothorax developed during the course of COVID-19 pneumonia. *Korean J. Radiol.* **2020**, *21*, 541–544. [CrossRef]
17. Tucker, L.; Patel, S.; Vatsis, C.; Poma, A.; Ammar, A.; Nasser, W.; Mukkera, S.; Vo, M.; Khan, R.; Carlan, S. Pneumothorax and Pneumomediastinum Secondary to COVID-19 Disease Unrelated to Mechanical Ventilation. *Case Rep. Crit. Care* **2020**, *2020*, 6655428. [CrossRef] [PubMed]
18. Elhakim, T.S.; Abdul, H.S.; Pelaez Romero, C.; Rodriguez-Fuentes, Y. Spontaneous pneumomediastinum, pneumothorax and subcutaneous emphysema in COVID-19 pneumonia: A rare case and literature review. *BMJ Case Rep.* **2020**, *13*, e239489. [CrossRef]
19. Noppen, M. Spontaneos pneumothorax. Epiemiology, pathophysiology and cause. *Eur. Respir. Rev.* **2010**, *19*, 217–219. [CrossRef]
20. Schramel, F.; Meyer, C.J.; Postmus, P.E. Inflammation as a cause of spontaneous pneumothorax and empyema like changes. Results of bronchoalveolar lavage. *Eur. Respir. Rev.* **1995**, *8*, 397s.
21. Connors, J.M.; Levy, J.H. Covid 19 and its implication for thrombosis and anticoagulation. *Blood* **2020**, *135*, 2033–2040. [CrossRef] [PubMed]
22. Poissy, J.; Goutay, J.; Caplan, M.; Parmentier-Decrucq, E.; Duburcq, T.; Lassalle, F.; Jeanpierre, E.; Rauch, A.; Labreuche, J.; Susen, S.; et al. Pulmonary Embolism in Patients with COVID-19: Awareness of an Increased Prevalence. *Circulation* **2020**, *142*, 184–186. [CrossRef] [PubMed]

MDPI
St. Alban-Anlage 66
4052 Basel
Switzerland
www.mdpi.com

*Reports* Editorial Office
E-mail: reports@mdpi.com
www.mdpi.com/journal/reports

www.ingramcontent.com/pod-product-compliance
Lightning Source LLC
LaVergne TN
LVHW070620100526
838202LV00012B/691